VOICE QUALITY

The first phonetic description of voice quality production in 40 years, this book provides a new framework for its analysis: The Laryngeal Articulator Model. Informed by instrumental examinations of the laryngeal articulatory mechanism, it revises our understanding of articulatory postures to explain the actions, vibrations and resonances generated in the epilarynx and pharynx. It focuses on the long-term auditory-articulatory component of accent in the languages of the world, explaining how voice quality relates to segmental and syllabic sounds. Phonetic illustrations of phonation types and of laryngeal and oral vocal tract articulatory postures are provided. Extensive video and audio material is available on a companion website. The book presents computational simulations, the laryngeal and voice quality foundations of infant speech acquisition, speech/voice disorders and surgeries that entail compensatory laryngeal articulator adjustment, and an exploration of the role of voice quality in sound change and of the larynx in the evolution of speech.

JOHN H. ESLING, FRSC, is Professor Emeritus of Linguistics at the University of Victoria, British Columbia, Canada.

SCOTT R. MOISIK, PhD, is Assistant Professor in the Division of Linguistics and Multilingual Studies at Nanyang Technological University, Singapore.

ALLISON BENNER, PhD, is Humanities & Fine Arts Co-op Coordinator at the University of Victoria, British Columbia, Canada.

LISE CREVIER-BUCHMAN, MD, PhD, HDR, is a Senior Research Fellow with the CNRS, Université Sorbonne Nouvelle Paris 3, and Head of the Voice, Speech & Swallowing Lab, Head & Neck Surgery Department, Hôpital Foch, Suresnes, France.

In this series

CAMBRIDGE STUDIES IN LINGUISTICS

Voice Quality

VOICE QUALITY

THE LARYNGEAL ARTICULATOR MODEL

JOHN H. ESLING
University of Victoria

SCOTT R. MOISIK
Nanyang Technological University, Singapore

ALLISON BENNER
University of Victoria

LISE CREVIER-BUCHMAN
CNRS, Université Sorbonne Nouvelle Paris 3

CAMBRIDGE
UNIVERSITY PRESS

CAMBRIDGE
UNIVERSITY PRESS

University Printing House, Cambridge CB2 8BS, United Kingdom

One Liberty Plaza, 20th Floor, New York, NY 10006, USA

477 Williamstown Road, Port Melbourne, VIC 3207, Australia

314-321, 3rd Floor, Plot 3, Splendor Forum, Jasola District Centre, New Delhi - 110025, India

103 Penang Road, #05-06/07, Visioncrest Commercial, Singapore 238467

Cambridge University Press is part of the University of Cambridge.

It furthers the University's mission by disseminating knowledge in the pursuit of
education, learning and research at the highest international levels of excellence.

www.cambridge.org
Information on this title: www.cambridge.org/9781108736039
DOI: 10.1017/9781108696555

First published 2019
First paperback edition 2022

A catalogue record for this publication is available from the British Library

Library of Congress Cataloging in Publication data
Names: Esling, John H., 1949– author. | Moisik, Scott R., 1983– author. | Benner, Allison, author. |
    Crevier-Buchman, Lise, author.
Title: Voice quality : the laryngeal articulator model / John H. Esling, University of Victoria,
    British Columbia ; Scott R. Moisik, Nanyang Technological University, Singapore ; Allison
    Benner, University of Victoria, British Columbia ; Lise Crevier-Buchman, National Scientific
    Research Centre (CNRS).
Description: United Kingdom ; New York : Cambridge University Press, 2019. |
    Series: Cambridge studies in linguistics ; 162 | Includes bibliographical references and index.
Identifiers: LCCN 2019003350 | ISBN 9781108498425 (hardback) |
    ISBN 9781108736039 (paperback)
Subjects: LCSH: Voice–Physiological aspects.
Classification: LCC QP306 .E85 2019 | DDC 612.7/8–dc23
LC record available at https://lccn.loc.gov/2019003350

ISBN 978-1-108-49842-5 Hardback
ISBN 978-1-108-73603-9 Paperback

Contents

Figures

Tables

Preface

This book presents a revised approach to phonetic voice quality description through the introduction of the Laryngeal Articulator Model, a new approach to vocal-tract articulatory function. Our model supersedes the simple glottal phonation paradigm of the lower vocal tract that has guided a century of phonetic and linguistic research. The Laryngeal Articulator Model presents the larynx as a complex articulator that shapes resonances and generates multiple vibration sources. This model has important consequences for the interpretation of basic places of articulation as well as for how voice quality interacts with the other elements of speech.

Our aim is to provide the groundwork for generating new hypotheses for experimental phonetic and linguistic research into speech-sound production in the lower vocal tract. We introduce new structures and movements to clarify and simplify the process we identify as laryngeal constriction. We present many examples of speech production (phonetic, extralinguistic, paralinguistic, and linguistic) to demonstrate how the laryngeal articulator works and case studies that illustrate the application of the model to linguistic analysis. The model is particularly relevant to the analysis of voice quality, as the lower vocal tract is the primary shaper of sound quality that is transferred through the rest of the vocal tract. This work is part of an ongoing attempt to construct an auditory portrait of what the laryngeal articulator produces.

The account of the structure of voice quality settings presented here follows the phonetic theories of Abercrombie (1967) and Laver (1980). The major and novel difference is in how the vocal tract is described. Rather than defining the larynx as only the glottis, generating phonation types but not articulations, with an open pharynx above it in which the tongue is the main articulator, the Laryngeal Articulator Model (LAM) introduces the 'two-part vocal tract', comprising a laryngeal and an oral articulator (Esling 2005). The glottis is still the opening from the lungs, bronchi and trachea into the vocal tract, but instead of it being the only site at which periodic energy is generated as a function of vibrating tissues, the laryngeal articulator contains multiple sites of potential vibration. The role of the tongue is also redefined. Instead of the tongue being the principal articulator in the laryngeal vocal tract, the epilaryngeal tube, incorporating the ventricular folds and aryepiglottic folds, is identified as the 'first articulator' above the glottis, which exerts changes, together with lingual retraction and larynx raising, on the shape of the rest of the pharynx and of the oral vocal tract. Above the velopharyngeal port, the nasal tract acts primarily as a resonating cavity rather than as an articulator. The oral articulator, from the uvula to the lips, generates the complex articulations and resonances that characterize most sounds in the world's languages. The important distinction in the LAM lies in the interaction between the laryngeal and oral regions, affecting the balance of overlapping secondary articulation and sequential coarticulation. In order to define linguistic, paralinguistic, and extralinguistic phonetic sound qualities, this auditory balance must be dissected and attributed to the relevant regions of the vocal tract.

In the simplest deconstruction of the Laryngeal Articulator Model, the vocal tract is divided into two parts – the laryngeal vocal tract and the oral vocal tract. At the next level of complexity, the vocal tract can be divided economically into five major articulators: larynx, velopharyngeal port, tongue, jaw, and lips. The model is relevant at any level of phonetic description, but our primary aim is to demonstrate how the laryngeal region of the vocal tract shapes the longest-term construct of speech – voice quality. In describing a speaker's voice quality, the five articulators can serve as a checklist to identify the key settings or postures that best characterize each region. The laryngeal articulator is considerably larger in the LAM than in previous models of vocal-tract function. This is telling for phonetic theory. The larynx in the LAM incorporates the pharynx, that is, those multiple cavities between the glottis and the uvula, and, in a departure from previous models, the larynx is an articulator. The laryngeal articulator is critical for speech acquisition by infants, as well as having implications for the origin of speech and for the rehabilitation of speech in the event of speech disorders and surgical repair. The number and types of sounds that can be produced by the articulating structures in the larynx are far greater than in traditional interpretations, and they are more closely co-related to the articulations produced in the oral part of the vocal tract than previously thought. The articulatory decision at the velopharyngeal port is basically whether a sound is nasal (with an open port) or oral (with a closed port), with gradations that are important when distinguishing the segmental, dynamic, and long-term strands of accent. The tongue is arguably the primary articulator of the majority of sound contrasts across the languages of the world, making up the large repertory of lingual sounds evident in the various tableaux of speech sounds, including the official chart of the International Phonetic Association (IPA 2005) and the charts in the *iPA Phonetics* app, derived from Esling (2010). Significantly linked with lingual articulation is the action of the jaw, which determines the openness of vowels (and of voice quality) in the front part of the vocal tract. The final determinant of voice quality is labial configuration, significantly coordinated with lingual articulation. This reanalysis of the vocal tract prompts a fundamental research question: how does the laryngeal articulator interact with the articulators in the oral vocal tract (and vice versa)? The material presented in this book – voice quality categories, simulation of articulatory interactions, illustrations of auditory qualities, phonological mapping of articulator relationships, characterization of infant speech, description of clinical interventions, and discussions of where laryngeal articulation and voice quality fit within larger phonetic debates – provides an articulatory and auditory framework for addressing that research question. (An inventory of voice quality descriptors, to which this volume makes reference, can be found in the *iPA Phonetics* app on the Apple Store (Coey et al. 2014, Esling et al. 2015).) Audio files of settings on the Voice Qualities page can be compared with videos of articulatory postures at each place along the Consonant Chart.

Notation for the transcription of voice quality has expanded somewhat since Laver (1980: 162–165), mainly in the clinical context. Ball et al. (2000) increased symbol designations to accommodate the description of disordered speech. Ball et al. (2018) expanded and reorganized the inventory and re-evaluated phonation-type symbols to be more compatible with laryngeal articulator behaviour as described in the LAM. Some of these categories are incorporated in the expanded Consonant Chart in the app.

These notes describe material that can be accessed online. A set of media files accompanies this book to illustrate canonical voice quality categories from Chapters 1 and 2, case studies and simulations from Chapter 3, linguistic, paralinguistic, and extralinguistic illustrations from Chapter 4, qualities of infant speech in the progression of ontogenetic phonetic development from Chapter 6, illustrations of voice qualities in disordered speech and post-surgery from Chapter 7, and quality-related phenomena from Chapter 8. The video, audio, and text companion files accompanying each chapter are available on a Google Drive site with a link from CUP. Examples of canonical voice quality categories are also available within the *iPA Phonetics* app.

Acknowledgements

We are grateful to a number of people, as research collaborators, linguistic consultants, and supporters, whose assistance and input helped to make this work possible. We would like to thank Jerold A. Edmondson, Jimmy G. Harris, and Zeki Majeed Hassan for their fieldwork expertise, their collaboration in carrying out experimental phonetic procedures, their astute ability to identify contrasts in articulation and quality across a range of disparate languages, and their contribution of data to the illustration of articulatory production and quality distinctions in this volume and online. We are grateful to Li Shaoni (李绍尼), to Ziwo Lama (拉玛兹倔), and to Cécile Padayodi for participating in phonetic experimentation and contributing their linguistic expertise and data samples. We are also grateful to Chakir Zeroual for his participation on our research projects and for facilitating the collection and analysis of infant vocalizations from Morocco. We thank Michael Mawdsley and Michael Ross for attending laryngoscopic examinations. We owe a debt of gratitude to Thomas M. Hess, Geoffrey N. O'Grady, and Barry F. Carlson for their expertise in understanding the sound systems of Indigenous languages and for the inspiration and encouragement they provided over the years towards the analysis and description of phonetic patterns in many languages of the world. We are especially appreciative of the contribution of Katherine E. (Katie) Fraser and George Louie in providing linguistic data and interpretation, and we acknowledge the participation of Arne Foldvik in early laryngoscopic research, together with James K. F. (Tony) Anthony at the University of Edinburgh, and for providing data. We appreciate and acknowledge the contributions of Mihoko Teshigawara, Izabelle Grenon, and Lisa Bettany to our research projects and in the evaluation of voice quality and infant speech, and the contribution of Christopher Coey for providing technical support in data collection, programming, and post processing.

We have enjoyed the support of the Laboratoire de Phonétique et Phonologie, UMR7018, at the Université Sorbonne Nouvelle Paris 3, and the active sponsorship by Jacqueline Vaissière of the Canadian research team in Paris in

2006 and of the LABEX lecture series in 2014. We thank the ORL teams at the Hôpital Laennec and the Hôpital européen Georges-Pompidou – Daniel Brasnu, Ollivier Laccourreye, Stéphane Hans, and Madeleine Menard – for their research collaboration in laryngeal surgery and anatomical/pathophysiological classification. We are grateful to Philippe Halimi for supporting our experimental phonetic MRI investigations at the Hôpital européen Georges-Pompidou and to Angélique Amelot for data processing, and we acknowledge the material shared by Didier Demolin on comparative laryngeal anatomy. Bernard Harmegnies has supported our approach to investigating voice quality at the Université de Mons since 1989. We are indebted to Leonardo Fuks and Milton Melciades Barbosa Costa at the Universidade Federal do Rio de Janeiro for facilitating an innovative experimental investigation of laryngeal postures, and to Ian Stavness, Sidney Fels, John Lloyd, Peter Anderson, Antonio Sanchez, and Bryan Gick, among many others at UBC for the use of ArtiSynth, their work on the ArtiSynth platform, and enabling the development of a model to illustrate the action of the laryngeal mechanism.

For contributing linguistic data from a variety of languages, we would like to thank Gedung Jungney, Gugsa Tekle, Châu Văn Nguyễn, Akiyo Pahalaan, Signe Eggers-Weber, Thomas Jensen, Ivan Omari, Rhoda Spinks, Alex Sherwood, Margaret Sherwood, Pauline Flett, Mohamed Hassan Mohamoud, and John Nyok. For her management of our field site in Yunnan, China, and for facilitating the collection of infant vocalizations, we would like to thank Duan Jianying (段剑英).

We owe much of our conceptual outlook and auditory formulations to the mentorship of Ian Catford, David Abercrombie, Bill Labov, Bill Wang, and Michael Dobrovolsky. For contributing their time and encouragement in productive discussion over the years, we would like to thank John Laver, John Local, Paul Johnston, Francis Nolan, Asher Laufer, Tom Baer, Sandra Whiteside, Dennis Preston, Nina Grønnum, Gert Foget Hansen, Craig Dickson, Henry Warkentyne, and, in particular, Ewa Czaykowska-Higgins for her collaboration in formulating the Phonological Potentials Model.

We would like to acknowledge the Social Sciences and Humanities Research Council of Canada for the funding that made our instrumental research, data analysis, travel and conference participation, and the preparation of reports, of articles, and of this book possible. A series of SSHRC Research Grants – 410-93-0539, 410-2000-901, 410-2003-1624, 410-2007-2375, 410-2011-0229 – supported our research on voice quality and phonatory effects, laryngoscopic and other instrumental experimentation, and our study of the acquisition of the phonetic capacity by infants. Several General Grants from

SSHRC to the University of Victoria also supplemented this research. We also acknowledge Faculty Research Grants from the University of Victoria that supported our phonetic research initiatives.

We owe the greatest debt to the indulgence of our families: to Kazimiera for her belief, patience and support, and to Natalia for inspiring many aspects of this work; to Carly and Azula for their love and support; to Anna and Loucas for their ongoing support and contributions to the study; and to Louis, Lionel, Elena, and Pamela, for their unfailing support – heartfelt gratitude.

Abbreviations

AD	anterior digastric muscles
AE	aryepiglottic (muscles or folds)
AFPL	anterior frontal partial laryngectomy
+ATR	plus advanced tongue root
–ATR	minus advanced tongue root (i.e. retracted tongue root)
CHEP	cricohyoidoepiglottopexy
CHP	cricohyoidopexy
CN	cranial nerve
CT	cricothyroid muscles
EGG	electroglottography (electroglottogram)
EL	electrolarynx (voice)
EMA	electromagnetic articulography
EMG	electromyography
EV	esophageal voice
f0	fundamental frequency
F1	first formant
F2	second formant
FG	Feature Geometry
FLPL	frontolateral partial laryngectomy
GGA	anterior genioglossus muscles
GGM	medial genioglossus muscles
GGP	posterior genioglossus muscles
GH	geniohyoid muscles
HBB	human beatboxing
HG	hyoglossus muscles
(o)IA	(oblique) interarytenoid muscles
(t)IA	(transverse) interarytenoid muscles
ISP	inter-speech posture
LAM	Laryngeal Articulator Model
LCA	lateral cricoarytenoid muscles

LI	longitudinalis inferior muscles
LS	longitudinalis superior muscles
LTAS	long-term average spectrum
LVT	lower vocal tract
MRI	magnetic resonance imaging
NMM	neuromuscular module
OO	orbicularis oris muscles
OOIm	orbicularis oris inferior marginalis
OOIp	orbicularis oris inferior peripheralis
PCA	posterior cricoarytenoid muscles
PD	Parkinson's disease
PPM	Phonological Potentials Model
RLN	recurrent laryngeal nerve
rtMRI	real-time magnetic resonance imaging
SCHLP	supracricoid hemilaryngopharyngectomy
SCPL	(horizontal) supracricoid partial laryngectomy
SG	styloglossus muscles
SGPL	supraglottic partial laryngectomy
SLLUS	Simultaneous Laryngoscopy and Laryngeal Ultrasound
SLN	superior laryngeal nerve
TA	thyroarytenoid muscles
TE	thyroepiglottic muscles
TEV	tracheoesophageal voice
TH	thyrohyoid muscles
TL	total laryngectomy
TMJ	temporomandibular joint
UES	upper esophageal sphincter
UFT	Unified Feature Theory
UVT	upper vocal tract
VFP	vocal fold paralysis
VPA	Vocal Profile Analysis
VVFC	Vocal-ventricular fold coupling

1   *Voice and Voice Quality*

This chapter presents voice quality as a long-term component of accent. We describe in detail the Laryngeal Articulator Model (LAM), defining key terminology and providing a unified account of laryngeal anatomical structure and physiological function. We present observations of lower-vocal-tract phonetic phenomena that have often been portrayed in inconsistent, confusing, and incorrect ways in the literature on speech physiology and in describing the sounds of the world's languages. Prior to the methodology described in this text, the structure and functions of the laryngeal articulator, and hence of voice quality, were poorly understood, partly because of the difficulty in visualizing the articulator producing its full range of sounds as they occur in the world's languages. Categories are presented in order from the lower to the upper vocal tract, paying specific attention to laryngeal categories.

1.1   Voice Quality Defined

Voice quality, in its broadest theoretical sense as a phonetic descriptor of accent, refers to the long-term characteristics of a person's voice – the more or less permanent, habitually recurring, proportionately frequent characteristics of a person's speech patterns (Abercrombie 1967, Laver 1980). A parallel term denoting how we recognize a person's voice is 'long-term quality' (Nolan 1983). As a property of accent, voice quality refers to all of the habitual, long-term background, or holistic characteristics perceived as the most constant or persistent over time in a person's speech. Perceptually, it is the longest-term phonetic strand of the aural medium for language. The other two strands, the voice dynamics (prosodic) strand and the segmental strand, are progressively shorter term. Segments (vowels and consonants) last for tens or hundreds of milliseconds, voice dynamics (e.g. intonation) components can occur over a stretch of syllables or words, while voice quality, as Abercrombie (1967: 91) put it, 'refers to those characteristics which are present more or less all the time that a person is talking: it is a quasi-permanent quality running through all

1

the sound' of a person's speech. Elements of all three strands can be shared characteristics acquired as a part of the person's regional or social upbringing. Individual anatomy has a part to play, and some characteristics are learned and adopted idiosyncratically by the individual, but most characteristics of all three strands of accent are acquired remarkably similarly by members of the same linguistic community in a given generation. Still, the 'accent' of a place should not be assumed to be absolutely uniform across all speakers. In assessing the voice quality common to a regional or social group, the identification of those voice quality traits that are preponderant within selected sociolinguistic samples of speakers determines the extent of their distribution.

The term 'voice quality' has been used in another sense. In what could be called colloquial phonetic usage, 'voice quality' is applied narrowly to the kind of voicing produced at the glottis, specifically by the vocal folds. In voice quality theory, this narrower usage is more precisely termed the description of 'phonation type' or 'phonatory quality'. In somewhat intermediate phonetic usage, the term has also been used to designate the short-term effects, or 'register' effects, that originate within the larynx, in the lowermost part of the vocal tract in general. They are generally syllabic in duration and linguistically contrastive in the particular sound system or phonology in which they occur. We shall often use the cover term 'vocal quality' in referring to these shorter-term auditory effects produced by vocal-tract configurations, especially those produced within the laryngeal articulator.

Whether in its broader or narrower sense, the sound generated at the glottis, primarily by the vocal folds, is considered the source or the first element that shapes a person's speech. When we recognize a person by the sound of their voice, voice quality in the broader sense is generally what we mean. We are responding to speech cues that are the most persistent, habitual or long-lasting in the accent of the person whose voice we are hearing. These speech cues can be perceived in short portions of speech precisely because they are properties incorporated to varying degrees into the rapidly changing short-term vowels and consonants that make up the rapidly fluctuating segmental level of speech. In the broader sense of long-term voice quality, the vibrations originating within the larynx constitute the phonation type that is the background heard throughout the voiced sounds that a speaker produces. This provides a holistic unity to the auditory character of the voice despite the variation found in the segmental and voice dynamic strands. Components of the speech signal generated in the laryngeal articulator are particularly amenable to long-term functionality, since vibrations are inherently sustained relative to more momentary articulatory gestures and because articulations in the lower vocal tract are generally slower than those in the oral vocal tract. The laryngeal source signal is then modified through the shapes created by the positions of the articulators in the rest of the laryngeal articulator and through the upper vocal tract, producing characteristic resonances. These spectral characteristics are more telling when the source is voiced (due to periodic vibrations) rather than voiceless (when the glottis is open); but laryngeally voiceless sounds can also have spectral frequencies associated with them as a result of turbulence (friction/noise) generated by articulatory postures in the laryngeal vocal tract before the speech signal is further modified by actions of the oral articulators. To the extent that the laryngeal source signal and consequent vocal tract modulations persist throughout the sounds that an individual speaker produces, they can be identified auditorily as quasi-permanent (Abercrombie 1967) or long-term (Laver 1980, Nolan 1983) elements of voice quality. Because these characteristics are present more or less all the time that a person is speaking, they come to typify the sound of the person's voice.

Change in language is endemic, and the different phonetic components of speech interact in the process of sound change. This may apply especially to voice quality as a vehicle for sound change, because the longest-term strand of accent carries fewer attributes of contrastive linguistic meaning than voice dynamics patterns or segmental articulations. We do not yet know exactly how the other strands depend on voice quality characteristics to carry their contrastive meaning. To know this, we should have to discover how changes to voice quality settings affect each particular segment or intonational pattern in a phonology. Of course, it remains possible that changes in voice quality setting will have no appreciable effect on the nature of segments or prosodic patterns as they express linguistic meaning. Still, we hypothesize that subtle changes in parallel strands of accent are a potential agent of sound change; that is, altered longer-term qualities on a given segment, segmental string or prosodic pattern can shift the meaning-carrying attributes of that sound sequence. For example, combinations of secondary qualities influencing primary segmental (or syllabic) articulations can facilitate the development of a new primary category. Secondary pharyngealization on uvular segments has been described as a potential vehicle for uvulars to diffuse lexically to pharyngealized uvulars and to become primary pharyngeal segments, as they are reported to have done in Wakashan languages (Carlson and Esling 2003). Such processes are inherently auditory – a function of acquisition in context. With the requisite experience, it is common for listeners with regional linguistic familiarity to be able to identify what particular region a speaker comes from or social group a speaker belongs to by their accent. Our heuristic process is equally auditory – developed through the association of speech articulation with the auditory identification of resulting sound patterns. Our aim in this volume is to present the background for those associations, to characterize the auditory quality of these sounds, and to offer illustrations of cases (individuals, linguistic communities, and linguistic contrasts) where those auditory qualities occur.

The comprehensive description of voice quality presented by Laver (1980) reviews the concept of voice quality in phonetic theory, presents the categories and labels for analysing voice quality settings, and summarizes the articulatory, acoustic, and auditory research relevant in defining each category. Laver also makes a pertinent observation about voice quality as auditory background – the relatively stable 'ground' against which the 'figures' of rapidly fluctuating consonants and vowels move in a 'figure-to-ground' relationship (1980: 5). He describes a triad of levels of meaning: linguistic (the figures), paralinguistic data, and voice quality (the extralinguistic background). His approach reflects Abercrombie's (1967) partitioning of the aural medium, in which the timing of auditory/physiological processes is emphasized. Voice quality, as the shifting 'overall timbre' of the voice, was also explored by Pike (1967: 525–527); but he considered it a 'subsegmental' phonemic unit for signalling contrastive meanings, in the sense of attitudinal expression, rather than a suprasegmental layer. What the theories share is the view of articulatory postures and movements over varying time periods creating auditorily recognizable settings of the vocal tract. Therefore, it is of critical importance to define a model that relates all the elements of the vocal tract in a coherent way. A linear 'source-filter' vocal tract model, where the larynx is only a sound-source modulator and the tongue, jaw and lips the principal consonantal and vocalic articulators, has its limitations. It has no way of elegantly linking glottal shape and oral articulation with the postural configurations (of whatever duration) that occur between them – all of which are interdependent. It is in effect missing a piece – the complex of sources and resonators that is the larynx.

1.2   The Laryngeal Articulator

In the model we have developed, the 'Laryngeal Articulator Model' (LAM), the lower part of the vocal tract contains a complex articulator equivalent to the tongue in the oral vocal tract. This replaces the ideas that the pharynx is an empty space controlled only by the muscles around its walls, that the tongue is the articulator that produces pharyngeal sounds, and that the epiglottis is an active articulator or the closing mechanism of the airway. All 'pharyngeal' and 'epiglottal' sounds, pharyngealization effects, epiglottalization effects, laryngealization, glottalization, and an array of lower-vocal-tract volume effects are produced by the action of the aryepiglottic constrictor mechanism together with associated tongue retraction and larynx raising. The locus of stricture is the upper border of the epilaryngeal tube. The aryepiglottic folds are the active articulator, and the epiglottis is the passive articulator. The model elaborates the larynx as an articulator rather than just a source of vocal fold vibration (Esling 2005, 2010). It also redefines the relationship between vibratory structures in the laryngeal space and identifies a set of resonating cavities that shape spectral energy in ways that are predictable based on the inherent folding properties of the articulator. The tongue is given a new relationship to the laryngeal articulator, as the tongue is no longer the primary articulator of pharyngeal/epiglottal sounds.

Our research has focused on observing what occurs within the lower vocal tract, in what we generally refer to as the 'laryngeal constrictor'. This mechanism as a whole is responsible for constriction at the glottis (which cannot be said to constrict on its own) and for increasing degrees of constriction that affect the shape of resonating cavities in the lower vocal tract and create new points of vibration. We have examined the principles that link the laryngeal region (which the airstream passes through first) with the oral region of the vocal tract and how this laryngeal region is used in various languages to signify meaning. Figure 1.1 presents a graphic two-dimensional representation of the two-part Laryngeal Articulator Model. The laryngeal articulator itself is depicted within the laryngeal vocal tract – the space beneath the dotted line, from the glottis (vocal folds), through the epilaryngeal tube, in front of the aryepiglottic folds at the top of the tube, up behind the hyoid bone, through the upper pharynx to the back of the tongue and beneath the uvula. Retraction of the tongue is related to laryngeal articulation, as is larynx raising. Other movements of the tongue (raising and fronting) define states of the oral vocal tract, as do movements of the velopharyngeal, mandibular, and labial articulators. Full constriction of the laryngeal articulator (also called the laryngeal constrictor mechanism or the aryepiglottic sphincter) defines the physiological process of airway closure (Esling 1996). It is important to note that while the laryngeal articulator could be viewed as a 'pseudo' or 'functional' sphincter (and we often refer to it, and the aryepiglottic folds specifically, as such), it is not an anatomical sphincter (Fink 1974a, 1974b).

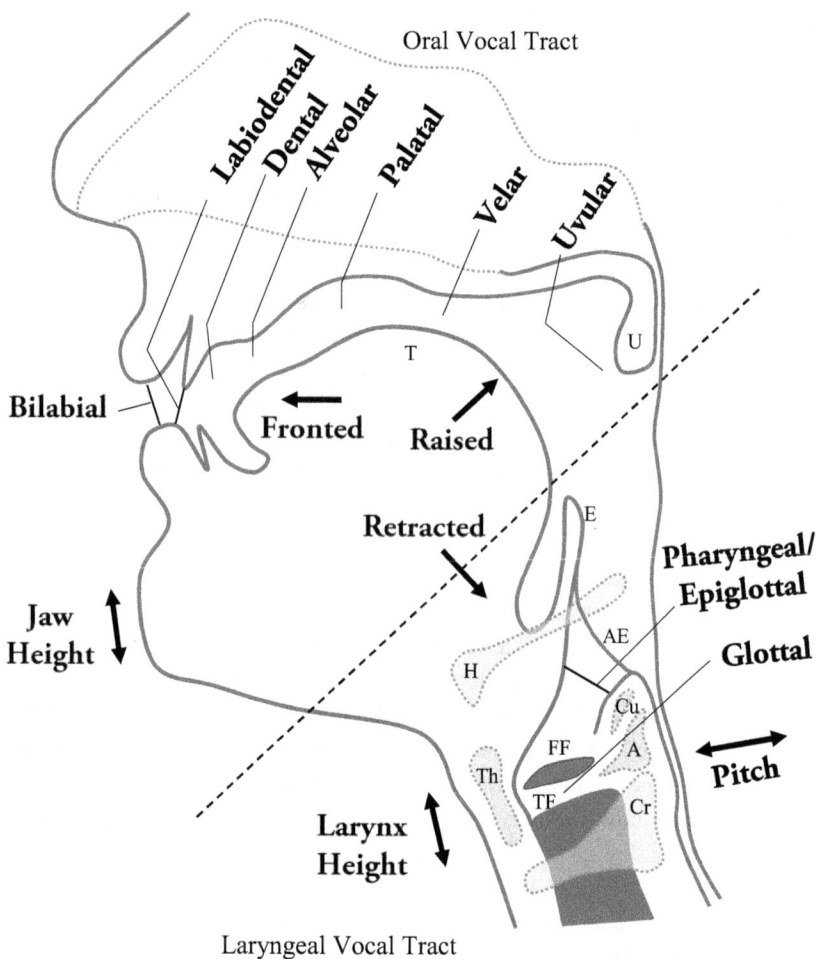

Figure 1.1 *The Laryngeal Articulator Model, or the two-part vocal tract*
T = tongue; U = uvula; E = epiglottis; H = hyoid bone; AE = aryepiglottic
folds; Cu = cuneiform cartilage; A = arytenoid cartilage; Th = thyroid
cartilage; FF = ventricular (false) folds; TF = vocal (true) folds;
Cr = cricoid cartilage.

Figure 1.1a in the accompanying media files illustrates the three stages of the compression or 'folding' behaviour of the vocal tract model in Figure 1.1. The laryngeal mechanism is shown, from left to right, from open, to closing, to almost closed. With progressive closure, as the constrictor mechanism folds in tighter on itself, tongue retraction and larynx raising also increase.

The model serves as the background guiding the interpretation of the voice quality strand of accent. Our designation of laryngeal activity as articulation reconciles the narrow notion of voice quality as phonation or vibratory register with the broader description of voice quality as a set of configurational postures throughout the vocal tract. The multitude of vibrations the laryngeal articulator can generate is a function of its pattern of constriction, related to its articulatory shaping of the lowest resonating chambers in the vocal tract. These resonances are a function of the volume of the epilaryngeal tube, of the degree of tongue retraction into the pharynx induced by aryepiglottic fold tightening and consequent vertical compaction, of the height of the larynx (distance below the hyoid bone) during these events, and of changes in the dimensions of the piriform fossae. Normally, the larynx is raised during laryngeal constriction, compressing the epilaryngeal tube and shortening the vocal tract through the pharynx. With accompanying tongue retraction, the pharynx is also compressed vertically, and resulting pharyngeal volumes are smaller. These effects are produced deep in the vocal tract, earlier than other resonance or noise components generated in the upper (oral) vocal tract. As a result, the laryngeal constrictor mechanism exerts a profound effect on the production and perception of voice quality throughout the entire vocal tract. Understanding that the larynx is an articulator and not just the location of vocal fold vibration makes it easier to grasp the ambiguity of voice quality as laryngeal phonation in counterpoint to voice quality as the long-term setting of the articulators. The laryngeal articulator contains and combines both of these actions at the same time, and there is no clear-cut physical boundary between the posture of the mechanism for generating a particular phonation type and for generating a resonance with spectral (formant) characteristics that might otherwise be termed vowel quality and attributed solely to a dominant lingual posture in the oral vocal tract. In fact, the interlaced relationship between vowel quality, tonal quality, and phonatory quality as components of voice quality is a fundamental principle underlying the Laryngeal Articulator Model of speech production in phonetic theory.

Although voice quality in its narrower sense is taken to refer only to phonation produced by the vocal folds at the glottis, sources of periodic vibration are not restricted to the glottal level alone. There are three main sets of folds within the laryngeal mechanism that can generate periodic energy: the vocal folds, the ventricular folds, and the aryepiglottic folds (Edmondson and Esling 2006). The vocal folds are the most efficient source of voicing, but the ventricular folds can add to the aerodynamic/mechanical action of vocal fold vibration, as in harsh types of phonation (cf. Esling 2005) or in some Tibetan chanting or throat-singing styles (Fuks et al. 1998). The third level of stricture in the larynx – the aryepiglottic folds – represents the sphincteric pursing of the top of the epilaryngeal tube. It is the primary place of articulation at which pharyngeals are produced. Sounds labelled as epiglottals are also produced at this same place of articulation, since there is no other 'place' that forms stricture in the lower vocal tract. Distinctive periodic signals, different from vocal or ventricular vibration, are generated when a particular configuration of the laryngeal constrictor mechanism allows the aryepiglottic folds to trill (vibrate) against the epiglottis. All three levels of laryngeal folds generate periodic signals that can be taken as a 'source'. Besides the three main sets of folds within the larynx, other tissues can also be made to undulate when aerodynamic flow is sufficient, including tissues in the walls of the epilaryngeal tube and the pharynx, the tip of the epiglottis, and even mucosal accumulations that build up in narrowed passages of the airway.

As an articulator, the larynx adds a complex of possibilities to the formulation of how each of the three strands of accent is constructed. It also lends a new phonetic interpretation to how linguistic, paralinguistic, and extralinguistic meaning relate. Inherent in the model is the principle that pharyngeals are primary in the formation of voice quality, both in its narrow sense and in its broader sense. That is, vibratory patterns that can be associated with voicing (phonation) reflect the same vibratory possibilities associated with pharyngeal articulatory contrasts, for example, pharyngeal/epiglottal trilling. This has important consequences for voice quality theory. It means, firstly, that the articulatory mechanism for producing pharyngeal sounds is more complex than previously considered. The auditory distinctions and descriptive categories that have proliferated to account for the many distinctions in this region have been justifiable and insightful (IPA 1989) but were not well explained by the vocal tract model available at the time. Pharyngeal articulations are essentially laryngeal, since epilaryngeal-tube stricture and the aryepiglottic fold constriction that occurs at the top of the epilaryngeal tube are at the same time responsible for protective airway closure and for the generation of sounds labelled 'pharyngeal' or 'epiglottal'. This implies that there are not two separate, linearly organized places of articulation for the category pharyngeal/epiglottal, which is not independent of the larynx (see Esling 1999). Furthermore, instead of laryngeal sound production being restricted to glottal events (attributed to the vocal folds and shaping of the glottis), laryngeal sound production includes both glottal events and pharyngeal/epiglottal articulatory possibilities through the epilaryngeal tube and past the aryepiglottic folds at its superior border. These structures are depicted in Figure 1.2. Describing

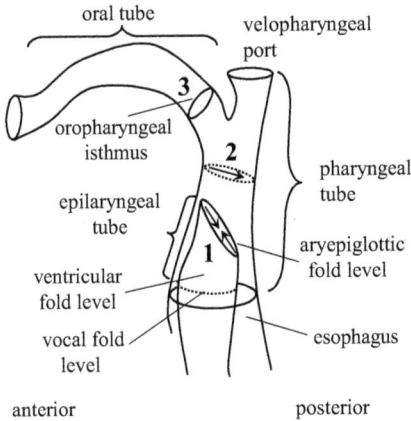

© 2018 Scott R. Moisik

Figure 1.2 *The epilarynx as a tube-within-a-tube*
The tube-shaped epilarynx is found at the bottom of the pharynx tube;
together these two regions define the lower vocal tract (LVT). The broad,
mostly independent actions of these tubes are (1) epilaryngeal constriction
and (2) pharyngeal constriction. The anterior boundary of the LVT is
delimited by (3) velic sphinctering at the oropharyngeal isthmus.

pharyngeal articulations as a function of the laryngeal mechanism also has the consequence that pharyngeals precede other places of articulation in vocal tract geography and occupy a preeminent place in the chronological acquisition of speech sounds, so that the description of pharyngeal/epiglottal articulations figures at the core of voice quality description when infants are first learning to speak (addressed in Chapter 6).

1.3   Origins of Voice Quality Theory

The comprehensive history of voice quality presented by Laver (1975, 1979, 1980, 1991) chronicles the earliest origins of the concept of voice quality in phonetic theory. Laver (1975: 90) credits Wilkins (1668) with being the first in English to identify different linguistic communities as having generalized speech characteristics as a product of the different ways of rendering the basic set of speech sounds and the preponderance of certain sounds. Wilkins called individual speech sounds 'letters' and the generalized characteristics the 'pronunciation' – the differences in 'pronunciation' between languages depending 'upon the nature of those letters, of which they do chiefly consist and are framed' (1668: 381). In the nineteenth century, Henry Sweet at Oxford, whom many credit with being the inspiration for George Bernard Shaw's character Professor Henry Higgins in *Pygmalion* (cf. *My Fair Lady*) but which was more likely directly inspired by Daniel Jones (Collins and Mees 1998), explored 'the quality of the voice' in contrasting languages (1877). Sweet used the term 'organic basis' (1890: 69, Henderson 1971: 182–187) to refer to the long-term quality specific to a given language, although it is likely that others in the nineteenth century, such as Alexander Graham Bell (1908) shared the same concept. Paul Passy and Daniel Jones fostered this view of the 'indexical' nature of accent (see Laver 1968), inspiring Beatrice Honikman at University College London to explore 'articulatory settings' in the accents of various language groups (1964). Abercrombie's (1967: 89–95) definition of 'voice quality' is the most cogent placement of the concept within phonetic theory as having a general, relatively non-fluctuating quasi-permanent character, distinguishing it temporally from rapidly fluctuating segmental (vowel and consonant) articulations and middle-duration dynamic (prosodic) patterns.

A long-standing hypothesis in voice quality theory has been the premise that the long-term postural setting of the articulators predisposes and facilitates the performance of the more rapidly fluctuating segmental articulations. A corollary of this hypothesis is that adopting the long-term postural setting of a new target language makes it easier to perform the shorter-term segmental (and perhaps dynamic) articulations of that language. This was Honikman's goal in describing the articulatory settings most characteristic of the speech of contrasting languages (see also Esling and Wong 1983). As Sweet put it: 'Every language has certain general tendencies which control its organic movements and positions, constituting its organic basis or basis of articulation. A knowledge of the organic basis is a great help in acquiring the pronunciation of a language' (1890: 69). These claims have proven difficult to demonstrate empirically, although they provide a theoretical argument that remains attractive. Chomsky and Halle drew attention to a preparatory state of the articulators before speaking, with the vocal processes adducted in preparation for voicing, which they called the 'neutral position'. As Chomsky and Halle observed, citing cineradiographic studies of speech, 'just prior to speaking the subject positions his vocal tract in a certain characteristic manner' (1968: 300). There was initial scepticism that a physiological posture acquired over time could be universal rather than a function of cultural development (Annan 1972). And research into voice quality has demonstrated that the 'neutral position' of the articulators is language specific, that is, it exhibits a configurational bias depending on the speech patterns in the language variety a speaker has learned (Gick et al. 2004). Kedrova and Borissoff (2013) have summarized the treatment in the Russian literature of the principle of 'articulatory base' as a 'summation' of phonetic movements distinguishing specific languages.

Studies have gradually established some of the configurations proper to specific language varieties, for example, sociophonetic research on social stratification (Knowles 1974, Trudgill 1974, Esling 1978, 1991) and long-term average spectral research (Harmegnies 1987, Harmegnies et al. 1989, 1994, Esling et al. 1991) which assesses the distribution of energy peaks in the spectrum integrated over time. The importance of Harmegnies' contribution is enhanced by the attention to phonemically balanced texts as a basis for comparing long-term settings, in order to reduce the biased effect of recurring segmental articulations on algorithms that measure average spectral energy over time. Other important studies have included acoustic research on bilingual speakers (Bruyninckx et al. 1994), Vocal Profile Analysis (Laver et al. 1991, Laver and Mackenzie Beck 2007, Stuart-Smith 1999, Mackenzie Beck and Schaeffler 2015), acoustic research across language varieties (DiCanio 2009, 2012, Garellek 2012), ultrasound research (Schaeffler and Scobbie 2010), perceptual studies of ethnicity (Trent 1995), and research into gender styles and speaker identity (Podesva 2007, Podesva and Callier 2015). It has been more common to identify linguistic predispositions at the level of basic or simple phonation types, e.g. creaky voice and falsetto, although some products of the laryngeal constrictor, e.g. harsh voice, have been identified. This is likely the result of both the basic role that phonation plays in giving the voice its fundamental nature and the familiarity that the description of phonation type has enjoyed in linguistic research (as well as its close association to pitch). Some studies specify larynx positioning, for example, applications of the Vocal Profile Analysis in sociophonetic, mother–child, or disordered speech contexts (Mackenzie Beck 1988, 2005) or in socioforensic voice comparison (Foulkes and French 2012, San Segundo et al. 2016, 2018), in which, for example, Panjabi English in the UK has been described as lowered larynx, denasal, and lingually raised (velarized or uvularized) (Wormald 2016). A promising approach to identifying habitual articulatory settings throughout the vocal tract during rest and speech-ready positions by quantifying automatically extracted images from real-time magnetic resonance imaging (rtMRI) has been begun by Ramanarayanan et al. (2013).

Descriptive phonetic labels that have articulatory referents are distinguished by Laver (1974, 1980) from popular 'impressionistic' labels for voice quality. Descriptive (auditory) phonetic labels differ from popular usage, since they are shared by a community of phoneticians who have learned and applied them with reference to self-produced and observed articulatory production. This derives from the phonetic principle that a normal human vocal tract generates predictable auditory and acoustic outcomes when particular articulatory gestures are produced and that phoneticians trained in the same descriptive paradigm share a common set of referents. Agreement, however, is a function of training and time on task. Although Catford (1977a) argues that proprioceptive mechanisms underlie the ability to hear differences in sound states and to associate them with the movements of one's own articulators, it cannot be said that all phoneticians will share the same perceptions, or indeed articulatory productions, even though they were trained in the same school. Nevertheless, when an auditory system attains wide acceptance by the academic community, linguists tend to accept phoneticians' or fieldworkers' notation that a vowel has an [i] quality or an [u] quality, for example, or that one vowel is modal and that another is non-modal. Our approach follows primarily the methodology of auditory description. Our model, as it is applied to voice quality analysis, endeavours to make at least one auditory distinction clear – the difference between constricted and unconstricted laryngeal states, and their articulatory origins. In the Edinburgh phonetic tradition, the realizations of long-term phonation type and of long-term articulatory setting are referred to as an individual's 'voice quality settings' (Laver 1980). Research is invited to test the acoustic consequences of contrasting laryngeal settings and whether particular settings facilitate the articulation of specific segmental targets. Experimental techniques to examine long-term postures of the oral vocal tract and of laryngeal articulator movements in particular can be expected to contribute larger sample sizes of data to address the 'facilitative posture' hypothesis in voice quality research (a term we prefer to 'ease of articulation').

Beyond individual differences, we are able to distinguish auditorily if a person has a cold, or laryngitis, or various chronic conditions from the characteristic long-term qualities affecting the person's normal speech. Within a national community, we can often tell where a person comes from based on the shared voice quality settings peculiar to any given region, depending on our exposure and experience. Social class is also marked by a preference for particular settings, but these also depend on regional standards of accent. Nasal voice, for instance, carries high social prestige when associated with certain accents (viz. RP, Standard Edinburgh English) but stands out as an undesirable feature to many listeners when associated with other accents (see Esling 2000). Attributions of status are quite subjective. Tracing the incidence of voice quality traits, and people's reactions to them, however, is a valuable tool in sociophonetic research (cf. Preston 2006). Language attitudes, and even the desire to modify one's own accent when learning a second language, can be dependent on identities and feelings of self-esteem signalled by differences in voice quality settings (Gobl and Ní Chasaide 2003).

Paralinguistically, changes in setting over short periods of time give an indication of changing stylistic choices or emotional states of the speaker. These are referred to as 'register shifts'. Although some aspects of the vocal expression of emotion may be physiologically universal, interpretations of subtle vocal cues are culturally conditioned (Laver and Trudgill 1979, Scherer 2003). Listeners may be tempted to extend interpretations of emotion to ascribe fixed psychological traits to a speaker. The cultural contexts of this kind of stereotyping have been explored through phonetic analyses of the production of various voice types by professional voice actors and by evaluating listeners' perceptual responses to a range of vocal character-role portrayals (Teshigawara 2003, Teshigawara and Murano 2004, Moisik 2012).

1.4   Articulatory Parameters

1.4.1   Phonation Types

In the following sections, voice quality categories are described auditorily with their articulatory correlates, beginning with the production of phonation types (vibratory sources) in the larynx, then the discrimination of resonance or noise or vibratory characteristics within the laryngeal vocal tract, and finally the identification of resonance or noise or vibratory characteristics through the oral vocal tract. The categories are updated from Laver (1980), where the majority of descriptive information can be found, but instead of dividing the vocal tract into laryngeal and supralaryngeal parts, we include as phonation all vibrations that can occur within the laryngeal articulator. Our descriptions concentrate on the configuration of the laryngeal constrictor mechanism.

Phonatory laryngeal categories include the distinction between *breath*, which generates noise through friction, and *voice*, which generates a quasi-periodic vibratory signal. This fundamental distinction was described by Wilkins in the seventeenth century (1668), where breath was associated with *mute* consonants and voicing with *sonorous* consonants (cf. the French usage *sourde* vs. *sonore*). The terminology remains useful, because even twentieth-century phonetic descriptions sometimes use the term *voicelessness* for breath, which is only one of a number of voiceless states of the glottis. Breath and voice constitute a crucial phonetic means of distinguishing consonants in the stream of speech, but they are not adequate to account for all of the subtle modifications that the laryngeal constrictor mechanism can bring to voice quality. Another voiceless state of the glottis (or, more properly, state of the larynx) is *whisper*, which resembles breath at the level of the glottis but which is laryngeally constricted through the epilaryngeal tube above the glottis, generating enhanced friction and therefore greater noise. The unconstricted laryngeal posture for breath and the constricted laryngeal posture for whisper represent phonetic options for the realization of voiceless consonants (or vowels) in a sound system. Varying from individual to individual, increased whisperiness can be thought of as an enhancement of the basic breath state that gives the voiceless consonants in the stream of speech more friction and therefore a cumulative *whispery* quality. Degrees of breathiness and whisperiness lie along a continuum of openness to tightness of the aryepiglottic constrictor mechanism that distinguishes different speakers' voices.

The same principle applies to the voicing of vowels and consonants. If a speaker's phonation is neutral – the most usual kind of voice – it is described as *modal voice*, in the sense of the mode of a distribution. Hollien attempted to define modal in terms of normal frequencies used in speaking and singing (1972, 1974: 126). Laver disputed the reliability of pitch as a definition and considered 'the neutral mode of phonation' only a description of voicing 'when no specific feature is explicitly changed or added' (1980: 95). Laver deferred to aerodynamic-myoelastic studies such as Catford's (1964: 32), who, like many others, used the term 'normal' for modal voicing (which may not, however, be the norm for any given linguistic community). What our model contributes to the debate is a definition of laryngeal constriction – the progressive folding or buckling of the aryepiglottic constrictor mechanism – causing a departure from modal phonation. Adding increased laryngeal constriction to otherwise modally voiced components of speech will alter the quality of phonation in one of two ways. Either the voicing will take on the phonatory characteristics of *harsh voice* or pitch will lower to what is termed *creaky voice*, since laryngeal constriction also shortens the vocal folds (increasing their effective mass per unit length) and lowers pitch (in addition to its effect on phonatory quality). Of course both could happen. Either one of these effects could be termed 'laryngealization' and designated broadly in IPA notation with the subscript tilde [̰]. This example demonstrates two principles in voice quality analysis: (1) that an articulatory modification in a critical part of the vocal tract can have multiple effects, pitch being a significant variable; and (2) that the modification can have related effects on both voiceless and voiced segments. It would be unusual for the addition of increased laryngeal constriction in a voice to affect only the voiced components of speech and not the voiceless components. A likely phonatory effect of constriction would be increased whisperiness on the voiceless segments and increased harshness on the voiced segments.

Voiced phonation can also take on breathy or whispery characteristics. *Breathy voice* is the state where vibration for voicing occurs at the anterior end of the glottis while air is escaping at the wider posterior end of the glottis. The parallel laryngeally constricted state of *whispery voice* has the same glottal configuration as breathy voice but with a narrowed epilaryngeal tube over the top of the glottis creating greater turbulent friction and noise and affecting the character of voicing. A voice might be encountered that realizes voiceless segments as breath and voiced segments as breathy voice; or a voice might realize voiceless segments as whisper and voiced segments as whispery voice. Varying degrees of *whisperiness, harshness,* and *creakiness* can be combined, all being functions of laryngeal constriction. The descriptive convention is usually to specify whether the constituent elements are present to a slight, moderate, or extreme degree. Thus, a voice could demonstrate varying degrees of the constituents of *harsh whispery creaky voice.* By contrast, breathiness reflects an open (unconstricted) laryngeal posture – where the aryepiglottic constrictor mechanism is in its unfolded position. In the pitch domain, stretching the glottis in the antero-posterior direction (known as longitudinal tension and the opposite of low-pitched creaky voice) changes the voice component towards the *falsetto* end of the pitch continuum. The same auditory qualities that occur during constriction can also be realized at high pitch as degrees of *harsh whispery creaky falsetto,* although the articulatory mechanisms may differ. The detailed relationships between pitch and laryngeal articulator postures are not yet well understood, underlining the need for further research into the articulatory correlates of auditory voice quality settings.

1.4.2 Elaborations of the Laryngeal Articulator

Harshness is a function of the laryngeal constrictor mechanism – a complex quality that interacts with pitch in unique ways. Harsh voice quality is identified when the voicing frequency becomes irregular or aperiodic (jitter in acoustic terms), amplitude begins to vary (shimmer in acoustic terms), and as the vocal folds and ventricular folds are compressed in a narrowing supraglottic space by the overarching tightening of the aryepiglottic folds. When pitch is low (i.e. when there is little antero-posterior longitudinal tension to stretch the vocal folds), the aryepiglottic folds themselves can be induced to vibrate. This quality is what occurs in a growl. This is referred to as *aryepiglottic trilling,* a form of harsh voice usually at *low pitch.* Harsh voice, at *mid pitch* for the sake of comparison, is the neutral state of harshness and has less likelihood of aryepiglottic fold trilling, as the laryngeal structures are more compacted from bottom to top. When glottal length is increased, as for falsetto, but tight supraglottic laryngeal constriction is maintained, the stretching mechanism and the constriction mechanism create an isometric tension that keeps the glottis closed unless a forceful airstream is used to generate phonation. This type of harsh voice occurs at *high pitch*. The quality is strained, often called *pressed voice* in speech-science contexts, and resembles articulatorily a glottal stop with air being forced through it. The auditory quality is characteristic of phonating during heavy lifting, alternatingly holding the breath. All categories of harshness are related by the presence of laryngeal constriction – an action that tightens the epilaryngeal tube and compresses vibrating structures vertically, interfering with the glottal vibration pattern.

Aside from phonatory or vibratory effects, the laryngeal constrictor mechanism generates resonances through changes in pharyngeal volumes that have distinctive auditory correlates. *Raised-larynx voice* – the auditory label defined by Laver (1980: 24–29) – is the archetypal quality resulting from a shortened pharyngeal volume due to aryepiglottic constriction, tongue retraction, and larynx raising. Relative pitch needs to be high in order for this auditory quality to be realized. Otherwise, if relative pitch is low, the same constricted posture of the laryngeal/pharyngeal resonators for raised-larynx voice generates an auditory quality that is termed *pharyngealized voice*. Both settings require the laryngeal constrictor to actively narrow the epilaryngeal tube. The primary parameter differentiating the two qualities – pitch – requires cricothyroid contraction to lengthen the vocal folds for raised-larynx voice and thyroarytenoid activity to shorten and bunch the vocal folds for pharyngealized voice. Achieving low pitch by lowering the larynx is antagonistic to the larynx raising that reflexively accompanies laryngeal constriction, resulting in pharyngealized voice sounding more strained to produce than its more reflexively natural counterpart, raised-larynx voice.

The muscular mechanism for raising the larynx is one of the three principal components of the laryngeal constrictor mechanism. The muscles responsible for elevating the larynx in the settings of both raised-larynx voice and pharyngealized voice – the suprahyoid group and, critically, the thyrohyoid muscles – are the same muscles used in swallowing, which involves lifting the tongue up and forwards and then backwards as aryepiglottic constriction occurs, the tongue retracts, and the larynx raises to protect the airway. It is critical to our approach that raised-larynx voice quality be viewed not just as a product of lifting the laryngeal cartilages (together with the hyoid bone or not). Lifting the larynx up to the hyoid bone is part of a recruitment chain that entails other parallel actions, namely, engaging the aryepiglottic constrictor and retracting the tongue. Since the hyoid bone is suspended muscularly between the mandible and the thyroid, with no articulation with any other bone, the natural reflexive action of laryngeal constriction recruits the hyoglossus muscles to pull the tongue down to the hyoid bone (the anchor bone of the tongue) at the same time that the larynx as a whole is lifted towards the hyoid bone by the thyrohyoid muscles. Larynx height is the most manipulable of the three components of laryngeal constriction. It is possible to pull the larynx downwards while the aryepiglottic constrictor narrows the epilaryngeal tube, but this is not a reflexively natural manoeuvre; whereas either retracting the tongue to its hyoid base or raising the larynx up to the hyoid bone will reflexively trigger the aryepiglottic mechanism to engage. To assume that the acoustic consequence of raising the larynx is that all spectral formants should rise does not take into account the mechanics of the laryngeal constrictor. Although Sundberg and Nordström's (1976: 38–39) phoniatrician and singer subjects controlled larynx height, resulting in elevated formant frequencies, Nolan (1983: 182–187) cites a number of results for raised-larynx voice where F1 increases but F2 decreases, concluding that some form of pharyngeally constricted configuration is responsible. Our explanation for this quantum coming together of F1 and F2 (as well as for unexplained F3 and F4 effects depending on vowel quality) is that aryepiglottic constriction of the epilaryngeal tube is occurring during raised-larynx voice, with accompanying tongue retraction. Moisik (2013: 293–308) presents a detailed acoustic analysis of the influence of larynx height on formant structure, measured using laryngeal ultrasound, showing the effect to be complex, with raised-larynx voice generally associated with lowering of F2 and F3. We further contend that aryepiglottic constriction during raised-larynx voice explains the results of Nolan's and Laver's productions and that this articulatory combination is the normal reflexive pairing for this voice quality type. Nolan's (1983: 183) radiographic tracings of contrasting larynx heights illustrate the narrowing of the epilaryngeal tube that occurs in the raised mode. The examples we present in Chapter 2 and Chapter 4 reflect this pairing, and we contend that the average speaker (not trained professionally in voice to suppress these relationships) would produce the canonical qualities of raised-larynx voice and of pharyngealized voice with active laryngeal constriction. Even in the case of a professionally trained singer, we suspect that the ability to suppress laryngeal constriction during larynx raising will result in other compensatory articulatory effects. This would explain why F1 did not increase and F2 increased substantially for close front vowels for Sundberg and Nordström's subjects, but F1 increased and F2 did not increase as much for open vowels; open vowels being more integrally susceptible to the action of the laryngeal constrictor.

To stretch and relax the muscles used in raising the larynx and constricting the epilaryngeal space, the opposing set of infrahyoid muscles, particularly the sternothyroid muscles, contract to lower the larynx. This is what happens in a yawn. The quality of voice generated is called *lowered-larynx voice*. This auditory category is accompanied by low pitch. Otherwise, if pitch is high, the same lowered posture of the larynx generates what is recognized auditorily as *faucalized voice* (Esling et al. 1994), when the 'faucal pillars' of the palatoglossus and palatopharyngeal muscles are visibly stretched at the back of the mouth, due to the larynx descending and pulling them downwards. Larynx height is not an explicit parameter in the chart of the IPA. The effect of lowering the larynx has been described from cineradiographic data as an 'expanded pharynx', correlated with advancing the tongue root, which contrasts in Kwa languages with a 'constricted pharynx' (Lindau 1975, 1979). Our model classifies the latter as laryngeal constriction, correlated with retracting the tongue root and raising the larynx, and its associated effects. Acoustically, reducing cavity volume within and around the epilaryngeal tube raises spectral frequencies; but concomitant tongue retraction enlarges other resonating spaces so that F2 and F3 are lowered, as in an open vowel. For this reason, laryngeal constriction typically yields a high F1 and low F2. The lowered-larynx setting, as the polar opposite of constriction, naturally moves the tongue forward as the airway opens and pharynx volume expands, lowering spectral frequencies. These contrasting articulatory configurations generate different resonances and predispose opposing phonatory effects. The raised-larynx setting predisposes narrowed-tube whisperiness or harsh effects such as aryepiglottic trilling. The lowered-larynx setting predisposes opening of the airway and breathiness; hence its correlation with yawning. These postures are traditionally described as supralaryngeal longitudinal settings (Laver 1980). Localizing them within the larynx and defining the degree of laryngeal constriction relative to larynx height, following the Laryngeal Articulator Model, allows parallels to be drawn between vocal tract resonances and related phonation types, the articulatory postures that generate them, and their auditory correlates (Esling 2005).

For lowered-larynx settings, the sternothyroid muscles pull the thyroid cartilage directly towards the sternum. The sternohyoid and omohyoid muscles may contract during lowered-larynx voice and faucalized voice, but this may not be necessary for all speakers in normal speaking style. The thyrohyoid muscles do not contract. If they did, approximating the thyroid cartilage and the hyoid bone, synergistic laryngeal constriction would ensue, and the resulting quality would acquire the attributes of pharyngealized voice or of raised-larynx voice. The acoustic effect of lowering the larynx is, in general, to decrease formant frequencies, due to the expansion downwards and increased volume of the epilaryngeal cavity and upper pharyngeal cavity. It is important that an expanded pharyngeal cavity is also a function of an open, unconstricted epilaryngeal tube. The setting for raised-larynx, by contrast, is opposite in all of these respects: the tongue is retracted, pharynx spaces are shortened and narrowed medially, and the epilaryngeal tube is shallow and narrow and pushed anteriorly and upwards so that it is tucked up under the tongue and epiglottis. It is important to note that in almost every sagittal image or tracing in the literature, the epilaryngeal tube and other laryngeal articulator structures are absent, and the space between the epiglottis and vocal folds is empty. Figures 1.1 and 1.2 identify their location. The diagonal angles of the laryngeal constrictor mechanism make it difficult to image instrumentally. We nevertheless emphasize that existing data on the larynx and pharynx should be reinterpreted using the parameters of the LAM. The phonetic characteristics of each laryngeal state will be examined in detail in Chapter 2, with imaging depicting laryngeal articulator movement presented in Chapter 3.

Video 1.1 illustrates the difference between the neutral larynx posture of falsetto and lowering of the larynx for faucalized voice, maintaining high pitch. Nolan's (1983: 183) x-ray tracing of lowered larynx demonstrates how the epilaryngeal tube deepens and widens, how it is pulled posteriorly, and how the pharyngeal space above it is expanded vertically and widened due to the relatively unretracted tongue posture. The full extent of the effects on glottal voicing of exerting longitudinal tension for high pitch while at the same time lowering the larynx (as in faucalization) remains understudied.

1.5   Supralaryngeal Categories

1.5.1   Velopharyngeal Settings

Above the laryngeal articulator, along a line intersecting the tongue and the uvula, at what can be called the right angle of the vocal tract, the oral articulator begins. The nasal tract also branches off at this point. Behind the uvula, the quality of *nasal voice* is generated when an open velopharyngeal port couples the nasal tract to the other resonators. Nasal resonance differs from laryngeal and oral articulatory adjustments since the shape of the nasal cavity does not change articulatorily, but the degree of nasality is influenced by the size of the velopharyngeal opening. Because of this, the quality of nasal resonance is often thought of forensically as a useful marker of individual identity, with fewer anatomically varying elements than other, more manipulable, settings (Dickson 1980). The prevalence of nasality in a voice, reflecting the degree of velopharyngeal port opening and the proportion of time it is opened, can vary as a consequence of social accommodation in acquiring a language. The degree of acquired nasality is under a speaker's control and remains a powerful indicator of social or regional background. Altering the shapes of the cavities below the velopharyngeal port, such as raising or retracting the tongue or raising or lowering the larynx, will also have an effect on the quality of nasal resonance. Such lingual postures play a role in *denasal voice*, which is an interesting combination of tongue raising and nasal airflow in juxtaposition to the denasalization of segments that are normally nasal, such as [m] becoming [b] or [n] becoming [d]. This illustrates how long-term voice quality can be defined by its interaction with the segmental strand of speech.

The muscles that open the velopharyngeal port are the palatoglossus muscles, linking the soft palate and the tongue near the back of the oral cavity. These muscles define the first (more lateral and anterior) 'faucal pillars' that can be seen at the rear of the oral cavity. The palatopharyngeal muscles form the second (more medial and posterior) faucal pillars and may also assist in lowering the velum. However, since the port is open during quiet nasal breathing, to produce a nasal sound it is sufficient simply not to close the port. Gravity assists in maintaining an open port in upright positions. Nasal closure could therefore be considered the active acquired articulation for oral speaking. In efficient adult speech, the speed of segmental articulation requires that the velopharyngeal musculature shifts quickly between oral and nasal components, within the limits of long-term voice quality and depending on the phonotactic distribution of nasality in the particular language. In cases of rapid transition, the muscles for closure and the muscles for opening will alternate actively. The palatal levator muscles, descending from the temporal bone of the skull, close the velopharyngeal port, commonly by the 'coronal' or 'trapdoor' method of closure (Gick et al. 2013). The palatal tensor muscles and uvular muscle assist with stiffening the velum for closure.

1.5.2   *Lingual Settings*

The tongue is the principal oral articulator. Its temporal interaction with the movements of the jaw and the lips defines most segmental sounds along the parameters of place and manner of articulation, from labial to uvular. The long-term postures of these articulators are salient accompaniments to the segmental stream of speech, providing the background noise, resonance, and perturbations perceived as voice quality settings. While the tongue retracts as a reflexive complement to laryngeally constricted sounds, the tongue raises (upwards and posteriorly) to produce uvularized or velarized sounds. Persistent raising of the tongue in this way, where the lingual dorsum habitually approximates or frequently returns towards the soft palate yields *uvularized voice* or *velarized voice*. Uvular approximation is as far as the tongue can go back into the upper pharyngeal cavity without retracting towards the laryngeal articulator. Velar approximation occurs further forward, about where the soft palate joins the hard palate. Both tongue raising (uvularization and velarization) and tongue fronting can be accompanied by tongue retraction as a secondary quality or as a consonantal or vocalic gesture, and it is physically possible to raise the tongue up and back and to front the tongue at the same time.

Palatalized voice results from the fronting of the tongue, with the tongue tip down, so that the body of the tongue fills the top of the oral cavity. There is some indeterminacy in voice quality theory as to how much of the time the tongue body spends in a lifted posture when the auditory quality is palatalized vs. how frequently palatal articulations occur. In most cases, movements of the tongue tip and jaw depart from the centre of gravity of the tongue body to perform various segmental articulations, but the positioning of the 'centre' also depends on where the other parts of the articulators are positioned. In extreme cases of palatalized voice, all segmental articulations can be produced with the tongue tip anchored behind the lower incisors. The detection of a preponderance of palatalized sound would lie at the extreme end of a perceptual continuum that can decline to moderate or slight. *Palato-alveolarized voice* is a quality resulting from a more fronted posture of the tongue body that can also have a tongue-tip-anchored lingual posture. When the tongue body moves forwards, and closer to the hard palate due to the downward sloping angle of the hard palate through the alveolar ridge to the teeth, *alveolarized voice* or *dentalized voice* can result. These places of articulation are closely related to how tongue-front consonants are produced, so there may be more overlap of the positioning of the tongue body with the activity of the tongue tip. But persistent fronting of the tongue tip to or through the teeth gives a distinct long-term percept of dentalization (as in Dutch-accented English). The habitual orientation of the tongue tip has given rise to the categories *tongue tip articulation (apical)*, *tongue blade articulation (laminal)*, and *retroflex articulation*, the last of these being the most distinct in both articulatory and peripheral auditory terms. It could be postulated that the posture in which the tongue body is oriented lends a more uniform impression of persisting quality, while the activity of the tongue tip conveys an impression of long-term quality through the frequency of repeatedly articulated consonants in a particular direction. In general, tongue-fronted, tongue-raised, and tongue-retracted postures reflect the three main contractile directions of the extrinsic lingual musculature. There is synergy between the muscles, so all may participate in holding the tongue body in a relatively fixed orientation, varying in the proportion of contractile strength. For any given speaker, the propensity of the musculature to pull in a particular direction over time defines the preferred locus or centre of gravity of the body of the tongue. Clearly delineated auditory qualities are easiest to detect when the 'centre' posture is exaggerated, as in canonical phonetic illustrations, while individual speakers may not emphasize a single locus so clearly in their language. Numerous key illustrative tokens of each category are offered in Chapter 4.

The Laryngeal Articulator Model has implications for the design of the vowel space. Fronted vowels and raised vowels can be isolated, with retracted vowels separated from the other two directions since they are implicated in pharyngealization and laryngealization manoeuvres. Figure 1.3 depicts the variably dependent role of retraction – the mediating link between vowel quality and laryngeal quality. The spatial notions of high-low and front-back are therefore replaced in our terminology by fronted, raised and retracted, with open vowels being distinguished from close vowels at the front of the vowel space by the opening of the jaw. Fronting, raising, and retracting are lingual parameters, while opening and closing are mandibular parameters. The basis for redrawing the vowel chart is explained in Esling (2005).

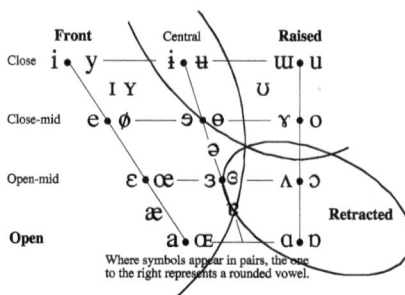

Figure 1.3 *An adapted IPA vowel chart*
This demonstrates three directions of major lingual pull (front, raised, retracted), the action of the jaw at the front of the mouth (close–open), and the affinity of retracted vowels to laryngeal constriction.

The tongue is retracted by the hyoglossus (HG) muscles. It is raised (pulled up and back) by the styloglossus (SG) muscles. The three parts of the genioglossus muscles – posterior (GGP), medial (GGM), anterior (GGA) – are responsible for moving the tongue for front gestures, as well as synergistic stabilization. Harris et al. (1992) analyse the participation of these muscles in the shaping of a set of American English vowels, based on electromyographic (EMG) readings. For [i], major activity is recorded in the GGA to pin the tongue tip behind the lower teeth and the GGP to front the tongue body. For [e ɪ ɛ], there is important GGA activity but little GGP activity. All front vowels register activity of the geniohyoid (GH) muscles for lowering the jaw, while [æ] shows maximum GGA and GH activity. Small proportions of HG activity and smaller proportions of SG activity accompany front vowels, as stabilizing forces. For [ɑ], there is maximum HG activity, with stabilizing by GGA, GH, and SG. In their study, [ɔ] has maximum SG activity, pulling the tongue back, with HG participating strongly in positioning the tongue. The close back vowel [u] registers very strong SG activity, with reduced participation of the other muscles, while [ʊ] shows weak activity in HG and SG. This could be due to the nature of /ʊ/ in the American vowel set, which would not be expected to be as close and back as Cardinal [ʊ]. Honda (1996) represents the tongue-control muscles as two pairs of antagonists to explain tongue-body positioning in a four-corner vowel space: GGP for tongue fronting, HG for tongue retraction (down and back), GGA for tongue lowering (down and front), SG for tongue raising (up and back). EMG results confirm that GGP activity is prominent for the [i] corner of the vowel space, HG activity is highest for [ɑ], GGA activity peaks for [i] and [æ] (with jaw opening presumably accounting for [æ]), and SG activity peaks for the [u] corner of the vowel space. Antagonistic position-ing of the tongue implicates some SG activity for [ɑ], although it could be that the American target vowel moved closer to Cardinal [ɔ], and some HG activity for [æ], which from a laryngeal constrictor perspective demonstrates the inherent susceptibility of [æ] and [ɑ] to retraction.

This presents a picture of the tongue moving in three principal directions in the oral cavity, balanced by the forces of the extrinsic lingual muscles, with hinged jaw opening as the principal parameter at the front. To obtain dental-ized, alveolarized, palato-alveolarized, and palatalized lingual voice quality settings, we posit that GG, particularly GGP, contraction predominates to front the tongue. To obtain velarized and uvularized lingual voice quality settings, we posit that SG contraction predominates to raise the tongue (likely aided to a substantial degree by intrinsic lingual muscle contraction), keeping it in that position so as to produce a noticeable effect on articulations that naturally move away from the raised back part of the oral cavity. The voice quality parallel to GGA anchoring of the tongue tip for vowel [i] would extend to palato-alveolarized and palatalized voice, where tongue blade articulation could be expected to occur, but not necessarily to dentalized and alveolarized voice, where tongue tip articulation might be expected (but neither is obligatory). Tongue tip articulation involves interaction between the longitudinalis superior (LS) muscles to lift the tip and the longitudinalis inferior (LI) muscles to lower the tip, for which the front of the tongue must be free from excessive GGA activity in order to retain rapid mobility. Retroflex articulation of the tongue tip requires considerable longitudinalis superior contraction to hold the tip in a curled-back posture or to return to that position from other articulations that cannot be represented accurately when retroflexion is present. Retracted settings of the tongue body, when HG is active, are reflected in laryngeally constricted postures: pharyngealized voice and raised-larynx voice. The tongue cannot be retracted very far independently of the reflexive contraction of the aryepiglottic sphincter, usually with larynx raising. Therefore, HG contraction accompanies a series of actions involving not only the tongue but primarily the entire laryngeal constrictor mechanism.

Hardcastle (1976) depicts the location of each muscle group for all of the articulatory regions discussed here and contains a detailed illustration of how the intrinsic lingual muscles, particularly the transverse and vertical muscles, participate in the articulation of a fricative such as [s] (pp. 134–137). A considerable amount of research is still needed to determine the role of the intrinsic lingual muscles in shaping the contours of the front of the tongue and in forming medial sulculization to achieve delicate differences in sound quality such as those that occur in Dutch or Greek varieties of /s/. Ladefoged and Maddieson (1996: 145–164) refer to some of the fine differences in fricative production that require exceptional diacritic marking to convey their quality.

1.5.3   Mandibular Settings

Jaw posture has a noticeable impact on voice quality perception. One salient reason for this is the effect jaw opening has on vowel quality, which is why vowels in the IPA chart are labelled from close (pronounced /klos/) to open (rather than high to low). It is the jaw that opens to produce an open vowel, as can be demonstrated by producing an [i ~ æ] alternation without moving the tongue from its body-fronted tip-down configuration but only displacing the jaw. In terms of lingual articulatory possibilities, the element of jaw movement also explains why there is no fourth parameter of tongue-body movement to lower the tongue – only fronting, raising, and retracting. There is greater potential for tongue retraction to occur (down and back) as the jaw opens for an open [æ] vowel, but there is no specific lingual muscle lowering the tongue (other than the body-fronting and tip-anchoring muscle contractions that may occur for front vowels as a set). As long-term, quasi-permanent postures, or preferences, the contrasting close and open configurations are generalized as *close jaw voice* and *open jaw voice*. Close jaw voice might sometimes be rendered as clenched jaw, which is an extreme version of close jaw. The muscle groups effecting closure by lifting the jaw are the masseter and temporalis muscles, while opening the jaw is achieved by the anterior belly of the digastric (AD) and the geniohyoid muscles (Laver 1980: 65–67). The internal (medial) pterygoid muscles can assist in closure, and the external (lateral) pterygoids in opening. The pterygoids generally lever the jaw by pulling forwards towards the sphenoid bone, and are therefore the primary agents of jaw protrusion. Dropping the mandible from the temporomandibular joint (TMJ) occurs among elite singers to enhance resonance (Nair et al. 2016), presumably achieved by a combination of suprahyoid and external pterygoid activity. It is instructive to clench the jaw while articulating a full set of vowels, compared with opening the jaw wide while articulating the same set, in order to calibrate the effect of voice quality setting on individual vowel quality and to get a sense of which vowels are most susceptible to the effects of each setting. In addition to the up-down dimension, the jaw also moves in the front-back dimension. Named for the approximation of the upper teeth to the lower lip, *labiodentalized voice* (mandibular retraction) contrasts with *protruded jaw voice* (mandibular protrusion). Each setting has its own constraints on what labial configurations can accompany it.

Protruding the jaw (with the lower teeth and lip) is due to internal (medial) pterygoid contraction, pulling the mandible forwards by its rami, assisted by masseter/temporalis contraction upwards, and balancing antagonistically with anterior digastric and geniohyoid contraction downwards as to how far the jaw is opened during speech. Given the synergism of the internal pterygoids and the jaw-closing musculature, it would be more likely for protruded jaw to occur together with a close jaw posture than with an open jaw posture. In labiodentalization, the maxillary-to-mandibular positioning involves the anterior suprahyoid musculature (AD, GH) and tongue-floor musculature (mylohyoid) in balance with masseter/temporalis stabilization, pulling the jaw back so that the upper teeth extend beyond the lower lip. Contracting the levator labii superior muscles adds a lip-raising accompaniment, baring the upper teeth. Both labiodentalized and protruded settings are subtle postures to achieve and not uncommon as articulatory settings. If, however, the jaw-opening musculature were engaged more dramatically with external (lateral) pterygoid contraction, pulling the condyloid processes of the mandible forwards, levering the jaw downwards, an unusually open, gaping mouth would result. This would be an unusual speaking posture, exerting pressure on the TMJ.

1.5.4   Labial Settings

Labial postures are not only auditorily but also visually salient in voice quality perception, even more than tongue-front behaviour. *Close rounded voice, open rounded voice* (which also implies jaw opening), and *spread lip voice* are maximally distinctive. Articulatory rounding or protruding of the lips lengthens the vocal tract, while labial spreading shortens the vocal tract, with predictable acoustic/auditory effects. Saying a phrase, or counting 'one, two, three, four, five . . .' with close rounding vs. spreading, demonstrates the scale of the effect on the vowels and consonants spoken with these sustained postures.

Close rounding refers to the labial setting in which the lips are relatively close (rather than open), rounded (rather than spread), and where the jaw is also close (rather than open). This is the labial posture also described as 'rounded' for consonants such as [w] or for close vowels such as [u] or [y] or for close-mid vowels such as [o] or [ø]. Over a stretch of speech, during which consonants and vowels fluctuate, not all sounds will have the same degree of rounding. The effect of close rounding is naturally relative. Some segments, such as [i], which is canonically unrounded, are more susceptible to its effect than others, such as [u], which is already rounded; however, it is possible for [u] to be more rounded during the application of a close rounded setting than it otherwise would be, and [i] can become rounded during the application of a close rounded setting without necessarily becoming [y]. The concept of a quasi-permanent long-term setting is an abstraction: an averaging of the effect of the posture on all of the segments in the stretch of speech. A speaker with a habitually close rounded setting has on average more segments that are more rounded than they would be in the comparable speech of another speaker, in the same language or in another language. The muscles implicated are the orbicularis oris muscular complex (OO), which rings the mouth, and the muscles for closing the jaw: the masseter and temporalis.

Open rounding refers to the labial setting in which the lips are relatively open (rather than close), rounded (rather than spread), and where the jaw is also open (rather than close). This labial posture is also the 'rounded' feature of open vowels such as [ɒ] or [ɶ] or for open-mid vowels such as [ɔ] or [œ]. The muscles implicated are the OO, and the muscles for opening the jaw: the anterior digastric and geniohyoid. Not all segments in a stretch of speech can change their labial specification to open rounded without interfering with the linguistic meaning conveyed by that segment. The strong effect of open rounding may therefore limit its prevalence in many sound systems. There are two types of rounding that can be achieved by the labial muscles which are not adequately described by the terms 'close' or 'open' rounding. These are (1) anteriorly, the activity of the marginal layer of the orbicularis oris inferior muscles (OOIm) inducing sphincteric lip closure, and (2) the activity of the peripheral layer of the orbicularis oris inferior muscles (OOIp), with the depressor labii inferior muscles, enabling lip protrusion, as in tightening a purse-string (Honda et al. 1995b, Stavness et al. 2013). Varying degrees of marginal and peripheral activity can result in labial closure with or without protrusion, depending on the amount of OOIp contraction. Sweet's (1877) 'outer rounding' and 'inner rounding' (Henderson 1971: 63) attempted to capture this articulatory distinction.

Labial spreading as a voice quality setting could be described paralinguistically as smiling while speaking. As with the paralinguistic interpretation of 'smiling', the posture is an abstraction, where the 'smile' or spreading can be distinguished more readily during some segmental articulations rather than others. As with all other long-term settings, it is quasi-permanent, i.e. a muscular adjustment that is relative to the other muscular adjustments that are required to produce each segmental articulation. The muscles implicated are the risorius muscles, which pull back the corners of the mouth, and also the zygomatic muscles, pulling up and back on the sides of the mouth, when the effect is more extreme.

Some settings demonstrate asymmetrical postures, either unilaterally or as upper-lip effects. The lips and the front of the tongue are the most malleable and subtle of the articulators. They are also among the least well defined in IPA usage (see Esling 2010). Both the settings of the lips and settings of the front of the tongue are affected by the position of the jaw. Opening or closing or protruding the jaw affects the shape of the lips or, at least, can serve as a platform against which the lips can operate. Similarly, the positioning of the tongue front operates on the platform of the positioning of the jaw, so that front vowels, for example, are more determined by jaw opening than by tongue-front movement. Rounding or spreading of the lips is one parametric alteration that does not capture fully the range of movements that the lips can achieve. Independent movement of the lower or upper lips extends beyond the limits of the traditional taxonomy for labial settings. Furthermore, the movement of the lower (mandibular) lip is more dominated by the position of the jaw than is the upper lip. So a protruded jaw implies also a protruded lower lip; and the difference between close rounding and open rounding is primarily a function of jaw opening. The upper (maxillary) lip is more independent of jaw movement in average speaking circumstances. That is, in normal phonetic production (the average range of phonetic usage), settings of the upper lip are more likely to vary as a function of accent over the long term than movements of the lower lip, which will fluctuate more in response to jaw movement. It is therefore important to elaborate on the traditional description of what the lips can do together, to include descriptions of the settings of the upper lip and the lower lip independently.

A setting of the upper lip that is under close control and which can be manipulated in a longer-term role and superimposed on consonantal and vocalic articulations is the raising of either side of the upper lip. Raising one side of the upper lip as a dominant articulatory posture may favour particular segments (e.g. close vowels) in the phonological inventory, or raising both sides of the upper lip uniformly may correlate with a distinction in the segmental inventory that would be obscured were it not for the enhancement of the labial posture (see Section 4.2.5.4). Upper-lip elevation is achieved by levator labii superior muscular activity, with bilateral levator anguli oris accompaniment if it is more pronounced. Unilateral levator anguli oris contraction (left or right) is responsible for asymmetrical raising of the upper lip. Both postures can occur together with labial spreading.

1.6   The Pharyngeal Argument

1.6.1   *How the Pharynx Relates to the Larynx*
In the Laryngeal Articulator Model, the laryngeal articulator is the pharyngeal articulator, and it is the key to understanding voice quality. All manners of pharyngeal/epiglottal articulation are produced by aryepiglottic sphincteric stricture with associated tongue retraction and larynx raising. The action of the aryepiglottic folds at the top of the epilaryngeal tube has been attested through laryngoscopic observations of a great number of languages whose sound inventories contain consonants, vocal qualities, or tonal register qualities produced in the throat. Two places of articulation in traditional phonetic theory – 'pharyngeal' and 'epiglottal' – are both a function of this mechanism; that is, they represent the same place of articulation. A range of manners of articulation can be produced at this single place of articulation, through the narrowing of the epilaryngeal tube, through vibrations of structures above the

vocal folds, and through raising or lowering the larynx as a whole. Glottal articulations occur immediately below the bottom of the epilaryngeal tube (beneath the ventricles), which means, in effect, that glottal, pharyngeal, and epiglottal sounds are all components of the laryngeal articulator. For voice quality theory, this signifies that the manners of articulation articulated at the laryngeal constrictor (pharyngeal) place of articulation are fundamentally connected to the mechanism for producing phonation type. This means that some pharyngeal/epiglottal articulations are also states of the larynx and that phonation types and states of the larynx are not restricted to the glottis.

Many researchers' observations have led to the development of the LAM. As Laufer and Baer recall (1988: 184–185), a number of early phoneticians had been able to identify many of the components in the production of pharyngeals. The involvement of the epiglottis and the arytenoids was noticed by Brücke (1860). Panconcelli-Calzia surmised correctly in 1924 that backing of the epiglottis, raising of the larynx, and general constriction of the pharynx (although he assumed that the pharyngeal constrictor muscles constricted rather than the aryepiglottic sphincter muscles) are active in producing pharyngeals. Tur-Sinai (1937) made a correct analogy to swallowing and the production of pharyngeals. In the more recent literature on pharyngeals, numerous terms hint at the action of the laryngeal articulator mechanism as explained in our model. Hockett wrote of a '*pharyngeal catch*' 'in the lower pharyngeal region' (1958: 66). Catford, in his review of articulatory possibilities, advanced the term 'epiglottopharyngeal' to characterize 'extreme retraction of the tongue, so that the epiglottis approximates to the back wall of the pharynx' (1968: 326). He doubted whether a stop articulation could be performed at this location 'since it seems to be impossible to make a perfect hermetic closure between epiglottis and pharynx wall – stop-like sounds produced in this way appear to involve glottal closure as well as epiglottopharyngeal close approximation'. This was correct, as even though the tongue and epiglottis can approximate the posterior pharyngeal wall, they cannot effect the kind of seal that the aryepiglottic mechanism makes, and we do not consider their retraction possible without prior epilaryngeal closure. There are reports of the tongue closing against the posterior pharyngeal wall in some compensatory disordered speech (Honjow and Isshiki 1971), but this cannot be called the usual 'pharyngeal stop' commonly found in linguistic sound systems (see Sections 2.3.6 and 4.3.2). Catford identified, however, that 'epiglottopharyngeal *fricative*, *approximant* and possibly *trill* can be produced' (1968: 326), bolstering the argument that the place of articulation is below the lingual root area. Delattre (1971) identified acoustic characteristics of pharyngealization and framed vowel qualities in German, Spanish, French, and American English in terms of their parallels to the pharyngeals of Arabic. This interpretation is instructive because it introduces the notion that constriction in the pharyngeal region can accompany a variety of backed sounds even in languages that do not have pharyngeals per se. In early fibreoptic laryngoscopic work, Fujimura and Sawashima (1971) suspected that [tʔ] finals in American English can involve adduction of the ventricular folds, suggesting that 'glottalization' may involve stricture above the glottis. Catford also identified a 'ventricular or strong glottal stop ... [ʕ͡ʔ]' in contrast with [ʔ] (1977a: 163). This sound is what Gaprindashvili (1966) called a 'pharyngealized glottal stop' (cited in Catford 1977a: 163) and which has sometimes been called a 'pharyngeal stop' in the Georgian literature (Catford 1977b: 289). A second sound identified by Catford as [ɦʕ], 'with occasionally "bleat-like" ventricular trill plus ventricular turbulence' (1977a: 163), suggested that other manners of articulation could be produced deep in the pharynx, in contrast to Arabic [ħ] or [ʕ]. Laufer and Condax used laryngoscopy to observe the activity of the epiglottis in the production of Semitic pharyngeals [ħ] and [ʕ] and concluded 'that the articulation is between the base of the epiglottis and the top of the arytenoids' (1979: 52). Laufer and Baer (1988) identified the retraction of the tongue in a constriction in the lower part of the pharynx, implying that compression of the pharyngeal walls plays little role in pharyngealization and is at least not independent of tongue/epiglottis retraction. As for the role of larynx height, Nolan (1983: 182–187) cited acoustic, radiographic, and physiological evidence to associate pharyngealization with elevation of the larynx. Nolan's x-ray tracings (1983: 183) show clearly that the posture for raised-larynx voice both alters the angle and constriction of the larynx tube and involves the tongue (and epiglottis) filling more of the lower pharyngeal space. All of these descriptions focus on the pharynx in an attempt to explain how it is linked to the voice production mechanism in the larynx.

A number of studies have focused more particularly on the larynx. In their pioneering applications of laryngoscopic technology, Williams et al. observed a progression of constrictions consisting of 'narrowing of the whole laryngeal vestibule from sphincteric action of the aryepiglottic folds, epiglottis and even the lateral pharyngeal walls' (1975: 310). Their observation of aryepiglottic fold activity predates other mentions, at a time when the majority of research considered only pharyngeal wall or epiglottal compression. Their experimental approach laid the groundwork for establishing that the aryepiglottic constrictor mechanism is the basis for producing pharyngeal quality. Roach also observed that 'glottal closure' for certain glottalized consonants 'is in fact made with

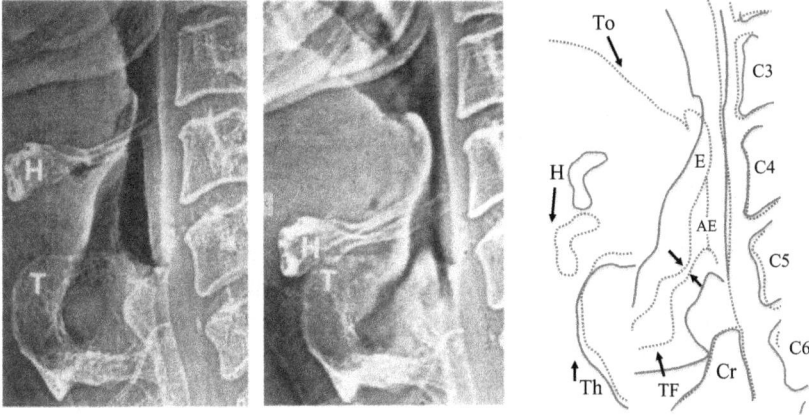

Figure 1.4 *X-ray photographs of the lower vocal tract by Tony Traill*
The images compare a neutral vocal tract posture with the posture of a vowel
with 'strident' phonation in !Xóõ. The image on the left shows the neutral
vocal tract (an open breathing larynx) with a wide pharynx and unconstricted
epilaryngeal tube. The image on the right shows a 'sphinctered' state of the
laryngeal articulator with a narrowed pharynx and constricted epilaryngeal
tube to generate aryepiglottic trilling.
H = hyoid bone; T/Th = thyroid cartilage; Cr = cricoid cartilage; TF = vocal
(true) folds; AE = aryepiglottic folds; E = epiglottis; To = tongue; C =
cervical vertebrae.
(Traill 1986: 126, Ladefoged and Maddieson 1996: 311). Reproduced with permission.

closure not only of the true vocal folds but also of the false vocal folds and the
aryepiglottic folds' (1979: 2). Gauffin noted that the protective closure of the
larynx is performed by all the constrictor muscles of the larynx to constrict
'larynx tube opening', characterizing a glottal stop as a 'reduced protective
closure' (1977: 308), referring to the primary anatomical mechanism that we
refer to as the laryngeal articulator and implying that 'full' protective closure is
associated with an airway-blocking pharyngeal stop, i.e. epiglottal stop. X-ray
photographs comparing a neutral vocal tract posture with a 'strident' vowel
posture in Khoisan (Traill 1986: 126), which also appeared in Ladefoged and
Maddieson (1996: 311), very clearly illustrate a simultaneous narrowing of the
pharynx behind the epiglottis, raising of the larynx, approximation of the
arytenoid cartilages to the base of the epiglottis, and vibration of the aryepiglottic folds against the tubercle of the epiglottis. Traill's images are reproduced
here as Figure 1.4, showing an open breathing larynx contrasted with 'strident'
or 'sphincteric' phonation. Traill identifies the 'laryngeal sphincter' as a

phonatory mechanism, differentiating !Xóõ 'plain voiced', 'murmured', and 'sphincteric' vowels [a a̰ a̰] (1986: 125). Fibreoptic laryngoscopic photographs support this description, showing very clearly the voicing mode and the breathy voicing mode at the glottis in contrast with pharyngealized laryngeal constrictor mode (1986: 124). The detailed account presented by Traill (1985: 78–79), in which he comments on the balance between constricted aryepiglottic folds at the same time as an apparently abducted glottis and open supraglottal lumen, resembles most closely the configuration for the voiceless pharyngeal/aryepiglottic trill in our work. Painter described the laryngeal constrictor mechanism in detail as part of the swallowing process, whereby 'approximating the cuneiform cartilages and aryepiglottic folds . . . the epiglottis is drawn backwards over an already closed airway' (1986: 330). Painter's description of the components of the basic 'effort and swallowing gestures' as a sequence of vocal fold adduction, ventricular fold adduction, cuneiform cartilage and aryepiglottic fold approximation, and epiglottis retraction (in conjunction with general tongue retraction) conforms very well with the model that we have put forward.

Studies that have focused on the singing voice also offer insights into the role of aryepiglottic postures in the production of distinctive voice qualities. Yanagisawa et al. (1989) used laryngoscopy to demonstrate that a range of auditory targets correlate with contrasting degrees of aryepiglottic fold closure and with contrasting larynx heights for some target qualities. Titze and Story (1997) further support the notion that the 'epilarynx tube' has a facilitative effect on vocal fold vibration and an influence on the mode of vibration as well as a determining role in shaping spectral formants. Titze (2008) identifies the epilarynx as the key modulating vocal tract structure in nonlinear source-filter acoustic coupling. Honda et al. identify a 'tightening of the larynx tube, or the aryepiglottic space [for opera, as] an effective gesture for producing a ringing voice quality used for producing loud and bright sounds' (1995a: 36). In conjunction with 'a forward shift of the hyoid bone while maintaining a low-larynx position for opera quality', they identify 'a bending and a stricture of the aryepiglottic space'. Studies that focus on the pharynx and those that focus on the larynx ultimately weave a connection between the two: an integration of pharyngeal and laryngeal behaviour, described as an action of the aryepiglottic sphincter in Esling (1996) and later as a laryngeal articulatory mechanism with multiple source, resonance, and noise-generating properties (Esling 2005).

1.6.2   Methods of Observing the Pharynx and Larynx

Direct oral and nasal endoscopy provides a tool for phoneticians to observe visually the structures of the pharynx and larynx during articulation. Our initial instrumental research employed techniques developed by Williams et al. (1975) using experimental laryngoscopic equipment developed by Sawashima et al. (1967). We began by examining phonetically controlled articulations to establish a baseline of pharyngeal articulatory possibilities. This canonical modelling approach was then extended to catalogue the articulatory and phonatory possibilities of the whole larynx. Then, we observed laryngoscopically native speakers of a wide array of languages to investigate the articulatory correlates of pharyngeal and laryngeal strictures and qualities. Languages were chosen in which phonological contrasts in the lower vocal tract are implicated or controversial.

Laryngoscopic images of the pharynx and larynx were obtained using a Kay Elemetrics Rhino-Laryngeal Stroboscope 9100B with a dual halogen (fixed) and xenon (strobe) light source. Recordings were made at the University of Victoria between 1996 and 2016, using a Kay 9106 70° rigid fibreoptic endoscope with a 35mm lens affixed to an integral continuous-fibre light cable attached to a Kay RLS 9100B light source to illustrate the range of possible canonical phonetic states in the laryngeal articulator. Initially, images were captured with a Panasonic KS152 camera and Mitsubishi S-VHS video cassette recorder BV-2000 (30 frames/sec) and later digitized. Later recordings were captured with a three-chip Panasonic GP-US522 camera and a 28mm lens for optimal wide-angle framing of laryngeal mechanisms during nasendoscopic filming of unimpeded speech production. Video recordings were captured directly to a Sony DCRTRV17 Mini-DV Digital Camcorder (30 frames/sec) and postprocessed with Adobe Premiere 6.5. The subject in the observations of basic canonical states was the first author, using the rigid Kay scope, placed at an angle over the tongue to view the laryngeal structures. The posture adopted during transoral observation was a close variety of schwa [ə̝], since the rigid tube in the mouth precludes the production of vocalic contrasts. Recordings of linguistic consultants were made with an Olympus ENF-P3 flexible fibreoptic laryngoscope to illustrate the incidence of laryngeal behaviour in various languages. The challenge in transnasal laryngoscopy is to see beyond the apex of the epiglottis with enough light and a clear enough field of view during anything but a close front vowel [i]. Other instrumental methods include cineradiography, ultrasound, and MRI. The phonetic categories established using these techniques and the operation of the laryngeal mechanism are discussed in Chapter 2, and case studies and simulations are elaborated in Chapter 3. The various contrasts that languages can exploit within the laryngeal articulator are illustrated in Chapter 4.

1.6.3   Categorization of Pharyngeals and Their Relationship to the Larynx

A common misconception about the larynx and how it interacts with the tongue, in medical science and phonetics, is that the epiglottis is pulled back over the larynx to close off the airway. This view fails to capture the subtlety and versatility of the laryngeal constrictor mechanism. To close the airway, the larynx and aryepiglottic folds are pulled up and forwards towards the tubercle at the base of the epiglottis by the internal and external portions of the thyroarytenoid (TA) muscles, possibly aided by bulging of the folds produced by the sparse aryepiglottic muscles (Reidenbach 1997, 1998a, 1998b, Moisik and Gick 2017), recruiting the hyoglossus muscles to stabilize the hyoid bone and retract the tongue and epiglottis, and the thyrohyoid muscles to raise the larynx as a whole up towards the hyoid bone. In this buckling manoeuvre, many muscles participate in a complex set of reflex arcs to achieve a series of gradational postures culminating in full, effective, multiplanar sealing off of the airway. This was clear to the innovative surgeon and anatomist Victor Negus in the 1940s, who wrote that in the human larynx, as well as in that of dogs and many other omnivores, 'it is evident that protective closure is at the level of the upraised aryteno-epiglottic folds, and not at the glottis, which in this instance is bounded by the inferior division of the thyro-arytenoid fold' (1949: 60). He contended that this higher-level valve evolved to prevent passage of air through the larynx in species with independent use of the forelimbs (1949: 102), but this remains a matter for further interdisciplinary investigation. Fink (1974a, 1975) referred to the 'folding' ('plication') of the laryngeal mechanism, and to vertical 'coupling'. Fink's (1975) comprehensive account of the history of laryngeal anatomy reminds us that the multiple-valvular nature of laryngeal closure, inherent to the LAM, had been described physiologically by Czermak (1861) in a flurry of research initiated by García (1855).

Another popular but erroneous concept is the notion that the tongue performs all articulations as the active articulator from dentals to pharyngeals, excluding glottal sounds. This view does not capture the breadth or importance of the laryngeal mechanism in producing sounds in the pharynx. The valves of the larynx are concisely described in Pressman (1954), including the notion of the 'aryepiglottic sphincter', and Edmondson and Esling (2006) have demonstrated that pharyngeals and pharyngealization are a product of the valve action of Negus's 'aryteno-epiglottic folds' combined with tongue retraction and larynx raising, compressing the pharynx vertically from above and from below. Revising the phonetic description of pharyngeals as a function of the aryepiglottic constrictor has as its consequence the remapping of voice quality

Table 1.1 *Pharyngeal consonantal distinctions of the laryngeal articulator (including various parallel descriptions)*

[ʔ]	(voiceless) glottal plosive; glottal stop
[h]	voiceless glottal fricative; breath
[ʔ]	(voiceless) pharyngeal stop; epiglottal stop; aryepiglottic plosive; 'strong' or 'massive' glottal stop (in earlier usage)
[ħ]	voiceless pharyngeal fricative; voiceless epiglottal fricative; aryepiglottic fricative
[ʜ]	voiceless pharyngeal fricative with aryepiglottic trilling; voiceless pharyngeal trill; voiceless epiglottal trill
[ʕ]	voiced pharyngeal approximant; voiced epiglottal approximant; aryepiglottic approximant
[ʕ]	voiced pharyngeal approximant with aryepiglottic trilling; voiced pharyngeal trill; voiced epiglottal trill

categories in the lower vocal tract, giving rise to the LAM. The revisions to pharyngeal consonant descriptions introduced by Esling (1996) are elaborated in Table 1.1, as a basis for redefining phonation type and states of the larynx. It is important to note that the difference between [ħ] and [ʜ] is defined here as a fricative vs. a trill (of the aryepiglottic folds). The reason is that the distinction between 'pharyngeal fricative' and 'epiglottal fricative' is meaningless in our model, since they reflect the same place of articulation (which could also be labelled 'aryepiglottic'). There is, however, a need for symbols to represent trilling at this place of articulation. The difference between [ʕ] and [ʕ] is also defined here as an approximant vs. a trill (of the aryepiglottic folds), because it is uninterpretable to contrast a pharyngeal approximant and an epiglottal fricative, whereas it is logical to characterize a pharyngeal approximant becoming a pharyngeal trill through increased stricture and/or airflow. An enhancement in degree occurring at the aryepiglottic constrictor captures elegantly the contrast between fricative noise or approximant resonance and the addition of induced vibration with minimal change to articulator posture. It is entirely possible that a distinction in larynx height may lead transcribers to select [ħ] where the larynx is lowered and [ʜ] where the larynx is raised, based solely on the noise spectrum. While the distinction in noise frequency can play a role, either a more raised-larynx [ʜ] or a less raised-larynx [ħ] may also be susceptible to aryepiglottic fold trilling, which also generates contrastive sound quality at the pharyngeal/epiglottal place of articulation. The same argument applies to [ʕ] and [ʕ], although to a lesser extent, because lowered-larynx and raised-larynx approximant resonances are less clear to distinguish in voiced mode, and because there is a strong potential to trill a raised-larynx aryepiglottic approximant when glottal voicing is present. The degrees of stricture, modes of vibration, and resonance possibilities of the pharyngeal consonants bear a direct relationship to the range of voice qualities that the laryngeal articulator can produce. The same articulatory postures that shape pharyngeals govern the laryngeal qualities classified in Chapter 2.

2 Laryngeal Voice Quality Classification

Chapter 2 reorganizes the classification of voice quality in Laver (1980) with laryngeal categories derived from the Laryngeal Articulator Model. A number of phonation types in Laver's set are not primarily glottal but are a function of aryepiglottic stricture, namely whisperiness, creakiness, and harshness. These phonation types are related to one another according to the presence and extent of laryngeal constriction. We present an expanded set of states of the larynx, revising the earlier notion of 'states of the glottis'. Following our model, phonation is extended above the glottis to include other vibrating structures through the epilaryngeal tube. These states represent static conceptualizations of the possible configurations of the airway that can be associated with sound qualities generated in the larynx. Laryngeal stops are included in the set; these are also a function of laryngeal constriction and can be identified auditorily by their transitions. Drawings represent canonical vocal settings – 'cardinal' reference points defined by auditory theory in the same way that symbols in a phonetic chart reflect key points in the sound space between other symbols. Depicting states renders explicit the components that are posited to participate in the production of each auditorily designated value. In Chapter 4, these reference points are supported with evidence from individual voices and language examples to illustrate where the phonetic qualities are observed to occur.

2.1   States of the Larynx and Phonation Types

States of the glottis have been enumerated by Catford (1964, 1977a: 105–106) in the context of phonation types. The states refer to the shapes of the glottis that produce the sounds, and the sounds themselves are the types of phonation generated at the glottis, which was assumed to be the sole source and controller of phonation. In our interpretation, the states refer to the shapes of the many components of the laryngeal articulator that produce the sounds rather than only the shape of the glottis. That is, the source of initial energy for the speech signal is taken to have multiple components due to postures within the aryepiglottic constrictor mechanism rather than just being a function of glottal shape. Phonation types have enjoyed a broad interpretation historically, and they are given an even broader interpretation in our analysis from the perspective of the laryngeal articulator or what we have sometimes called the 'whole larynx' (Moisik and Esling 2011).

The notion of 'states of the glottis' is based on a source-filter model, whereby all qualities of the source of the sound-pressure wave are attributed to the configuration of the vocal folds at the glottis. In that view, the shape of the glottal aperture was taken to be responsible for all of the vibrations that generate a sound wave once airflow is applied through the glottis, without consideration of where the controlling configurations and tensions occur that account for that shape. This assumption differs in the LAM, in which the larynx is a multifaceted organ with numerous possibilities for producing resonance, noise, or periodicity. The airstream can cause vibration to occur not only at the glottis but at multiple points through and above the epilaryngeal tube; and varying the shapes of the various components of these structures has a direct impact on the complexity of phonation that results. In our view, it is preferable to refer to these structural postures as 'states of the larynx'. Although the relationship between elaborated laryngeal postures and phonation types is more comprehensive and accurate in this view, it increases the number of articulatory and aerodynamic components responsible for (or which potentially participate in) each phonation type. In the earlier view, when the larynx was not thought to be an articulator (with no active structural displacements against passive surfaces), glottal shape was a sufficient snapshot of the options for sound quality. Muscular control was not pursued beyond the intrinsic laryngeal musculature, and any postural modifications were viewed as filtering effects within a relatively straight pharyngeal tube. Therefore, the notion of states is less straightforward than before, but the proliferated set of gestures expands the combination of options that can participate in any sound generated in the lower vocal tract.

2.2   Canonical States and Movements

Auditory voice quality analysis is used in dialect and sociolinguistic research to identify and describe the indexical attributes of pronunciation and has been used as a focal point to illustrate differences between languages and as a guide to the learning and teaching of pronunciation (Honikman 1964, Esling and Edmondson 2011). Articulatory experimentation has used laryngoscopy (illustrated with photos and drawings in this chapter), ultrasound, cineradiography, and MRI to view the articulators and measure their excursion.

For each state elaborated here, laryngoscopic videos have been assembled to illustrate the articulatory postures that differentiate them. The aim is to draw attention to the main characteristics that accompany each phonatory target in the taxonomy. Drawings based on this data set are presented in the chapter to capture the abstraction or ideal conceptualization of each state. Videos also illustrate the various categories during the production of laughter. The sequence produced is 'imitated-laughter' with an opening/closing alternation, which in its unmarked form would consist of a breath+voice pattern: a voiceless glottal fricative being followed by laryngeal voicing (produced on a vowel in this case), i.e. [həhəhəhəhə]. The schwa vowel symbol represents the (approximate) oral quality of the sound during the voiced phase, the sound's phonatory properties being the ones directly relevant in the analysis of laughter – [ə] designating voicing, [ə̥] voiceless breath, [ə̤] breathy voicing, etc. Pitch declines over the performance of the syllable string, with the focus being on the alterations of laryngeal states during each laugh. That is, pitch is intended to be modified only as a result of varying states of the larynx. As an example of this principle, laughing in falsetto mode has high pitch as the target of voicing, but successive syllables are expected to decline in pitch. The methodology follows previous experimental procedures into glottal and overall laryngeal settings (Esling and Harris 2005), in which many languages have been investigated that make extensive use of the laryngeal articulator in segmental articulation, to carry register, or for secondary articulation.

Figure 2.1 identifies the structures visible through the nasendoscope. The open glottis is in breath position, bordered by the vocal folds, with the tracheal rings beneath. The ventricular folds lie above the vocal folds, at their anterior end, with

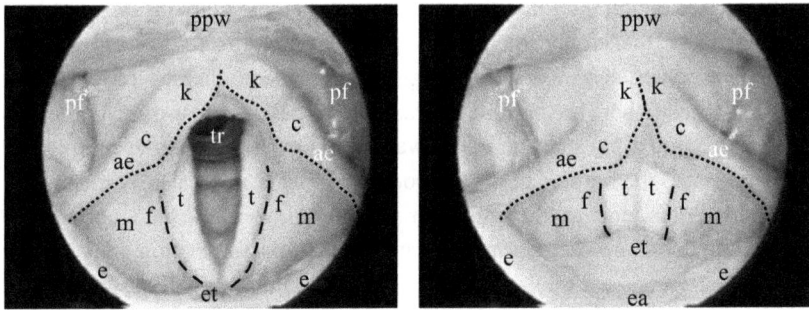

Figure 2.1 *The laryngeal articulator viewed through the fibreoptic laryngoscope, during breath (left) and voicing (right)*
Abbreviations: ae = aryepiglottic fold, c = cuneiform tubercle, e = epiglottis, ea = epiglottis (apex), et = epiglottis (tubercle), f = ventricular (false) fold, k = corniculate tubercle, m = inner mucosa of the epilarynx, pf = piriform fossa, ppw = posterior pharyngeal wall, t = vocal (true) fold, tr = trachea.
Lines: dashed line = medial edge of ventricular fold, dotted line = anterior edge of aryepiglottic fold (margin of upper epilarynx).

the space of the ventricles 'of Morgagni' between them. Critical to our approach is the identification of the upper border of the epilaryngeal tube (dotted line), which is lower posteriorly and higher anteriorly where the aryepiglottic folds reach the sides of the epiglottis. The round cartilaginous structures at the posterior end of the glottis are the corniculate tubercles at the tops of the arytenoid cartilages. The round tubercles visible within the aryepiglottic folds, above and lateral to the glottis, are the tops of the wedge-shaped cuneiform cartilages 'of Wrisberg' that give vertical stability, postero-anterior flexible mobility, and spring to the folds – identified originally by Camper (1779); see Fink (1975: 8).

2.3   Laryngeal Categories

2.3.1   Breathing/Inspiration

In *quiet breathing*, with normal resting tidal volume in the lungs, the glottis is relatively wide open, and the aryepiglottic folds are in their widest open state. In more forced inhalation, the glottal aperture widens even more, and the larynx may descend. Taking a deep breath in can therefore be characterized as the archetype of the non-constricted larynx, with widely separated vocal folds and widely separated aryepiglottic folds creating a maximally open epilaryngeal tube. It is important to remember that descriptions of glottal aperture that are based on mirror images may refer to the glottis as an 'inverted V'. In research using laryngoscopic imaging, where the view is not inverted but appears as if one were looking directly into the mouth and throat, the glottis is described as 'V-shaped'. In the laryngoscopic view, the aryepiglottic folds form a wide overarching inverted V, extending from the corniculate tubercles of the aryte-noid cartilages (where the oblique interarytenoid muscles cross over to join the aryepiglottic muscles) and running forwards and upwards along the aryepiglot-tic ligaments to the borders of the epiglottis. Figure 2.2 illustrates a moderately abducted glottis due to the muscular pull of the posterior cricoarytenoid muscles. In this stage, there is an absence of adductory constriction, the pharyn-geal space is open, and the larynx has neutral height or is slightly lowered.

Video 2.02 demonstrates the muscular pull of the posterior cricoarytenoid muscles to abduct the glottis during breathing. With full abduction, the larynx may lower slightly as air is breathed in. As air is breathed out, moderate adductory constriction occurs, as the glottis narrows to the state of breath, slight friction becomes audible, but the pharyngeal space and epilaryngeal tube remain open, with the larynx at neutral height. The glottis is wide open for inhalation and progressively reduces to a more adducted posture, more narrow than even the canonical state for breath.

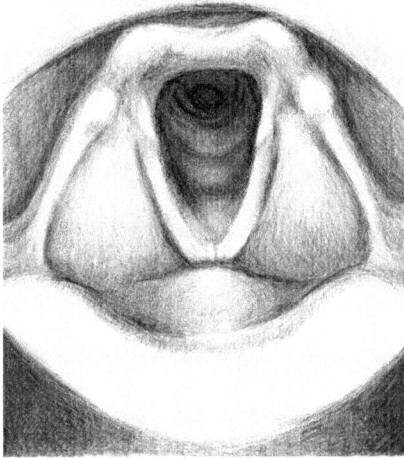

Figure 2.2 *The larynx during quiet breathing (inspiratory phase)*

2.3.2   Breath

Breath is a long-established term in the phonetic literature. Wilkins (1668) considered the modification of breathing to be responsible for the production of speech, in which sense he took breath to signify the air coming out of the lungs and through the mouth or nose. Wilkins had a very clear idea of the distinctive pairing of voiceless ('mute') vs. voiced ('sonorous') sounds, although not, apparently, as clear a notion of where voicing actually originates. His table of speech sounds (1668: 358) delineates voiceless/voiced pairs from the lips to the 'foremost palate' to the 'inmost palate'. He used 'breath' in the sense of 'continuant', whereas stops were classified as 'breathless'. His concept of 'tongue root' extended only to velar articulations, and 'h' sounds were classified with vowels as 'free' breathing. His etymological treatise (1668: 240) is interesting in classifying 'respiration' ('breathing, fetch wind, draw breath, take breath') together with 'snorting' ('snoring'), although his focus was more on nasal breathing than on anything occurring in the larynx. Wilkins (1668) is fascinating in that many terms used in contemporary phonetics and phonology were already in use at that time. Figure 2.3 illustrates that breath is more adducted in general than open respiration, certainly more than for inhalation. It could be called modified breathing for exhalation. It is marked

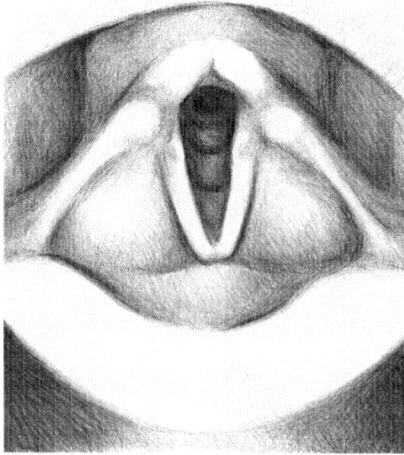

Figure 2.3 *The larynx in the state of breath (aspiration of a plosive; voiceless fricative)*

primarily by slight but effective parting of the vocal processes, with the corniculate tubercles typically remaining in contact with each other.

The breath state of the larynx is characterized principally by a V-shaped glottal aperture, although it is also associated with the functions of breathing (inhaling and exhaling) and lowering of the larynx rather than raising of the larynx. Catford (1964: 30) estimates the glottal area for breath at around 60 to 95 per cent of full glottal opening, but he was describing a range of apertures that produce aerodynamic turbulence and acoustic noise in general. We are distinguishing between 'breathing' as a variation in glottal aperture which may or may not produce turbulent noise, depending on rate of airflow, and 'breath', which is the state of the larynx for phonetic [h], aspiration as in [ʰp] or [pʰ], and in voiceless fricatives, when turbulent noise is identified with the speech sound. During breathing (Figure 2.2), the glottis is nearly fully open for normal inhalation but can narrow quite considerably, down to as little as 25 per cent, on exhalation. Since we are concerned more with the changing shape of the epilaryngeal tube and of the laryngeal constrictor than with the shape of the glottis per se, it is important to observe that, during inhalation, not only is the glottis wide open, but the structures surrounding the epilaryngeal tube are fully abducted; that is, the vocal folds are wide apart as the arytenoid cartilages are swivelled outwards by the action of the posterior cricoarytenoid

(PCA) muscles, the arytenoid cartilages are maximally separated atop the ring of the cricoid cartilage, and the corniculate cartilages and the cuneiform cartilages of the aryepiglottic folds are bowed outwards, away from centre, as far as they can go. During exhalation, aryepiglottic constriction can engage slightly, through slight contractions of the adductory lateral cricoarytenoid (LCA) muscles and interarytenoid (IA) muscles, causing the arytenoids and their corniculate tubercles to come together and the cuneiform cartilages to approach each other, towards centre, across the narrowed glottis. Fink (1974b) argues that corniculate contact stores elastic energy which is released in aiding the larynx to open wider (as in what he calls 'deep inspiration'). In breath (Figure 2.3) as phonetically defined, the glottis is open and relatively long, in a characteristic V shape, since laryngeal constriction is not present.

In Video 2.03a, breath can be observed as the [h] in the sequence [pʰə]. Our laryngoscopic evidence suggests that glottal aperture is around 50 per cent or less of full inspiratory opening during the production of [h], aspiration, or a voiceless fricative. Video 2.03b is an illustration of what could be broadly transcribed as [əɸə] (despite the presence of the rigid tube in the mouth), where the shape of the glottis, and of the epilaryngeal structures, during [ɸ] or any other voiceless fricative is the same as during [ʰ] in Video 2.03a. The aryepiglottic folds at the top of the epilaryngeal tube are not bowed inwards but straight, each one at a straight 180° angle across the cuneiform tubercle, from the corniculate tubercles at the apices of the arytenoids, forwards and upwards to the borders of the epiglottis. With each other, they form a nearly 90°-angle inverted V at the superior border of the epilaryngeal tube, over the V of the glottis at the bottom of the epilaryngeal tube. The state of breath can therefore be said to lack laryngeal constriction. Video 2.03x illustrates the intermittent occurrence of breath during an imitated-laughter sequence. The vocal folds are generally more abducted than in the canonical state of breath, and the noise generated is softer. Unlike laughter in a [haha] sequence with voiced vowels, the sequence here is [hh̥hh̥], with greater aerodynamic force on each second [h].

Related to the flow of breath through the vocal tract, voice quality schemata rarely include the notion of the control of aerodynamic flow. This is relevant when discussing the flow of breath through the glottis. When the airway is constricted, by the laryngeal constrictor mechanism, airflow is impeded and can be assumed to be reduced (e.g. in harsh voice). Even a higher rate of flow during constriction would produce greater turbulence and/or aperiodicity (e.g. in laryngeal constriction at high pitch, pressed voice). When the airway is not constricted and the flow of breath is relatively unimpeded, greater aerodynamic flow can act as a quality modulator, introducing characteristics of breath at susceptible points during the stream of speech. If habitual posturing of the articulators can be detected in the stream of speech, then the habitual presence of sustained, greater-than-usual airflow can also be detected as a quasi-permanent property of an accent, especially during segments that favour breathy flow (e.g. [h], other voiceless fricatives, fricativized [t]) and lengthened flow (e.g. vowels). In this way, duration interacts with positioning of the articulators to enhance aspects of setting (in this case, of the glottal abductors) to add an aerodynamic element to the articulatory description of voice quality.

2.3.3   Modal Voice

Catford describes *voice* as 'periodic vibration of the vocal folds under pressure from below (normal) or above (inverse)' (1968: 31). Normal refers to pulmonic egressive voicing, while inverse refers to pulmonic ingressive voicing (see Eklund 2008). Voice was described as 'sonorous' by Wilkins (1668: 358). Holder, with whom Wilkins had contact, recognized that the breath coming through a narrowing in the larynx which causes vibration to occur produces 'a Vocal sound or Voice' (1669: 23). For Wilkins or Holder, the breath was either 'mute' (voiceless) or 'breath vocalized' (voiced) (Holder 1669: 64). While we define breath as a subset of breathing, specifically related to speech sounds, we also recognize that it is the state of the larynx most closely associated with the opening of the airway (as in taking a breath). While these airway-opening manoeuvres represent a relaxing of the laryngeal constriction mechanism, the state of voice has some characteristics that relate it to the first stages of engaging laryngeal constriction. Figure 2.4 shows how the arytenoid cartilages and their corniculate tubercles are adducted by contracting the LCA muscles with support from the IA muscles (Hillel 2001). This action achieves medial approximation of the vocal processes of the arytenoids at the posterior end of the vocal folds, which come together at the midline as the muscular processes of the arytenoids swivel forwards. With airflow from below, the vocal folds begin to vibrate, producing *modal voice* when vibration is regular, there are no irregularities on the folds themselves, and no further constriction is added. Above the adducted arytenoids and vocal processes, the aryepiglottic folds are slightly bent, as the cuneiform cartilages have approximated each other slightly, but the laryngeal constrictor is still open.

Video 2.04x illustrates the intermittent occurrence of modal voicing during laughter. In the voicing of the vowel in [pʰə] (Video 2.03a), the onset of the vowel is influenced by the abduction for breath preceding it, so voicing starts as soon as the vocal folds come close enough together to begin vibrating in the airstream. In Video 2.04, the onset of voicing is more deliberate; there is a slight hesitation between the adduction of the glottal phonatory structures and the beginning of vocal fold vibration – a state which we call prephonation, as in Figure 2.5.

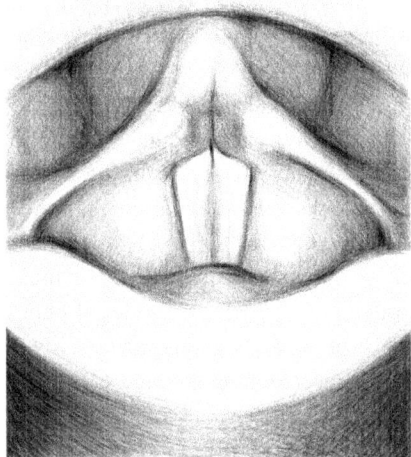

Figure 2.4 *The larynx in the state of voice (modal voice)*

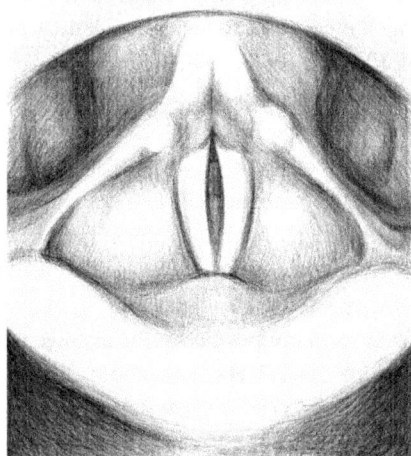

Figure 2.5 *The larynx in the state of prephonation*

The term 'modal voice' was proposed by Hollien (1972: 320) and adopted by Laver (1980: 95). Sweet (1906: 10) described voice as being produced in two ways. In the first way, the glottis is closed (let us say in the manner described above) so that airflow passes through in a series of rapid puffs. This most sonorous form of voice is what he called 'chest voice' or 'thick register'. In the second way, the vocal folds are stretched and brought close together without making a full closure of the glottis, producing a thinner quality of voice known as 'head voice' or 'thin register voice', the shrillest form of which Sweet (1877: 3) called *falsetto*. Modal voice is widely accepted to be produced through an undulating vibration of the vocal folds, which creates a pulsed output, the frequency of which is the interactive product of muscular and aerodynamic factors. In the aerodynamic-myoelastic model of phonation, the adducted vocal folds leave enough space for the pulmonic egressive airstream to pass through the narrowed glottis, accelerating the airstream and causing a drop in air pressure between the folds as a result of the Bernoulli effect, sucking the folds together to initiate the vibratory cycle of closing and opening (Laver 1980: 95–96). The myodynamic components involved in the adduction of the vocal processes of the arytenoids, orienting the vocal folds in place medially, are described in detail by Hillel (2001), who finds that minimal but optimal contraction in the interarytenoid muscles is usually sufficient to sustain the approximation of the vocal folds brought about by the initial contraction of the adductor (LCA) muscles. Following aerodynamic theory, the closure of the glottis resulting from the initiation of airflow through the approximated vocal folds causes an increase in air pressure subglottally which rapidly overcomes the myoelastic pressure holding the folds shut, whereupon they are blown apart, rapidly diminishing subglottal air pressure, leaving a pressure drop at the glottal borders, and sucking the folds back together again to begin a second cycle. According to Catford (1964: 31), the liminal pressure drop across the glottis in modal voice is of the order of 3 cm of water. Rates of flow vary according to types of voice 'register', from about 5 cl/s to a maximum of 23 cl/s for modal voice at 100 Hz. Since these are mean flow rates, rates in excess of these must occur, and since the glottal area is small, the general aerodynamic picture is of a series of high-velocity jets shot into the pharynx. Laver (1994: 193–194) reports that the recurring phonatory cycle for the average adult male is about 120 Hz, within a range of 50–250 Hz, and about 220 Hz for the average female, within a range of 120–480 Hz. Inverse flow (ingressive voice) is less efficient aerodynamically (Ohala 1983: 192–193), producing an irregular effect (Catford 1968: 318–319), but does occur in speech, essentially paralinguistically (Eklund 2008). The distinction between sounds made with breath and those made with voice appears to be universal among the world's languages.

2.3.4 Prephonation

The onset of voicing may occur in different laryngeal ways. The onset of the vowel in [pʰə], following breath/aspiration, starts as soon as the vocal folds come close enough together to begin vibrating in the airstream. In modal voicing not preceded by breath, the onset of voicing is more deliberate; there is a slight hesitation between the adduction of the glottal phonatory structures and the beginning of vocal fold vibration. We identify this state in our model as *prephonation*. The positioning of the arytenoids, their vocal processes, and the slightly bent aryepiglottic folds is the same as for voice, but the initiation of airflow which causes vocal fold vibration to begin is delayed. Figure 2.5 shows this state, in which voicing is ready to begin. The glottis is almond shaped, that is, the vocal folds remain bowed apart or concave before they start to vibrate. It is important to note that this state is not the same as glottal stop. In French, initial vowels may be preceded by breath or have a breathy onset. In languages such as German, glottal stop is the typical voicing onset for initial vowels. In English, initial vowels typically begin with prephonation – the intermediate state between breath and glottal stop.

In Video 2.05, the stricture (or oral closure) phase of [pə] is accompanied by prephonation at the glottis, before the onset of voicing for the vowel. In North American English and in Thai, this state of the larynx precedes an initial vowel in modal voice that is not heavily stressed; and it is the state of the larynx used during voiceless unaspirated oral stops and affricates.

Prephonation characterizes the oral closure phase of unaspirated stops before voicing begins, as in Figure 2.5. The articulatory stricture of an oral stop has traditionally been divided into three phases: (1) the closing (or onset) phase; (2) the stricture (or closure) phase; and (3) the release (or offset) phase. In the nineteenth century, Ellis (1869–89) and Sweet (1877) provided perhaps the best early European descriptions of these three phases. They called the three phases the on-glide, the consonant itself, and the off-glide. Abercrombie (1967: 140) and Laver (1994: 133) give good descriptions of the three phases of a stop. Laver clearly describes the overlap between the release (or offset phase) of an initial consonant and the onset phase of a following vowel. Unfortunately, since Ellis and Sweet, the state of the glottis during the articulatory stricture phase of initial voiceless unaspirated oral stops has been frequently confused with either a breathed (pronounced /brɛθt/) state of the glottis or a complete glottal closure. Harris (1987: 54–56) called it a weak glottal closure or a loosely closed glottis, implying that the glottis was neither completely adducted nor widely abducted. Catford (1964, 1968) makes no specific mention of the state of the glottis for voiceless unaspirated oral stops and affricates. In Catford (1977a), voiceless unaspirated stops and affricates are said to have a narrowed though not completely closed glottis that is restricted in cross-sectional area. However, Catford (2001: 56), quoting Harris (1999), calls this state of the glottis 'prephonation'. Our definition of this state of the larynx is a confirmation of Catford's (1977a, 2001) descriptions.

2.3.5   Glottal Stop

Glottal stop involves a greater degree of laryngeal constriction than breath, voice, or prephonation. Glottal stop is characterized by fully adducted arytenoids and aryepiglottic folds, postero-anterior pinching of the epilaryngeal tube so that the space between the arytenoids and the thyroid is shortened, variable vertical (upwards) compression of the distances between the three levels of folds, and consequently variable degrees of medial incursion of the ventricular folds. The degree of constriction which these characteristics demonstrate may vary on a continuum that differs from other stops. Oral stops are relatively simple in the structures that come together to achieve occlusion – the active articulator approximating the passive articulator. In the larynx, compression is not only postero-anterior but also vertical. The three levels of folds through the epilaryngeal tube interact in a continuous buckling man-oeuvre from the completely open posture for breathing to the maximally closed state of epiglottal stop. Glottal stop, in the middle of this manoeuvre, is a function of the immediately superior structures acting postero-anteriorly and vertically to impede the vibration of the vocal folds at the bottom of the epilaryngeal tube, causing them to stop vibrating, which we label as [ʔ]. The superior structures act as a braking system on glottal vibration (Moisik et al. 2015). The greater the degree of constriction, the longer the vocal folds are kept from vibrating.

In Video 2.06, glottal stop occurs as the onset of the utterance [ʔəː]. Although it is slightly stronger than the canonical glottal stop in Figure 2.6, as it opens into voicing, the white vocal folds and pink ventricular folds frame the characteristic state of glottal stop. In Video 2.07, glottal stop occurs as the coda of the syllable [əːʔ əːʔ] and is realized as a more forceful closure – ventricular stop. As the postero-anterior distance between the arytenoids and the epiglottic tubercle reduces, only the pink ventricular folds are visible.

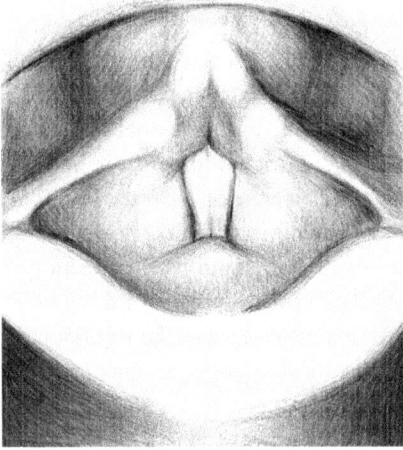

Figure 2.6 *The larynx in the state of glottal stop*

Defining how the stop is actually made has been a long-standing issue. Holder (1669: 60, 72) defined glottal stop as 'a stop made by closing the larynx'. A. M. Bell (1867: 46, 60) defined glottal stop as a glottal catch made with the glottis closed and a catch of the breath as in a cough, although he observed (astutely) that the linguistic effect of glottal stop is softer than in a cough. Sweet (1877: 6–7) also called glottal stop a glottal catch and defined it as a sudden opening or closing of the glottis, citing a familiar example of a glottal catch as in an ordinary cough. Heffner (1950: 125) and Jones (1956: 19) defined glottal stop as a closure and opening of the glottis. Jones added that the glottis must be tightly closed. Ladefoged (1975: 46, 1982: 50) referred to a glottal stop being made by holding the 'vocal cords' tightly together, also suggesting that glottal stops occur in coughs. Laver's definition of a glottal stop is a maintained complete glottal closure (1994: 187–188, 206). In our taxonomy, the stop occurring before expelling air in a cough is more occluded than a glottal stop, as Bell correctly surmised, unless the cough is very weak. Discussions of the role of the ventricular folds in the production of glottal stop can first be found in Lindqvist (1969) – the same researcher who later described glottal stop as 'a reduced protective closure' (Gauffin 1977) and whose work is reviewed by Lindblom (2009). This means that glottal stop is less massive and less efficient than the full protective closure of epiglottal stop, which is the more expected degree of closure preceding a cough.

In every instance of phonetic glottal stop we have observed, there is some postero-anterior narrowing of the epilaryngeal tube. Evidence shows that vocal fold adduction sufficient to produce glottal stop is aided by the lateral cricoarytenoid and thyroarytenoid muscles (Hirano and Ohala 1969). Since LCA (and IA) contractions are known to initiate adduction, we associate TA activity with narrowing the epilaryngeal tube. As constriction progresses into glottal stop, medial incursion of the ventricular folds increases, and the vocal folds beneath become increasingly obscured as their vibration is slowed and stopped. Garellek (2013) reports that 95 per cent of controlled productions of glottal stop exhibit at least some medialization of the ventricular folds, but only 17 per cent of the productions show firm midline contact of the ventricular folds, and vibration of the vocal folds tends to stop prior to maximum ventricular medialization. A weak glottal stop, illustrated in Figure 2.6, represents the next step on the closure continuum after glottal adduction – adequate to arrest voicing momentarily. There is some postero-anterior epilaryngeal narrowing and concomitant medialization of the ventricular folds, but the vocal folds are still visible. The aryepiglottic fold angle is about 140°. Figure 2.7 illustrates a stronger glottal stop, where the aryepiglottic folds bend to about 130°, and the

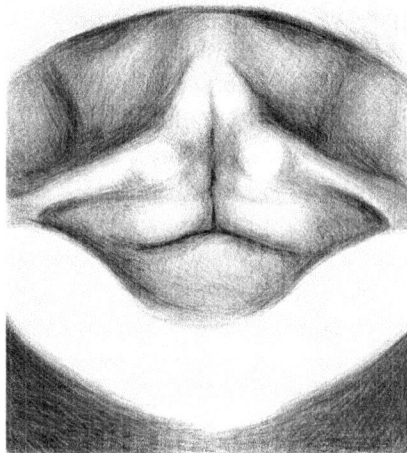

Figure 2.7 *The larynx in a strong (reinforced) glottal stop (ventricular stop)*

vocal folds are covered by the fully apposed ventricular folds, which also press down onto the vocal folds (like brake pads). This could be called a reinforced glottal stop or ventricular stop. Without the element of laryngeal constriction, whereby multiple structures act on vocal fold activity, there is no mechanism by which the vocal folds can cease vibrating on their own, except by abduction (opening to breath). Our research has shown that medial compression alone is insufficient for the glottis to close beyond prephonation to produce a stop, and the vocal folds have even been observed to remain slightly separated during stop-like gestures (as in the production of ejectives), indicating that medial compression is not the critical action (Moisik et al. 2015). Vocal-ventricular fold contact is the dynamic driver that causes the sudden changes in vibratory behaviour in the voiced sounds that surround a glottal stop (Moisik and Esling 2014).

2.3.6   Epiglottal Stop

Full respiratory arrest is the phonetic state of *epiglottal stop*. Epiglottal stop begins with the adductory actions for voice, progressing through the multiple postero-anterior and vertical compactions that produce glottal stop, and ending with complete aryepiglottic occlusion (with accompanying lingual retraction and vertical elevation of the larynx) that seals the airway. This is a massive buckling manoeuvre, which results in full protective closure of the respiratory system, allowing the cricopharyngeal sphincter behind the arytenoids to release and the esophagus to open for swallowing. These two sphincters of the larynx function inversely. When the aryepiglottic sphincter is open, the cricopharyngeal sphincter is shut, but when the cricopharyngeal sphincter opens, the aryepiglottic sphincter must close. In phonetic terms, when the aryepiglottic sphincter closes, the aryepiglottic folds moving forwards and upwards are the active articulator, and the epiglottis behind the tongue is the passive articulator. The main protagonists in this highly efficient manoeuvre are the forward and upward thrusting aryepiglottic folds, each bent at 90° pushing against each other medially and against the tubercle of the epiglottis anteriorly. The compacted space between the cuneiform 'elbows' of the aryepiglottic folds and the closure of each fold against the tubercle of the epiglottis can be seen in Figure 2.8 as well as the retracted tongue/epiglottis and the raised structures of the larynx (apparent by virtue of the larger size and brightness in the laryngoscopic light of the structures forming the upper border of the epilaryngeal tube).

Full engagement of the laryngeal constrictor for an epiglottal stop is what Catford termed a 'pharyngealized glottal stop' or 'strong glottal stop' in

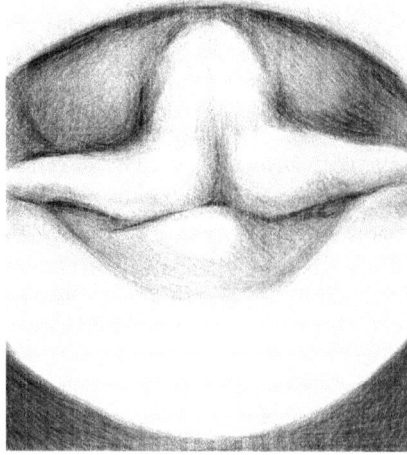

Figure 2.8 *The larynx in the state of epiglottal stop*

languages of the Caucasus, a 'pharyngeal stop' in Chechen (1983: 347), and a 'ventricular (plus glottal) stop' (1977a: 105). Early work by Stephen Jones at University College London (1934) influenced Catford to draw a relationship between increasing constriction and ventricular activity. Sapir and Swadesh described Ahousaht Nuuchahnulth pharyngeals as 'laryngealized glottals' (1939: 12–13). Jacobsen (1969: 125), citing Sapir's original description, called Nuuchahnulth /ʕ/ a 'pharyngealized glottal stop'. Gaprindashvili (1966) described a 'pharyngealized glottal stop', and Kodzasov (1987) described a 'strong glottal stop' in Nakh and Daghestanian languages. All of these descriptions imply a component added to glottal stop somewhere above the glottis. Hockett (1958: 66) recognized that 'a complete closure can be made in the lower pharyngeal region', and characterized /ʕ/ as a 'pharyngeal catch' in some dialects of Arabic, in parallel to his term 'glottal catch' for [ʔ]. However, he conceived of the root of the tongue closing against the rear pharyngeal wall, which parallels Pike's notion of the root of the tongue as a lingual articulator (1947: 21–22; see Laver 1980: 51) rather than as a concomitant to a laryngeal gesture, although Pike did postulate changes in vocoid quality due to larynx height. Catford's term, 'epiglottopharyngeal', is an auditory label implying stricture deeper than the lingual pharynx (1968: 326). Later terminology identifies more precisely the constricting action of the aryepiglottic folds

(Williams et al. 1975: 310). Roach observes that closure for certain glottalized consonants is 'made with closure not only of the true vocal folds but also of the false vocal folds and the aryepiglottic folds' (1979: 2). Gauffin comments that the protective closure of the larynx is performed by all the constrictor muscles of the larynx to constrict 'larynx tube opening' (1977: 308). Aside from its incidence as a speech sound, epiglottal stop closure is also the maximum stricture that occurs in gagging or in swallowing. A cascade of muscular contraction leads to full closure, but the primary muscles for reducing the postero-anterior space at the superior border of the epilaryngeal tube are the various strands and levels of the thyroarytenoid (TA) muscles. Other muscles implicated are LCA, tIA, oIA, perhaps AE, perhaps thyroepiglottic (TE), hyoglossus (retracting of the tongue), and suprahyoid (raising of the larynx) but also including thyrohyoid (TH). It is possible for the larynx to be lowered during the performance of epiglottal stop, but closure would be less efficient. The normal reflex is for the larynx to be raised during any gesture produced with laryngeal constriction. Raising also predisposes vocal-ventricular fold coupling (VVFC). When tighter degrees of constriction are applied, the ventricular folds compress onto the vocal folds, aiding in arresting their vibration in glottal stop and in epiglottal stop (Moisik and Esling 2014).

In Video 2.08, the laryngeal mechanism closes sphincterically to its maximum: epiglottal stop [ʔaːʔ]. Tongue retraction can be observed as aryepiglottic closure progresses, as can larynx raising (as the aryepiglottic folds become larger and brighter as they move towards the laryngoscope).

2.3.7   Whisper

Phonetic *whisper* is a state of the larynx that is distinguished from breath by the addition of laryngeal constriction. Auditorily, whisper generates more turbulent airflow, and therefore more noise, than breath. The source of this noise is the epilaryngeal tube, forming a narrow passage from the glottis through the aryepiglottic folds at the upper edges of the tube. The transition from breathing to breath to whisper can be thought of as an incremental narrowing of the airway from most open to moderately open to constricted. Aryepiglottic constriction does not close the airway as it does for glottal or epiglottal stop, because whisper requires continuous airflow and the glottis must remain open. In fact, whisper has the same abducted (or non-adducted) posture at the glottis as breath. The difference lies in the shaping of the tube above the glottis for whisper. The shape of the glottis itself for whisper

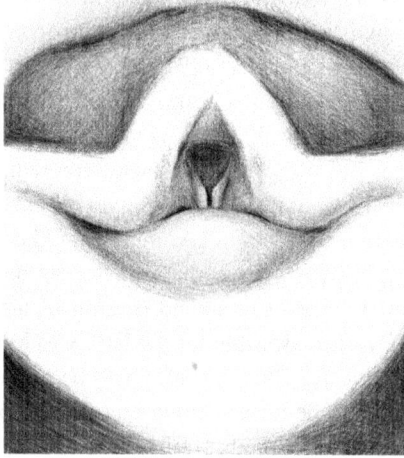

Figure 2.9 *The larynx in the state of whisper*

is non-controversial, as Laver (1980: 120–122) reports, often referred to as 'an inverted letter Y' (Luchsinger and Arnold 1965: 119), since the 'Y' was inverted in mirror images before the advent of laryngoscopic techniques. The shape of the glottis in Figure 2.9 is a posteriorly open 'Y', but that is not due to any independent alteration in glottal musculature from the state of breath. The change from the glottal 'V' shape to a 'Y' shape is due to the shortening and narrowing of the tube over the glottis. As in breath, the corniculate tubercles are in contact during this state. Aerodynamic descriptions of the turbulent aperiodic airflow in whisper (Catford 1964: 31, 1968: 319, 1977a: 96–98, 100, van den Berg 1968: 297) need to be interpreted in terms of the narrowing of the epilaryngeal tube (see Esling 1999, with epilaryngeal narrowing further supported by MRI evidence from Honda et al. 2010).

Different kinds of whisper have been posited in the literature, such as arytenoidal and ventricular whisper (Catford 1964: 33). In our schema, variations in the auditory quality of whisper can be explained by adjustments in epilaryngeal tube shape and larynx height. These two parameters have been largely ignored in phonetic classification but play a significant role in noise generation and formant structure. The phonetic description of whisper should not be confused with the conversational register of whispering. Whispering (speaking very quietly for secrecy or privacy) can be produced with the canonical phonetic state of breath or of whisper, allowing various modifications to the laryngeal structure to shape the noise component of whisper, or even using occasional voicing as in whispery voice (Section 2.3.9). Some speakers' whispering may be very soft and breathy, while others' may be whispery. Whispering may even be produced forcefully, though remaining voiceless, inducing epilaryngeal structures to vibrate (Section 2.3.14). Variations in the phonetic quality of whispering occur not only for social or idiosyncratic reasons but to preserve linguistic contrast in what is being said, for example, the preservation of tone in whispered Chinese (Gao 2002) or voicing contrasts in English (Mills 2009).

For whisper, as with any laryngeally constricted setting, the significant hallmark is aryepiglottic constriction, with forwards and upwards approximation of the aryepiglottic folds, lingual retraction, and the likelihood of larynx raising. Unlike voiced and stopped states, however, whisper has minimal or no glottal adduction. Therefore, the major action is the aryepiglottic folds bending at their cuneiform tubercles and pushing up against the epiglottis to either side of the epiglottic tubercle, away from the midline rather than pressing in medially. This movement gives them a slanted aspect over the glottis, each fold bending to about a 120° angle from its straight alignment during breathing, and allowing the glottis to remain open as a channel of air. This glottal aperture would produce breath if not for the aryepiglottically constricted tube, which generates whisper. A strong argument for this description is that [h] represents the archetype of breath, at the glottis, while pharyngeal [ħ] is simply '[h] whispered' (by adding a constricted epilaryngeal tube). Because the laryngeal constrictor is the mechanism for articulating pharyngeals, a strongly whispered [h] has the same configurational attributes as a voiceless pharyngeal fricative [ħ].

For whisper, in Video 2.09, the laryngeal mechanism can be seen to adduct into its constricted posture while the glottis remains open (essentially in the glottal state of breath). The aryepiglottic folds form the classic 'bent-elbow' shape, as air passes mainly through the cartilaginous glottis and partially through the ligamental glottis, but the vocal folds do not vibrate. The supraglottic musculature responsible for laryngeal constriction causes the glottis to be compressed into a 'Y' posture, beginning with breathing and breath, constricting for whisper, ending with release of constriction and opening as a continuum through breath and breathing as the enhanced noise dissipates. The parallel to other constricted states is the posture of the aryepiglottic constrictor, forming a narrowed epilaryngeal tube. The role of the tube in generating turbulent airflow is apparent in Video 2.09x of whispery laughter. Although there is adduction and abduction, the epilaryngeal tube maintains a constricted posture throughout.

2.3.8   Breathy Voice

Like breath, *breathy voice* is an unconstricted state. Both breath and whisper, distinguished by their contrasting noise profiles, can become voiced (sonorous) with the addition of vocal fold vibration, which combines a periodic signal with the characteristic airflow of each. The airflow in breathy voice is less turbulent than in whispery voice, because the laryngeal mechanism is open, allowing less impeded more linear airflow through the pharyngeal space; whereas in whispery voice, the epilaryngeal channel is constricted, adding friction and noise. The type of voicing that accompanies breathy voice and whispery voice also differs. Since breath is produced with an open supraglottic tube and whisper with narrowed channels above the glottis, the vocal folds in breathy voice experience less adductory constriction than in whispery voice. Breathy voice is symbolized in the chart of the IPA (2005) as the voiced glottal fricative [ɦ] or with a diacritic to mark the phonatory register of a vowel, e.g. [a̤]. In linguistic practice, it is possible that phonetic descriptions have used either [ɦ] or the [̤] diacritic when either breathy voice or whispery voice was observed. This usage is acceptable to signal a linguistic contrast, but the precise phonetic nature of phonation should be specified in greater detail for phonetic research.

Breathy voice is defined by Catford as 'breath + voice: glottis relatively wide open: turbulent airflow as for "breath" plus vibration of vocal folds' (1964: 32). Two familiar metaphors from Catford's definition are the 'sigh-like' quality and that the vocal folds 'flap in the breeze'. These auditory and mechanical characteristics are due to the open glottis between the arytenoids (the cartilaginous glottis) and to the open epilaryngeal tube that allows the vocal folds relatively free movement (along the ligamental glottis). The corniculate tubercles still come into contact despite arytenoidal separation. Abercrombie's (1967: 100–101) observation that 'breathy phonation' contrasts maximally with 'tight phonation' corresponds with Laver's (1980: 31) crucial observation that breathy voice and lowered larynx are auditorily and physiologically related. The opening of the airway and concomitant lowering of the larynx for breathing (and for the auditory quality of breathiness) are physiologically opposed to the 'tight phonation' and concomitant raising of the larynx which, along with tongue retraction, result from laryngeal constriction (Esling 1996, 1999). Laver (1980: 133), citing Fairbanks (1960: 179), also points out the relationship between breathy voice and low pitch. Two characteristics of breathy voice that relate to low pitch are the shortened length of vocal fold vibration and their relative separation and looseness. The vocal folds vibrate along only half the length of the glottis, as in Figure 2.10. The posterior half of

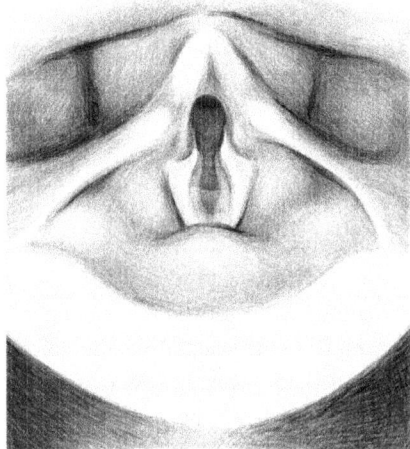

Figure 2.10 *The larynx in the state of breathy voice*

the glottis remains open, reminiscent of the abducted aspects of breath in Figure 2.3. The inherent opposition between abduction for breathiness and adduction for voicing restricts the distance along which the vocal folds can vibrate but allows greater vertical phase difference (freedom of the thick vocal folds to undulate slowly from bottom to top). The upper aryepiglottic border of the epilaryngeal tube maintains relatively straight lines.

Video 2.10 illustrates breathy voice. Adduction commences as for modal voice, stopping well short of full adduction of the arytenoids, as in the abducted state of breath, but the corniculate tubercles are apposed. Air passes relatively freely through the posterior gap in the glottis, while the vocal folds vibrate with wide excursions anteriorly. Many productions of breathy phonation could be expected to have even less postero-anterior compression than this example. In Video 2.10x of breathy-voiced laughter, the laryngeal constrictor is open and only shortens as pitch decreases towards the end of an episode.

Video 2.11 illustrates whispery voice, progressing from open breathing into whispery-voiced phonation (preceded by a brief stop) and into open breathing again. Like whisper, the laryngeal articulator adopts a constricted posture at the outset, forming a narrowed epilaryngeal tube, and as in breathy voice, the vocal folds vibrate along the anterior, ligamental glottis. In Video 2.11x of whispery-voiced laughter, the laryngeal constrictor is narrowed throughout and narrows even more as pitch decreases until the sphincter almost closes. Some harshness is induced, due to the tube narrowing required for whisperiness and because lowering pitch requires greater laryngeal constriction.

Video 2.11a illustrates the contrast between breathy voice and whispery voice (BV, WV, BV, WV). Whispery voice is marked by the sudden shift to a constricted posture of the aryepiglottic folds with raising of the larynx and consequent tubular formation above the glottis.

2.3.9   Whispery Voice

Whispery voice results from the addition of vocal fold vibration to whisper. With the aryepiglottic constrictor already engaged to create a narrowed tube above the glottis for whisper, the glottal adductory muscles contract to allow the vocal folds to vibrate. Or, starting from the state of breathy voice, progressive tightening of the laryngeal constrictor generates increasing degrees of whispery voicing. The main component of whispery voice is aryepiglottic constriction, as it is for whisper. The net effect is that glottal length is shorter postero-anteriorly in whispery voice than it is in breathy voice, medial compression is greater, and the potential for vertical compaction of the three levels of folds is greater. Vocal fold vibration in whispery voice is constrained postero-anteriorly, medially, and vertically by the tightening of the laryngeal constrictor. Tongue retraction and larynx raising also play concomitant roles, although these can vary. For example, the larynx normally raises with constriction, but it is possible (although anti-synergistic) to produce whisper or whispery voice with a lowered larynx, which changes the formant structure in the spectrum, expanding the depth of the pharynx and lowering F1 and F2. The state of the larynx in whispery voice is captured in Figure 2.11. The aryepiglottic fold angle is not as sharp in whispery voice as in voiceless whisper, each aryepiglottic fold bending to about 130° from its straight alignment during breathing, and the cuneiform cartilages do not push up as close to the epiglottis as they do in whisper. This configuration allows the glottis to remain open posteriorly, generating airflow through the channel of the epilaryngeal tube and becoming turbulent, with the vocal folds relatively free but sufficiently adducted to vibrate anteriorly.

Bell's category of 'whisper and voice heard simultaneously', which he called 'vocal murmur' (1867: 46), persists throughout the literature as 'whispery voice' (Catford 1964: 32, Laver 1980: 133–139). Sometimes the term 'murmur' is used to label voicing accompanied by noise, for example, to describe the 'voiced aspirated' stops of Indic languages (Abercrombie 1967:

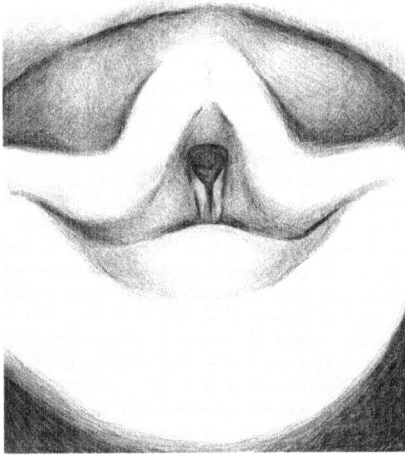

Figure 2.11 *The larynx in the state of whispery voice*

149, Ladefoged and Maddieson 1996: 58–62). However, the term 'murmur' is not phonetically precise, specifying a linguistic contrast that could refer to any number of positions along the continuum from breathy voice to whispery voice. Whispery voice is often explained as 'stage whisper', when actors give the impression of whispering by adding voicing so their voice will carry. Descriptions of whispery voice, such as Catford's (1977a: 99–101), uniformly locate the noise-generating source posteriorly between the arytenoid cartilages and voicing at the anterior end of the glottis or suggest that the vocal folds are relaxed and never close completely anywhere along their length, but none identify the role of the aryepiglottic constrictor mechanism until Esling (1996, 1999) and Esling and Harris (2003, 2005). Catford noted that 'Bell's further elucidation of this sound suggests, however, that he believed the whisper component to be produced in the pharynx' (1977a: 101). Bell's intuition is insightful in identifying where the noise originates in whisper and in whispery voice; the increase in turbulent airflow being a function of the narrowing epilaryngeal tube above the glottis, in the lower part of the pharynx, at the same articulatory place where pharyngeals are produced. Rather than explaining breath, whisper, breathy voice, and whispery voice as solely glottal phenomena, concentrating only on the shape of the glottal aperture, it is imperative to view whisperiness from the perspective of supraglottic constriction in which the shaping of the pharyngeal cavity is governed by the laryngeal mechanism of airway closure. From this perspective, whisper and whispery voice have parallel configurational relationships to other phonation types that share laryngeal constriction.

Laver points out that breathiness has limited combinatorial possibilities with other phonation types, while whisperiness can combine with harshness, creakiness, or ventricular voicing (1980: 133). The reason for these combinatorial affinities is their common articulatory basis in the laryngeal constrictor mechanism, while breathiness lacks laryngeal constriction. The similarity in the state of constrictor posture between whisperiness and stopping airflow can be seen by comparing the degree of laryngeal constrictor engagement for whisper, whispery voice, and glottal stop with that of epiglottal stop. The affinity of whispery states to creaky phonation and harsh phonation is also apparent in the shape of the aryepiglottic mechanism. In constricted states, there is an increased potential for structures other than the vocal folds to be set in motion. As airflow passes through the epilaryngeal tube, it affects the approximated soft tissues, which may be set in motion laterally of the cuneiform cartilages. The undulation of these structures can occur together with whispery voice because the narrowing of the constrictor mechanism required for whisperiness brings neighbouring structures into more medial, more anterior, and/or more vertically compressed positions where they can be affected aerodynamically by the flow of air through the narrowed and compressed tube. The more extreme the constriction along these three dimensions, the higher the probability that whisperiness will acquire traits of harshness (Section 2.3.12), whereas relaxing constriction diminishes the potential for harshness. The most salient contrast between breathy voice and whispery voice is the adjustment forwards and upwards of the aryepiglottic folds in whispery voice, causing the epilaryngeal tube to narrow. In breathy voice, airflow acts principally on the glottis, while in whispery voice, the airflow is channelled through the narrowed tube formed between the cuneiform cartilages and the base of the epiglottis, where the soft tissues adjacent to this channel can be set in motion.

2.3.10   *Falsetto*

Sweet describes *falsetto* as the thinnest and shrillest form of 'head' voice or 'thin register', which he interprets as the vocal folds being brought together only enough 'to enable their edges to vibrate, without any closure of the glottis' (1877: 3). Laver (1980: 118–120) reports a wide range of agreement in the literature between 1940 and 1980 in physiological accounts of the laryngeal mechanisms involved in producing falsetto. Hollien and Michel

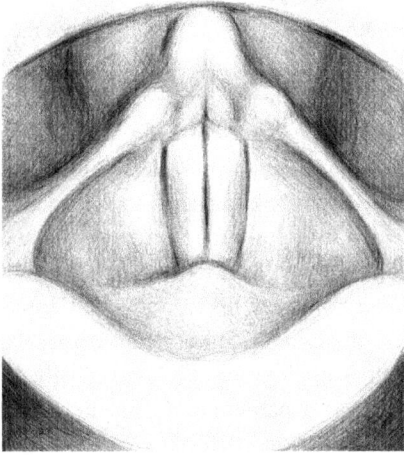

Figure 2.12 *The larynx in the state of falsetto*

(1968: 602) compare an average pitch range of modal voice in the adult male of 94–287 Hz with an average pitch range of falsetto of 275–634 Hz. The lower end of the falsetto pitch range overlaps with the high end of the modal range. Falsetto shares the same adductory traits as modal voice (both stopping short of aryepiglottic constriction), but the vocal folds are longer due to cricothyroid (CT) contraction and consequent tilting of the larynx. The vocal folds are stretched longitudinally so that they are thin at their edges, allowing only a portion to vibrate, while the remainder of the length of the vocal folds appears stiff and immobile. Figure 2.12 shows the vibrating portion of the folds to be just anterior to the vocal processes. The vocal folds are lengthened relative to modal voice (Figure 2.4). Falsetto is frequently accompanied by varying degrees of breathiness due to the escaping pulmonic airflow through the incompletely closed, non-vibrating portion of the glottis. Falsetto combined with audible breathiness is known as *breathy falsetto*. The propensity for these effects to combine arises because modal voice, falsetto, and breathiness are all functions of glottal adjustment rather than of laryngeal constrictor adjustment. As a result of general transglottal leakage, subglottal air pressure is typically lower in falsetto than in modal voice (Laver 1994: 197). The enhanced breathy quality of breathy falsetto results from increasing the intercartilaginous space (between the arytenoids), in the same way that breathy voice differs from modal voice. Another acoustic characteristic of falsetto is the much steeper slope of the spectrum of the laryngeal waveform for falsetto compared to modal voice (Monsen and Engebretson 1977: 988).

The laryngeal constrictor mechanism bears a relationship to the mechanisms for controlling pitch while speaking a language. Considering only pitch control, modal voice is in a low-mid part of the frequency range, falsetto is at the high end of the range, and creaky voice is at the low end of the range as a function of the narrowing constrictor. Lengthening and thinning the vocal folds to produce falsetto is achieved by contracting the CT muscles at the front of the two cartilages, bringing them closer together vertically and causing the vocal folds to be stretched between their anterior commissure and the vocal processes of the arytenoids. The thyroid may tilt forwards and downwards as pitch increases or, more usually, the cricoid and arytenoids rock backwards (van den Berg et al. 1960). Falsetto is not attested as a linguistically contrastive phonation type, but it sometimes has a paralinguistic function. Professional singers, in their range of pitch control in performing vocal registers, can overcome the articulatory anti-synergies that normally constrain the average speaker (Henrich 2006, Sundberg 2013). In our articulatory description, falsetto is a glottally adducted state with no epilaryngeal narrowing. The states classified as 'glottal' are therefore: breath, modal voice, breathy voice, falsetto, and breathy falsetto. Other adjustments are a function of the constrictor mechanism. It is somewhat counterintuitive that both breathy falsetto and whispery falsetto should occur, since breathiness and falsetto are glottal functions but whisperiness is a constrictive adjustment – the same mechanism for lowering pitch. However, CT stretching to increase pitch can occur together with constrictive supraglottic narrowing, in isometric opposition, as evidenced in Section 2.3.15. Whispery falsetto, and every other constrictive state that combines with falsetto, is therefore both a glottal high-pitch adjustment as well as an aryepiglottic constrictor adjustment. Whispery falsetto adds friction characteristics through the epilaryngeal tube beyond what is heard as pure breath. Creaky and harsh constrictive states add resonance and vibratory characteristics to falsetto that emulate the quality of those states at lower pitch.

Video 2.12 illustrates the state of falsetto. As for modal voice, beyond arytenoidal adduction for glottal voicing, the laryngeal mechanism remains unconstricted, so the epilaryngeal tube is open. Voicing can be seen to occupy only a thin short portion of the vocal folds just anterior to the vocal processes. Video 2.12x illustrates falsetto in laughter, which, like breath, modal voice and breathy voice, represents unconstricted laryngeal production.

2.3.11   Creaky Voice

Creaky voice, also called 'glottal fry' or 'vocal fry' (Hollien et al. 1966, Hollien and Michel 1968), has long been associated with low pitch (slow frequency of vibration) in particular accents (Abercrombie 1967: 101). Creaky voice, in contrast to falsetto, requires short, thick vocal folds, with a loose aspect, generally understood to be achieved by contracting the TA muscles from the borders of the arytenoids to the front of the epilaryngeal tube. Zemlin identifies the 'thyromuscularis portion of the thyroarytenoid muscle' as the main mechanism 'to draw the arytenoid cartilage forward, toward the thyroid, and thus shorten and relax the folds' (1968: 191). This results in a pattern where 'the closed phase occupies about 90 per cent of the vibratory cycle, and the opening and closing phases combined occupy about 10 per cent of the cycle' (1968: 197). While falsetto occupies the highest pitch levels, and modal voice occupies the mid-pitch range, the literature summarized by Laver (1980: 122) consistently reports that creaky phonation occupies the range below modal voice, typically below 100 Hz. Hollien et al. (1966: 247) remark on the participation of the ventricular folds and their possible influence on the vibrating mass, and Hollien (1972: 328) presents clear evidence that 'fry' involves vocal-ventricular fold contact. Catford's observation that only the ligamental glottis is involved (1964: 32–33) is consistent with Zemlin's physiological description of arytenoid fronting and with Catford's own categories 'ligamental' and 'arytenoidal', although his table does not admit the possibility that creak is 'ventricular'. Our research has confirmed that the ventricular folds can couple with the vocal folds during creaky phonation (Moisik et al. 2015). This vocal-ventricular fold coupling has four effects: (1) it increases the overall effective vibrating mass, lowering frequency; (2) it adds damping, making vibration more likely to cease; (3) it adds increased degrees of freedom to the system, encouraging irregular vibration; and, most importantly, (4) it perturbs the transmission of the mucosal wave by preventing its traversal across the surface of the vocal folds, causing the wave energy to be reflected back towards the midline earlier than what would occur for modal phonation (Moisik and Esling 2014).

It is critical to keep in mind that the vocal folds constitute a body-cover system (Hirano 1974). The body can become stiff through thyroarytenoid contraction (which, along with some collagen fibres of the ligament) makes up the body, while the cover (the mucosa and upper layers of the lamina propria) slackens. Deguchi et al. (2011) demonstrate with a finite-element model of the vocal folds that isolated TA contraction increases stiffness in the vocal fold body while simultaneously lowering stress in the cover. So it is incorrect to say that the vocal folds are 'slack' during creaky voice: they are simultaneously slack (cover) and stiff (body). The contraction of the TA helps thicken the body and increase effective mass per unit length, which should lower vibratory frequency, but tension cannot be entirely ignored. Given the increased mass and slackness of the cover, we would expect low frequency and irregular vibration, particularly if there is VVFC (which has the four effects described above). However, on occasion, the high stiffness in the TA required to generate epilaryngeal constriction may on occasion become manifest in paradoxically high-frequency vibration, offering an explanation for why glottal stop is sometimes associated with high tones (e.g. Coupe 2003) or why glottalization (often with creakiness) is also associated with the occurrence of high-pitched glottal squeaks (Redi and Shattuck-Hufnagel 2001, Hejná et al. 2016).

The literature identifies a single isolated burst, or set of aperiodic bursts, as simple 'creak' phonation (Catford 1964: 32, Laver 1980: 122–126). Such occurrences are treated as voiceless, since they do not represent periodic vibration. In so far as it is possible to generate isolated bursts, the state of the larynx would be the same as for creaky voice, differing only in timing. The laryngeal configuration would be one of glottal closure most of the time, opening only intermittently to emit a pulse. Occurring in succession, these are interpreted as creaky voice, which itself has a high (nearly 90 per cent) closed quotient (amount of the glottal cycle when airflow is blocked) (Zemlin 1968: 197). In laboratory settings, when creakiness is intentionally sustained, the frequency of pulses can be as low as 40 Hz (Catford 1964: 32), and between 24 Hz and 56 Hz, averaging 35 Hz (Michel and Hollien 1968). In casual speech the frequency of creaky voice at the ends of intonational phrases may be in the 60–80 Hz range, to contrast with modal production above 100 Hz. In this broad interpretation, the creaky-voice state of the larynx can be referred to as 'creaky', 'creakiness', or 'laryngealization'. Whether the burst or sequence of bursts being described is voiceless or voiced, research should focus on: (1) the glottal adduction mechanism for the positioning of the vocal folds; (2) postero-anterior epilaryngeal narrowing, complementing glottal adduction with added potential for related constriction events to occur; and (3) perturbation to the mucosal wave from VVFC.

Video 2.13 illustrates the shift from modal voice to creaky voice. As the laryngeal constrictor constricts, the tube narrows, and the vocal folds shorten and become bunched, pitch lowers. In this example, all of the characteristics of laryngeal constriction accompany creaky phonation. Video 2.13x illustrates creaky voice in laughter, where the aryepiglottic constrictor is nearly closed (as the cuneiform cartilages occlude against the base of the epiglottis) as is the case in whispery and harsh states.

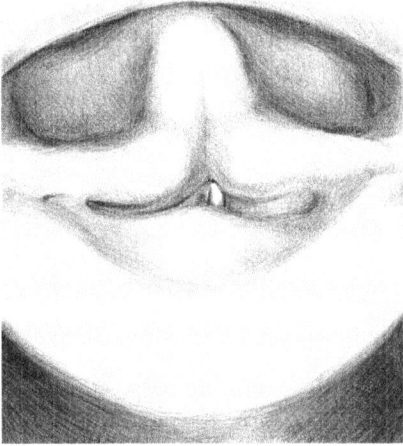

Figure 2.13 *The larynx in the state of creaky voice*

The action of the aryepiglottic constrictor is a salient aspect of creaky voice (as it is in whisper) as a tube-tensing device, to the point that the glottis is almost completely obscured beneath. Figure 2.13 illustrates the extreme degree of constriction that can be found in creakiness. The aryepiglottic folds are pursed to a 110° to 100° angle, and the epiglottic tubercle is very close to the advancing cuneiform tubercles. Tube constriction resembles more the state of epiglottal stop than glottal stop. Instead of focusing attention only on the size and shape of the glottal opening, it is important to concentrate on the structures immediately superior to the glottis, which have a direct effect on the airstream and glottal vibratory pattern. The role of the aryepiglottic mechanism in producing glottal stop and pharyngeal and epiglottal articulations is related to the production of creaky phonation, as often observed when creakiness (laryngealization) precedes or follows glottal arrest of the airstream (glottalization) in speech. Crucially, this implies a scalar relationship between the pitch mechanism and the laryngeal constriction mechanism. Falsetto, at high pitch, is an unconstricted glottal setting, where the CT muscles that stretch the vocal folds act perpendicularly to the adductory muscles that swing the folds into position for voicing. Creaky voice, at low pitch, is a laryngeally constricted setting, where the TA muscles that shorten the vocal folds comple-ment the adductory muscles that produce voicing. As a consequence of these pairings, within phonological systems, a constricted posture is less compatible with high pitch but more compatible with low pitch. These affinities do not preclude constriction from occurring at high pitch (see discussions of harshness below), nor do they preclude openness from occurring at low pitch (e.g. breathiness). However, the synergies within the pitch-constrictor relationship have implications for the potential arrangements of postures and sounds that carry linguistic contrast in a given language. For example, constricted registers may be less likely to occur on a high tone than on a low tone, or a creaky/breathy contrast may be more likely to occur on low tones.

The literature frequently discusses different degrees of creak in different linguistic contexts, distinguishing, for example, low-pitched phrase-final creak or 'pulsed voice' (Hollien and Michel 1968) from creaky voice or 'lax creaky voice' (Gobl and Ní Chasaide 2000) as sustained long-term phonatory settings (Infante Ríos and Pérez Sanz 2011). Garellek (2015) finds that phrase-final creak is perceptually distinct from creaky voice in within-word contexts in English. Gobl and Ní Chasaide (2000) recall Laver (1980: 124) citing Monsen and Engebretson (1977), who document variation in the glottal wave, including for creakiness, among speakers. This variation may arise from interspeaker differences in the deployment of laryngeal articulator parameters. The distinction between 'tight' and 'lax' creak might simply reflect the complex state of the vocal folds when the thyroarytenoid muscles tense, thereby thickening and increasing the effective mass of the body while simultaneously slackening the cover. Degrees of constriction, as well as of larynx height, may vary. Subglottal pressure could also play a role in differentiating these two regimes, with creaky phonation occurring at low pressures and harsher voice at higher pressures, meaning that as long as there is sufficient stricture for VVFC and perturbation of the mucosal wave and the pressure is low enough, creaky phonation will result.

Whisperiness and creakiness, because of their postural compatibility, are likely to combine and co-occur as *whispery creaky voice*. The vocal folds are shortened postero-anteriorly by the constrictor mechanism, an interarytenoid gap opens in the glottis (although the corniculate tubercles remain in contact), and the laryngeal constrictor is shaped into a tube that generates friction and noise. Here, one might ask whether a low-pitched phonation type like creak can be produced at the same time as a high-pitched phonation type, as in creaky falsetto or whispery creaky falsetto. Body-cover theory offers one answer. Another answer could be that it is more an issue of competing patterns. If high-pitched falsetto-range phonation is produced with intermittent vibratory characteristics that mimic creak (pulses of bursts detected at intervals), then we may call that type *creaky falsetto*. The addition of noise, due to tube shaping, would be *whispery creaky falsetto*.

2.3.12   Harsh Voice

From a glottal voicing perspective, there is wide agreement that *harsh voice* is a function of aperiodic irregularities in the acoustic waveform and noise in the spectrum (Laver 1980: 127). From a laryngeal articulator perspective, harsh voice obligatorily results from tightening the aryepiglottic constrictor mechanism, especially characterized by lower epilaryngeal tightening (ventricular adduction). VVFC with sufficiently high subglottal pressure also generates harshness (otherwise creaky phonation would result). Effects generated at the vocal folds are necessarily consequences of tightening the constrictor; narrowing the constrictor induces epilaryngeal structures to vibrate, and the narrow channelling above the glottis results in turbulence/noise in the signal. Descriptions of harshness in the literature reveal insights into the role of laryngeal constriction in shaping the vibratory patterns, noise-generating structures, and resonance cavities that give harshness its distinct but often disparate characteristics. Laver identifies adductive tension and medial compression as properties of harsh voice, but not longitudinal tension, since harsh voice is not usually high pitched (1980: 130). Catford created vocal-fold-based categories of phonation that correlate with harshness (and with whisper and creakiness) such as 'ligamental' and 'arytenoidal', but he was clear that 'ligamental stricture' is often accompanied by a pharyngealized quality that he attributed to 'upper larynx constriction' (1964: 33–34). We posit that the constriction he referred to is the aryepiglottic constrictor (the laryngeal articulator) and that its effect on quality is primarily due to articulatory action above the glottis rather than to an independent setting of the vocal folds. 'Rough' and 'hoarse' voice are common alternative terms, as are 'rasping', 'raucous', and 'strident' (Laver 1980: 127). For Fairbanks (1960: 171, 182–183), hoarseness combines the characteristics of harshness and breathiness. Kreiman and Gerratt (2000: 77–80) note that the terms hoarseness, harshness/roughness, and breathiness are common in describing pathological voices, but that perceptual categories often fail to correlate with physical measures. Laver (1980: 128) points out the anatomical relationship between vowel quality and harshness, and that open vowels are judged as more harsh than close vowels. Harshness increases progressively as vowels become more open and retracted, roughly in the order [i u] to [ɪ ʌ ʊ] to [ɛ æ ɑ ɔ], but varying according to consonantal and syllabic environments (Rees 1958). While acoustic correlates of aperiodicity (e.g. jitter, shimmer) have been widely researched, Laver reports that the only physiological correlate of harshness enjoying widespread agreement is 'laryngeal tension' (1980: 129). Various authors quoted by Laver associate this tension with 'the vocal folds', 'the throat and neck', 'the pharynx', and even 'the whole body'. Russell (1936) provides the useful observation that 'the red-surfaced muscles which lie above the vocal cords begin to form a tense channel' (cited in Laver 1980: 129, from Van Riper and Irwin 1958: 232). This could refer to the ventricular folds or indeed the entire narrowed aryepiglottic constrictor. With respect to vibratory frequencies, Van Riper and Irwin report that 'most harsh voices are relatively low in pitch' (1958: 232).

Our view focuses not only on the adductive structures around the glottis but continues up through the epilaryngeal tube to the aryepiglottic folds and the retracting base of the tongue, challenging the premises of what tension and compression and indeed constriction mean when referring to laryngeal behaviour. These forces need to be evaluated in terms of the entire vertical reach of the laryngeal mechanism, not just at the glottis. The references to laryngeal tension and to tense 'supraglottic' channelling can be explained by the action of the aryepiglottic constrictor mechanism, which reduces the epilaryngeal tube in volume, pursing it at the top and squeezing it between the base of the tongue and the elevating larynx. This affects the vibratory pattern of the vocal folds and adds the effects of other oscillators and airstream disruptors. The action of the constrictor in producing harsh voice, as with creaky voice, mirrors the mechanism for low pitch – TA muscle contraction for arytenoid fronting and vocal fold shortening. This relationship explains the correlation between harshness and low pitch. The parallel effect of the constrictor on glottal tension – vertical massing of vibratory structures associated with VVFC – gives the vibrations their irregular/aperiodic character, resulting from added degrees of vibratory freedom and perturbation to the mucosal wave. The complementary retraction of the tongue that occurs during constriction is consistent with the observation that open vowels demonstrate more harshness than close vowels. Open vowels are more susceptible to laryngeal constriction, as depicted in Figure 1.3, and opening the jaw is a concomitant aspect of efficient larynx closure. For instance, while the jaw closes reflexively in the first phase of swallowing to force food over the tongue, the jaw is free to open once the aryepiglottic constrictor closes, just as it opens reflexively during vomiting while still efficiently keeping the aryepiglottic constrictor closed. Vowels with jaw opening and lingual retraction are, therefore, most susceptible to the effects of harshness, imposed by the tightened constrictor mechanism. Adding Abercrombie's formulation of 'tight phonation' – allowing little air to escape, in opposition to breathiness where much air escapes (1967: 93) – and 'cartilage glottis firmly closed, the rest of the glottis in vibration, and constriction of the upper parts of the larynx' (1967: 100–101) – helps to localize the mechanism for harsh voice to the laryngeal constrictor and epilaryngeal tube above the glottis as the mechanism of compressing airflow, as in whisperiness and creakiness, and introducing tension to the larynx as a whole. We hypothesize that the noisy flow generated during harsh voice and the irregular periodicity ascribed to various sorts of harsh or hoarse voice originates in the channel formed by the epilaryngeal tube. Higher airflow from increased subglottal pressure (compared to creak/creaky voice) contributes to this noise. In our revised interpretation, whisperiness as a laryngeal state (as opposed to breathiness) is associated with harshness. The constriction shared between whisperiness and harshness explains Laver's original compatibility principle (1980: 19–20) in articulatory terms. While both are constricted, the distinction between harsh voice and creaky voice can be attributed largely to the more constricted laryngeal channel above the glottis and increased airflow in harsh voice (which can be enough to drive epilaryngeal vibrations).

Viewed from above, in Figure 2.14, the posture of the constrictor for harsh voice resembles that of creaky voice but with greater compaction of the epilaryngeal tube structures between the cuneiform cartilages and the

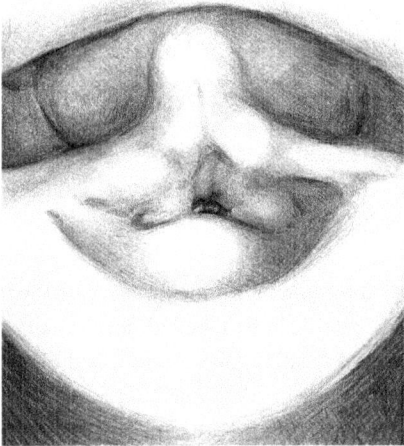

Figure 2.14 *The larynx in the state of harsh voice, at mid pitch*

epiglottis. Tension is posited postero-anteriorly due to the enhanced adduction of extreme laryngeal constriction. Due to these same stricture forces, compression is posited not only medially at the glottis but also vertically through the massed structures of the constrictor, undergoing both downward and upward pressure in the middle of the constriction manoeuvre. These hypotheses predicted by the model remain to be verified experimentally.

It has been shown that many pitch dependencies exist within the broad terminology of the taxonomy for voice quality (Esling et al. 1994), and harshness is a complex area of the taxonomy that requires differentiation of pitch correlates for effective interpretation. Frequency is a significant determiner in harsh voices because of the multiple effects introduced by the tightening constrictor mechanism, making the measurement of periodicity problematical for instrumental algorithms. Double peaks of different amplitudes in the electroglottographic (EGG) signal have long been indicative of introduced aperiodicity, characteristic of harsh voice (Esling 1978, 1984). EGG traces of creaky voice can yield double peaks of different amplitudes (Fourcin 2003). We interpret the double peaks auditorily as harsh creaky voice and articulatorily as indications of irregularity in the vibratory pattern due to vocal-ventricular fold coupling vertically through the constrictor (and possibly due to differences in subglottal pressure). VVFC, adding mass, damping, and degrees of freedom as constriction increases, perturbs the transmission of the mucosal wave, yielding irregular, aperiodic vibration that, with raised sub-glottal pressure, is classified auditorily as harsh phonation. The combination of massed vibration, generating periods of irregular amplitude, and a narrowed epilaryngeal tube with some glottal opening, generating friction and noise, creates *harsh whispery voice*. A combination of irregular amplitude peaks, noisy tube friction, and low-frequency or interspersed bursts over time yields *harsh whispery creaky voice*.

Just as laryngeal constriction generates harshness, transforming modal voice, constriction can generate harshness to alter falsetto mode. Overlaying falsetto with irregular, aperiodic, jittery phonation due to vertical compression within the constrictor, the voice may be called *harsh falsetto*. Irregularity in the time domain, where the pattern is intermittent, mimics creak, and together with vertical compression and elevated pitch can be labelled *harsh creaky falsetto*. A pattern of irregular amplitude peaks, noisy tube friction, and elevated pitch would be labelled *harsh whispery falsetto*. All four components – irregular amplitude peaks, noisy tube friction, interspersed bursts over time, and elevated pitch – would be labelled *harsh whispery creaky falsetto*. These compound phonation types, as presented in Laver (1980), remain auditorily

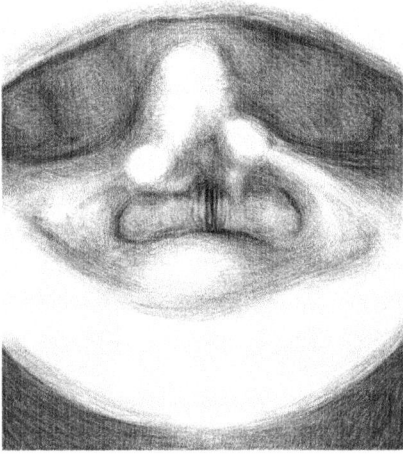

Figure 2.15 *The larynx in the state of ventricular voice*

constructed categories. Nevertheless, bringing the LAM into the equation provides a revised articulatory platform on which to base hypotheses about the correlates of harshness, whisperiness, or creakiness. Their articulatory relationship as aryepiglottically constricted productions introduces a premise for comparison, on which to design further perceptual and production research. In Chapter 4, we identify occurrences of each voice quality type discussed here in the voices of familiar, easily searchable speakers.

Video 2.14 illustrates all the hallmarks of laryngeal constriction generating harsh voice in a mid pitch range. Video 2.14x illustrates vibrations occurring through the epilaryngeal tube in the strong constriction of harsh laughter.

2.3.13 Ventricular Voice

In the absence of vocal-ventricular fold coupling, it is possible for the ventricular folds to engage in self-sustaining oscillation simultaneously with vocal fold vibration below, which is called *ventricular voice*. Auditorily, this phenomenon is a more extreme form of what occurs in harsh voice. Laver calls it 'severely harsh voice' (1980: 130), but visually differentiating the two modes of vibration in a laryngoscopic image proves difficult without sagittal corroboration. Ventricular voice presumes an active vibration of ventricular tissues, perhaps including the mucosal mass found between the ventricular folds and aryepiglottic folds. VVFC, important in achieving glottal stop or epiglottal stop and in producing creaky voice or harsh voice, is counterproductive to ventricular voice (Moisik and Esling 2014). VVFC is effective during tighter degrees of constriction when the ventricular folds compress onto the vocal folds to arrest their vibration in laryngeal stops, but for ventricular voice, VVFC would dampen the source-modulating free vibrations of the ventricular folds. Our prediction is that larynx lowering can be recruited to avoid the vertical compression that would inhibit ventricular fold vibration. This kind of control is highly specialized (and in the case of traditional throat-singing techniques requires years of training). No isolated, unvoiced ventricular vibration has been attested, presumably because the adduction and airflow necessary to drive ventricular voice also causes the vocal folds to vibrate.

Fuks et al. (1998), using high-speed glottography, have shown that the ventricular folds oscillate at half the fundamental frequency of the vocal folds (a frequency of f0/2) and sometimes f0/3 in vocal-ventricular voicing (as in the Tibetan chanting tradition). This is due to aerodynamic forces whereby glottal-flow pulses alternately sustain and attenuate the vibrations of the ventricular folds. This is called entrainment, where two oscillators that share the same energy source come to synchronize in period and phase lock in a ratio that reflects their natural modes (based on the masses and tensions involved). Fuks (1999) models this oscillation with two separate paired masses representing the vocal folds and another pair representing the ventricular folds. Sakakibara et al. (2004b) present evidence that in drone khöömei throat singing, both the vocal and the ventricular folds vibrate with the same periodicity but with a difference in phase. They observe that in kargyraa throat singing, the ventricular folds are looser and vibrate at half the frequency of the vocal folds. Their EMG experiments implicate the thyroepiglottic (TE) muscles, which closely parallel the LCA muscles, in constricting the epilarynx for both drone and kargyraa styles. TE activity is detected in drone style, but TE electrode readings are less active than for the vocalis muscles in kargyraa. Aryepiglottic (AE) muscle activity could not be measured. We would predict that the external TA muscles are implicated, since ventricular voice is not an open form but a laryngeally constricted form, and since the TE is actually part of the external/lateral TA with fibres extending upwards into the epilaryngeal mucosa towards but not reaching the epiglottis (Reidenbach 1998a, 1998b). Approaching EMG from the perspective of the laryngeal articulator implies that the involvement of the various bodies of the TA muscles should be tested, up through the level of the

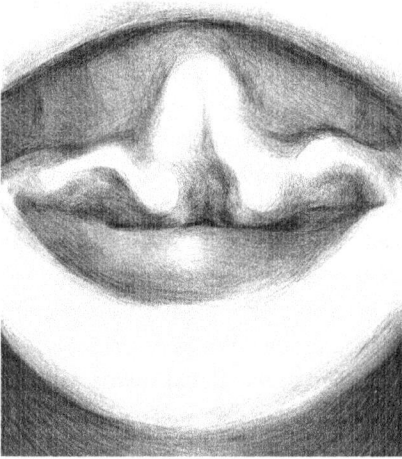

Figure 2.16 *The larynx in the state of harsh voice at low pitch (generating aryepiglottic trilling)*

AE muscles. However, the computational model of the larynx developed by Moisik and Gick (2017) confirms Reidenbach's (1997, 1998a, 1998b) assertion that full epilaryngeal closure is entirely possible without an AE muscle, and the sparseness, even rarity of AE fibres makes their EMG detection difficult experimentally. Even while testing the fine distinctions in TA fibres, the contribution of the musculature controlling larynx height (particularly lowering) to isolate the ventricular folds also needs to be tested. Auditory examples of ventricular voice are distinguished from harsh voice in Chapter 4.

Video 2.15 illustrates the constricted epilaryngeal tube and mucosal effects that characterize ventricular voice. We hypothesize that the vibration of the ventricular folds could be enhanced and more effectively isolated by lowering the larynx to reduce VVFC. The production of ventricular voice in the practised style of a Tibetan Buddhist chant master is illustrated in Section 4.1.2.5.

2.3.14 Aryepiglottic Trilling

When the laryngeal constrictor is engaged, as in the production of whisperiness, creakiness, or harshness, there is an increased potential for the aryepiglottic folds at the top of the epilaryngeal tube to respond aerodynamically to the narrowed channels of airflow and to vibrate. The vibration of the aryepiglottic folds is not the same as that of the vocal folds, since the vocal folds are paired with each other, while each aryepiglottic fold vibrates against a different side of the epiglottic tubercle. *Aryepiglottic trilling* can be called a variety of *low-pitched harsh voice*. The aryepiglottic folds assume a posture as in harsh voice, approaching the posture for epiglottal stop, where the cuneiform cartilages push up against the epiglottis, allowing air to flow medially through the glottis and between the pursed aryepiglottic folds as well as laterally between each aryepiglottic fold and the epiglottis, lateral to each cuneiform cartilage. Our illustration is voiced – colloquially a growl – but it could also be produced as a voiceless trill, with only the aryepiglottic folds trilling and glottal vibration absent. Vibration at this level of the laryngeal mechanism introduces, in effect, a competing sound source to the vocal folds. In ventricular voice, vibration is more closely tied to the glottal source, whereas aryepiglottic trilling is perpendicular to the folds beneath, and each fold can vibrate at a different frequency. In cases we have observed, the left aryepiglottic fold (image right) vibrates at the frequency of the vocal folds (around 110–120 Hz), and the right aryepiglottic fold (image left) vibrates at a frequency of 50–60 Hz (Moisik et al. 2010). The visual impression is of a long, straight, narrow channel from right to left through which airflow excites neighbouring soft tissues. Normally, the ventricular folds do not vibrate during voiced or voiceless aryepiglottic trilling, unless a speaker explicitly adds vocal-ventricular coupling to aryepiglottic trilling. Citing acoustic transition, EGG, and aerodynamic evidence, Sakakibara et al. (2004a) conclude that the vocal and aryepiglottic folds vibrate during 'growl' singing, but not the ventricular folds. The external fibres of the TA muscles are implicated in laryngeal constriction, supplementing and strengthening the LCA/IA muscle contraction that initiates the adductory process. Vocalis and thyroepiglottic muscle activity is identified by Sakakibara et al. (2004b) during 'growl' singing in their EMG experiments.

Constricted states of the larynx, especially epiglottal stop and aryepiglottic trilling, which involve extreme narrowing at the upper aryepiglottic border of the epilaryngeal tube, are closely related to physiological functions other than speech. The opposition between breath and laryngeal stops directly parallels airway control – open and closed. Full engagement of the constrictor parallels the fundamental physiological activities of swallowing and clearing the airway for the efficient integration of breathing with eating and drinking and, in the more recent evolutionary history of hominins, with the ability to speak. Tightening the airway while actively vibrating the aryepiglottic folds is the mechanism for 'clearing the throat', which in turn is accompanied by whispery-voiced vibration of the vocal folds, punctuated by epiglottal stop arrests of voicing. In throat clearing, the aryepiglottic constrictor is engaged throughout the manoeuvre, while glottal states fluctuate, generating variable flow patterns through the epilaryngeal tube. Although aryepiglottic constriction is largely a buckling manoeuvre rather than a sequence of independent muscle firings (Fink 1974a, Reidenbach 1997, 1998a, 1998b), myodynamic research can add to our knowledge of the relative contribution of TA/TE and AE activity in deglutition and linguistic contexts. The relationship of speaking to bodily function (of phonetics to physiology), specifically from the perspective of the laryngeal articulator, has a bearing on the investigation of the ontogeny of speech (the subject of Chapter 6) and on the phylogenetic origins of speech (discussed in Chapter 8).

Video 2.16 illustrates aryepiglottic fold vibration or trilling. The epilarynx is constricted, and both the vocal folds and the aryepiglottic folds are vibrating.

Video 2.16a demonstrates how aryepiglottic fold trilling facilitates clearing the throat. The extremely bent aryepiglottic folds (averaging a 90° angle from arytenoid to cuneiform tubercle to the lateral edge of the epiglottis) press up against the epiglottis, while the intercartilaginous opening of whispery voice can occasionally be glimpsed medially between the pursed cuneiform cartilages. Sometimes the vocal folds can also be seen, vibrating just under the epiglottic tubercle. As glottal voicing periodically arrests during the manoeuvre, the aryepiglottic folds continue vibrating as voiceless trilling. The manoeuvre begins with an epiglottal stop, and there are two epiglottal stops within the manoeuvre. At the end of the sequence, as aryepiglottic constriction releases and the vocal folds begin to abduct, voicing momentarily shifts from whispery to breathy, after which the vocal folds quickly separate and the glottis fully abducts for inhalation. Video 2.16x illustrates the extreme degree of cuneiform-epiglottis occlusion necessary for efficient aryepiglottic fold trilling (with glottal voicing) in a laughter sequence.

2.3.15 *Laryngeal Constriction at High Pitch*

Laryngeal constriction at high pitch is a final mode of laryngeally constricted phonation that can be considered a distinct state of the larynx. Whisperiness, creakiness, harshness, and aryepiglottic trilling all require constriction of the laryngeal constrictor, narrowing the epilaryngeal tube and increasing vertical compression, but each of these voicing types, as well as ventricular voice, has thus far been associated with lower pitch. This follows from our model, where tightening the constrictor mechanism enables the production of qualities we have labelled as 'constricted' and lowers the frequency of vocal fold vibration.

With the bunching and thickening of vibrating structures in creaky or harsh voice, aperiodicity or multiple periodicities increase, and oscillations decrease in frequency.

When the cricothyroid muscles contract to raise pitch at the same time that the laryngeal constrictor engages, distinctive qualities of phonation result. The effect is much as if glottal vibration were arrested, as in glottal stop, and then the vocal folds were stretched and made taut and air forced through the blocked passage. Longitudinal tension and aryepiglottic constriction are ostensibly opposite. Together, they produce an isometric tension whose net effect is to compress the airway while stretching the tight, thin vocal folds over a restricted length, generating a high frequency that differs auditorily from falsetto. The quality has similarities to harsh voice, and we have sometimes called it *high-pitched harsh voice* to indicate that the laryngeal constrictor is tightly engaged, in parallel to harsh voice at low pitch (aryepiglottic trilling) and harsh voice at mid pitch. Another label for this type of phonation in the clinical and singing literature has been 'pressed voice' (Bergan et al. 2004). Larynx height and pitch are variable parameters in how this unique combination of contractions is rendered. In phonation types where constriction is strong but without longitudinal compression, so that the vocal folds are not stretched and pitch is low, the larynx as a whole is generally raised. Pitch has also served to differentiate auditory qualities, i.e. pharyngealized voice and lowered-larynx voice have low pitch, but raised-larynx voice and faucalized voice have high pitch. In our present illustration of high-pitched harshness (pressed voice), the larynx is lowered, similar to its posture in faucalized voice, so that the length of the vocal tract is expanded. We offer this illustration because we feel it is the archetype of the isometric tightening and resulting strained quality of phonation in pressed voice. Just as it is possible to vary larynx height in combination with laryngeal articulator postures, the example of laryngeal constriction at high pitch could be produced with a raised larynx, which would make it a recognizable version of raised-larynx voice but with distinctly restrictive phonatory airflow. The raised-larynx posture is more reflexively consistent with Fink's 'effort closure state' when the mechanism is tightly folded (1974a: 126), suggesting that lowering the larynx might allow continuous phonation to flow more easily than when the larynx is near maximum closure. In either case, the ventricular folds are in contact with the vocal folds (VVFC), and this has a significant effect on vocal fold vibratory dynamics. The examples we present here are phonetically categorical, articulatory/auditory paradigms, intended as a theoretical model for empirical testing. Pushing phonetic parameters to the limit is not the usual experience of most language speakers, but it identifies the boundaries of articulatory performance in a systematic way that can be evaluated experimentally. We invite researchers to investigate the articulatory, acoustic, and biomechanical properties of the relationships we have identified within the laryngeal constrictor mechanism.

Video 2.17 illustrates a form of harsh voice (because of its laryngeally constricted state), which is often called 'pressed voice' because of its retention and measured release of subglottal air. When the vocal folds are visible, they are stretched and tight, resembling the glottal state of falsetto. As vertical constrictive pressure compacts the ventricular folds and the glottis is occluded, the image resembles the state of glottal stop. Here, the audio signal is clearly high pitched. Video 2.17x illustrates laughter with harshness from a tightly constricted laryngeal posture at high pitch. Because pitch is high, the length of the vocal folds (and concomitant arytenoid-to-epiglottis distance of the constrictor mechanism) is longer than in other constricted postures.

In Figure 2.17, the state of the larynx during laryngeal constriction at high pitch could be mistaken for glottal stop, as in Figures 2.6 and 2.7, except that the larynx is lowered and the vocal folds are more tightly stretched longitudinally and taut. The compression of the ventricular folds resembles their

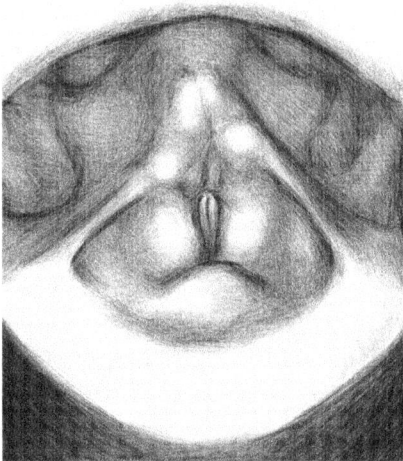

Figure 2.17 *The larynx in the state of harsh voice at high pitch ('pressed voice')*

configuration during glottal stop (more massed and medially adducted than for modal voice). The auditory impression is that of holding the breath and forcing the air out in tightly suppressed bursts. This most strained, ostensibly antagonistic combination of tight constriction with antero-posterior longitudinal tension exerts an effect on glottal phonation that neither mechanism could achieve alone. Neither the ventricular folds (although adducted close to the midline and pressing onto the vocal folds) nor the aryepiglottic folds appear to exhibit self-sustaining oscillations, and the tube is lengthened vertically, separating the laryngeal structures. When the pitch of this setting is increased to its maximum, the auditory quality reaches what Abercrombie called 'seal voice'. Laver associated this quality with 'ventricular falsetto' – 'very severe compressive effort of the whole larynx' (1980: 139). There are clearly many permutations of 'tight phonation' under the general label of harshness; and the LAM has identified aryepiglottic laryngeal constriction, larynx height variation, and the pitch factor as three dimensions of movement that must be taken into account in describing laryngeal articulation. While laryngoscopic observation and auditory comparison serve as a guide, with the model indicating how they relate to the articulatory behaviour of the constrictor, these productions invite further instrumental investigation.

2.4   Tense Voice and Lax Voice

Laver (1980: 141–156) has addressed 'tension settings' in detail. 'Tense voice' and 'lax voice' have been used as descriptors for high and low degrees of muscular tension generally throughout the vocal tract. In much of the literature reviewed by Laver, the identification of tension settings overlaps considerably with qualities that can be attributed to articulatory postures of the laryngeal articulatory mechanism. This applies to both phonatory qualities and resonance qualities (timbre). Tension labels can often be replaced by descriptions of phonatory effects generated within the laryngeal mechanism or by descriptions of qualities generated by configurations of the supraglottic structures of the laryngeal mechanism as it compacts towards closure or opens towards the respiratory state. In earlier research, 'tension' has often served as a generalized explanation to account for an increase in force, tightness, or effort at some unspecified location in the vocal tract. Many times, this vagueness results because the source-filter lingually-centred vocal tract is not an adequate model to account for the many tension adjustments that can occur in the laryngeal articulator of the lower vocal tract. In such cases, an understanding of how the laryngeal articulator works and what structural parts of the laryngeal mechanism can be made tighter or more closely squeezed together can yield more substantial explanations. By taking the 'whole larynx' (Moisik and Esling 2011) into account – oral and laryngeal vocal tracts – it should be possible to identify more accurately the sources of tension, which articulators are becoming tight relative to other structures, and the muscular contractions or synergistic actions involved.

2.5 Unconstricted vs. Constricted Laryngeal States

Gordon and Ladefoged (2001), focusing on the glottis, present a continuum of phonation differences from voiceless through breathy voiced, to modal voicing, and through creaky voice to glottal closure. Rearranging the laryngeal states we have looked at (and listened to) into a continuum from full openness to full closure within a multiplanar approach, as in Figure 2.18, adds perspective to the effect of the laryngeal articulator mechanism. Several linguistic realizations of laryngeal effects are more accurately visualized within a multiplanar approach, we believe. The full range of laryngeal effects needs to be expressed in a number of parallel views (see also Lindblom 2009: 151). Figure 2.18 depicts the transition from glottal openness (breathing), through breath and prephonation to modal voice, through glottal stop and reinforced (ventricular) glottal stop to epiglottal stop. Not all of these states are in the same plane. Breathing, at the left, has the lowest larynx position, and epiglottal stop, at the right, has the highest larynx position. As the larynx rises across the seven states, the laryngeal constrictor buckles inwards, and the buckling ary-epiglottic folds bend forwards, up and under the epiglottis. These idealized drawings are intended to compare differences between structures and do not reflect all dimensions of movement in the laryngeal constrictor; the actual motion of the constrictor mechanism is simulated in Chapter 3.

The fundamental distinction made in the larynx is between unconstricted and constricted laryngeal settings. Figure 2.19a compares three voiceless

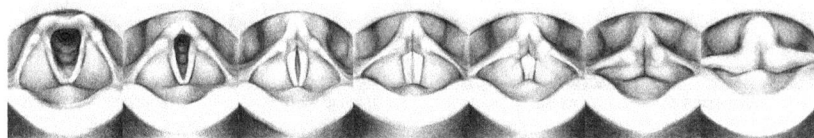

Figure 2.18 *Montage of laryngeal states on a continuum of openness from open to closed*

postures with three voiced postures, all of which are unconstricted. Each top image is equivalent to the image beneath, differing only in voicing. Figure 2.19b compares four constricted postures without voicing with their counterparts or near counterparts beneath. Breath, voicing, and whisperiness do not fit easily into the open-to-closed continuum, because this arrangement

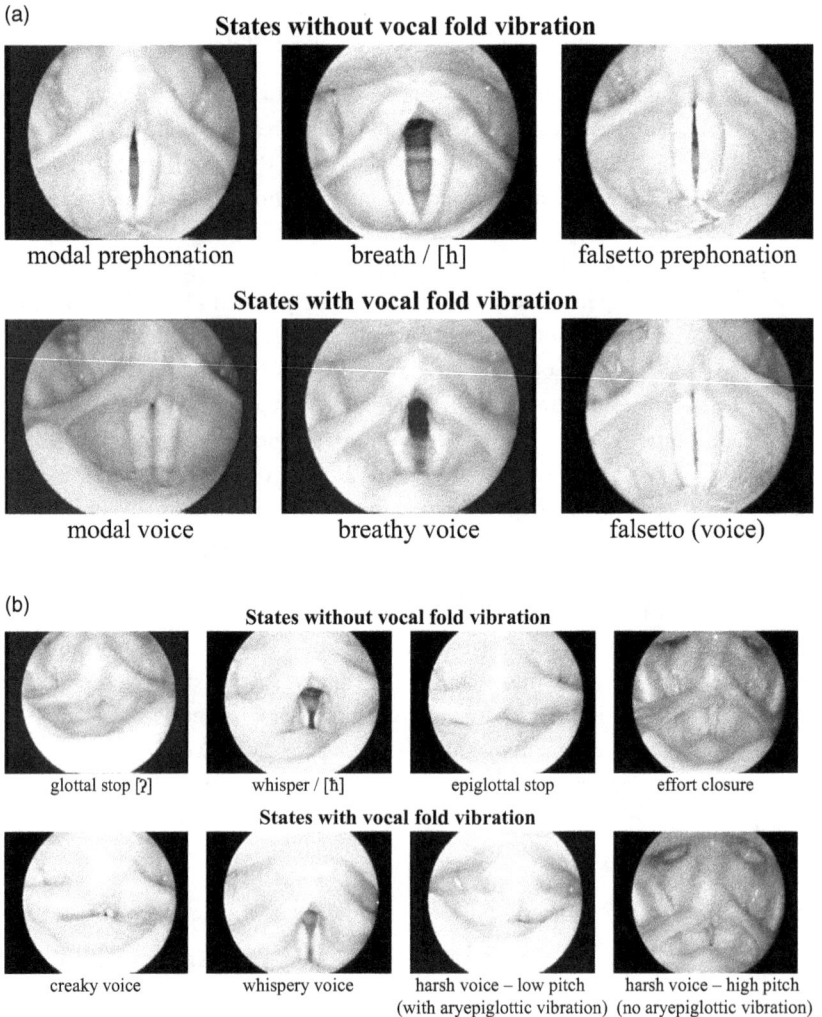

(a)

States without vocal fold vibration

modal prephonation   breath / [h]   falsetto prephonation

States with vocal fold vibration

modal voice   breathy voice   falsetto (voice)

(b)

States without vocal fold vibration

glottal stop [ʔ]   whisper / [h]   epiglottal stop   effort closure

States with vocal fold vibration

creaky voice   whispery voice   harsh voice – low pitch   harsh voice – high pitch
                              (with aryepiglottic vibration) (no aryepiglottic vibration)

Figure 2.19 *Comparison of laryngeal states by parameter*
(a) unconstricted epilarynx, (b) constricted epilarynx...

(c)

breath / [h] (unconstricted) whisper / [ɦ] (constricted)

little
to
modest
noise

breathy voice (unconstricted) whispery voice (constricted)

modest
to
high
noise

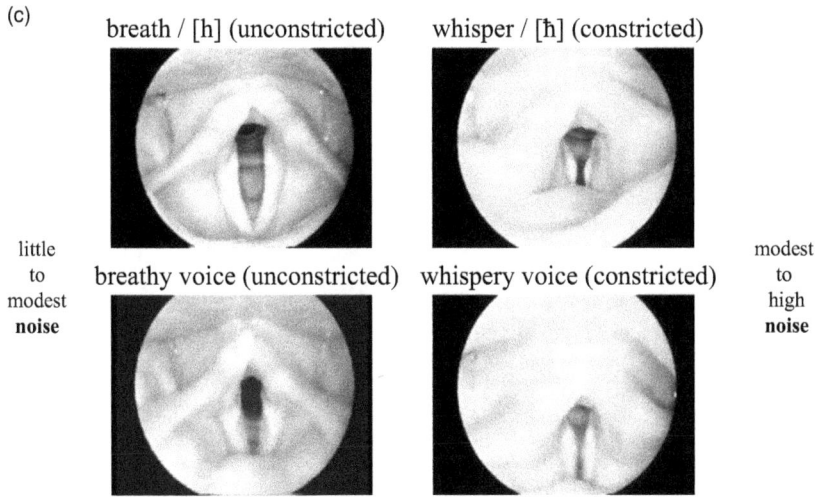

Figure 2.19 (*cont.*) ... *and (c) breathy vs whispery*

obscures their essential similarities and differences. The essential parameter of whisperiness is epilaryngeal constriction, as in epiglottal stop in Figure 18. Breathy and whispery states follow a parallel pattern, shown in Figure 2.19c. Starting with the open state of breath and adding voicing, breathy voice results. Adding constriction, whisper results. If both voicing and laryngeal constriction are added to breath, whispery voice results.

3 *Instrumental Case Studies and Computational Simulations of Voice Quality*

In Chapter 3, we present a survey of instrumental case studies along with several computational simulations that illustrate how the Laryngeal Articulator Model can guide empirical phonetic study. The purpose is to provide prima facie evidence for several key details of laryngeal behaviour in producing voice quality and associated segmental and phonatory phenomena. The range of different instrumental methods (high-speed laryngoscopy, cineradiography, simultaneous laryngoscopy and laryngeal ultrasound, MRI) and computational modelling techniques (lumped-element and finite-element modelling) is meant to provide a sense of the different avenues that can be explored. Each case constitutes its own sub-area. Further research is necessary to provide more generalizable results and to refine the model. However, these first exploratory steps provide the foundation for such work.

Although we begin the chapter with a brief survey of literature related to instrumental analysis of voice quality, we do not aim to provide an exhaustive summary of the literature on the broader topics that are relevant to the discussion (e.g. f0 control or the general use of instrumental techniques to examine laryngeal behaviour). Rather, we wish to draw attention to the nature of laryngeal constriction and to the absence of the epilaryngeal mechanism in the models that have guided instrumental research. Where appropriate, we point out the streams of the literature and particular examples that illustrate the knowledge gap about laryngeal constriction or that have served as precursors in developing our model.

3.1 Techniques to Examine Long-Term Voice Qualities

Acoustic techniques and various instrumental phonetic approaches have added quantifiable parameters to the definition of voice qualities. Acoustic long-term average spectrum (LTAS) analysis is an early quantitative acoustic approach to characterize long-term voice quality (Harmegnies 1987, Harmegnies et al. 1989, Esling et al. 1991, Bruyninckx et al. 1994, Harmegnies et al. 1994). LTAS captures both laryngeal and supralaryngeal effects but is especially useful as a non-invasive way of interpreting oral resonance postures. Electroglottography (EGG), or 'laryngography' (Fourcin 1974), has been used to identify differences in phonatory patterns and has contributed to distinguishing between pitch-related phonatory changes and constrictor-related vibratory phenomena (Esling 1984). Gick et al. (2004) used x-ray speech data of Canadian French and Canadian English drawn from a database assembled by Munhall et al. (1995). By measuring pixel distances within a set of stricture locations spanning the vocal tract but influenced primarily by the tongue and lips, they found that the speech rest position or inter-speech posture (ISP) differs by language. They argue that the ISP constitutes an active target, comparable to consonant or vowel targets, and probably needs to be learned as such. However, since they only measure the ISP, which was done to avoid the sort of segmental contamination of articulatory setting claimed to confound LTAS research, it is unclear if their findings generalize to the notion of articulatory setting (voice quality). The ISP could simply be the speech-preparedness target and not a property that pervades all of speech.

Following research by Gick et al. (2004), Wilson (2006) demonstrated the use of ultrasound to study ISP to identify language-specific articulatory settings (see also Wilson and Gick 2006, 2014). Several subsequent studies have also used ultrasound with this aim (Schaeffler et al. 2008, Mennen et al. 2010). More recently, electromagnetic articulography (EMA) (Święciński 2013) and MRI (Ramanarayanan et al. 2011, 2013, Benítez et al. 2014) have been marshalled to study articulatory setting, although acoustic techniques continue to be used (Lowie and Bultena 2007, Ng et al. 2012).

Phonetic, sociolinguistic, clinical, and forensic studies have used the Vocal Profile Analysis (VPA) scheme to evaluate individual and community voice quality attributes. VPA is an articulatory-auditory evaluation protocol (Laver and Mackenzie Beck 2007) employed by speech and voice professionals who share the same or similar training in phonetic listening (Mackenzie Beck 2005, Shewell 1998). In the forensic realm, expert voice comparison is an effective tool (Nolan 2005), and VPA has been usefully correlated with acoustic measures for speaker comparison (Foulkes and French 2012). The VPA scheme incorporates categories for supralaryngeal (oral) articulatory-auditory postures as well as lower-vocal-tract articulatory-auditory postures and is continually undergoing modification to accommodate developing theory (San Segundo et al. 2018). The instrumental identification of lower-vocal-tract behaviour and the reformulation of articulatory-auditory categories in the present work is intended to contribute to the continuing development of the VPA scheme.

3.2   Techniques to Image the Larynx

Imaging and measuring lower-vocal-tract articulation has been a long-standing challenge in phonetic research, with consequences for the description of voice quality. Electromyography (EMG) is highly invasive, and it is a challenge to sufficiently isolate desired muscle activity, especially the finer muscles of the epilarynx (Hillel 2001, Sakakibara et al. 2004b). EGG correlates laryngeal vibration in the horizontal plane (opening and particularly closing) with imaging data. The precise vertical location of where vibrations are occurring is not as easily distinguished, although double electrode pairs have been used to track vertical movements of the larynx (Rothenberg 1992). The Carstens Articulograph (3D EMA) tracks tissue movement using adhesive electromagnetic sensors, but attaching them deep enough in the lower vocal tract to collect data for pharyngeal or laryngeal motion has not been possible. Visual means of observing epilarynx behaviour, such as laryngoscopy, laryngeal ultrasound, x-ray, and MRI, can more easily evaluate epilarynx behaviour.

X-ray (usually cineradiography, i.e. video x-ray), popular in speech research from the 1960s to the mid 1980s, provides a two-dimensional projection of vocal tract structures. Because of the predominantly ventral-dorsal orientation of the vocal tract in the body, midsagittal imaging allows the sagittal profile of the epilaryngeal tube to be seen. In early linguistic experimentation, image intensifier technology placed strict limits on the diameter of the safely imageable area. Delattre (1971: 132) commented that 'if the lips showed, the pharynx did not, if the tongue tip showed, the tongue root did not'. However, x-ray images in Russell (1931) and Negus (1949: 147–148, figs. 160, 161) do show the entire vocal tract. Technological limitations may in part account for why the laryngopharynx is absent from many tracings, as depicted in Figure 3.1(a) below, precluding accurate evaluation of epilarynx state (see Esling 1996: 69, Edmondson and Esling 2006: 179–180). The tongue, because of its large, easily observable displacements, was the usual focus. Although Delattre's seminal x-ray study in 1971 increased the imageable x-ray footprint, only an outline of the laryngopharynx is indicated (Delattre 1971, Lindau 1975, 1978, Hess 1998) as in Figure 3.1(b). This type of trace permits evaluation of larynx height but omits the posterior border of the epilarynx, precluding evaluation of postero-anterior epilaryngeal narrowing.

The empirical limitations of x-ray data contributed to tongue articulation being taken as primary in describing pharyngeals and pharyngealization. Accounts of several language groups with lower-vocal-tract sounds illustrate this limitation: languages of the Caucasus (Dzhejranishvili 1959, Bgažba

(a) Gaprindashvili (1966, fig. 62):
[Hess 1998: 14]
Dargi [ʕ]

(b) Lindau (1978: 554, fig. 8):
American English [ɹ]

(c) Lindau (1975: 71, fig. 27):
Ateso [ɛ] ([−ATR] vowel)

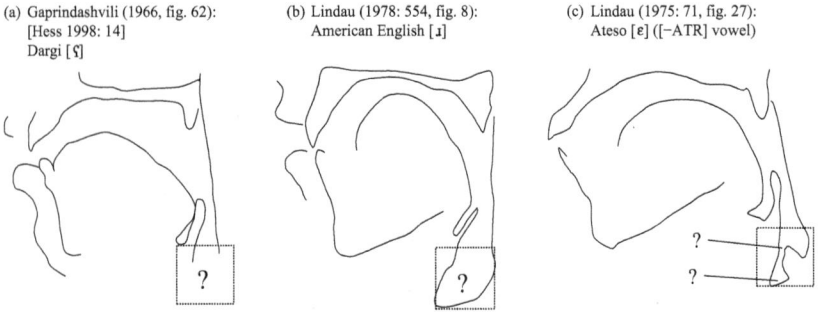

Figure 3.1 *Different styles of x-ray tracing*
(a) omitting the epilarynx entirely, (b) showing only the laryngopharynx, (c)
including an outline of the epilarynx but no clear indication of the
aryepiglottic folds or ventricular folds (symbolized with the question marks).
All images are retracings of tracings from the listed sources.

1964, Gaprindashvili 1966, Catford 1983: 348, Ladefoged and Maddieson 1996: 170, 308); the Tungusic language Even (Novikova 1960, Ladefoged and Maddieson 1996: 307); Niger-Congo and Nilo-Saharan languages with so-called tongue-root vowel harmony (Ladefoged 1964, Ladefoged et al. 1972, Painter 1973, Lindau 1975, 1978, Casali 2008: 506); and Arabic (Al-Ani 1970, 1978, Delattre 1971, Ali and Daniloff 1972, Ghazeli 1977, Boff-Dkhissi 1983). Most tracings of these data omit the epilarynx profile entirely, although there are some exceptions, illustrated by Figure 3.1(c). Popular phonetic texts reproduce these observations (Laver 1994, Ladefoged and Maddieson 1996), reinforcing the focus placed on lingual articulation in both phonetic and phonological research. For example, the feature [Advanced Tongue Root]/ [ATR] (Stewart 1967) reflects the emphasis on the tongue as controlling sound production in the lower vocal tract.

It is, nevertheless, possible to identify aspects of epilaryngeal stricture in some raw x-ray data. Traces as in Figure 3.1(c) permit evaluation of postero-anterior narrowing and vertical compaction of the epilarynx, though many aspects of epilarynx state still cannot be detected, such as latero-medial dimensions, the relationship between the ventricular folds and vocal folds, and the configuration of the aryepiglottic folds. Even in x-ray tracings that omit the epilarynx it is possible to extrapolate epilarynx state by the contour of the lower epiglottis and evidence of larynx raising. The existence of epilarynx activity is not wholly unknown in the research. In certain instances (e.g. Hess 1998) its presence is noted as a possible feature of some sounds. Generally, however, focus falls back on lingual position, as in Ladefoged and Maddieson's discussion of strident vowels (1996: 311–313), based on Traill's x-ray data imitations of !Xóõ (1985, 1986), and repeated in Pulleyblank's (2006: 17) conclusion that stridency in Khoisan languages is a specialized tongue configuration.

Fibreoptic laryngoscopy is a productive method of collecting visual data of lower-vocal-tract function. Early laryngoscopic visualization involved the use of a dental mirror, the resulting 'mirror image' being inverted. Fibrescopes first appeared in 1957, but the watershed in this research came in 1968 when flexible transnasal laryngoscopy was invented (Sawashima et al. 1967, Edmondson and Esling 2006: 160). It was at this time that Jan Gauffin (then Lindqvist) would visit the Research Institute of Logopedics and Phoniatrics at the University of Tokyo (collaborating with Osamu Fujimura, Masayuki Sawashima, Hajime Hirose, among others) and produce some of the first evidence of the functioning of the epilarynx for speech (Lindqvist 1969, Lindqvist-Gauffin 1972, Lindblom 2009). Two major limitations of laryngoscopy are that the epiglottis often obscures the view of the epilarynx, making [i] the ideal vowel for laryngoscopic examination and [ɑ] less viable (Williams et al. 1975: 305), and that vertical dimensions cannot be calibrated. Vertical epilarynx reduction and vocal-ventricular fold coupling are key axes of epilarynx action that are only interpreted subjectively using visual laryngoscopy. Larynx height can be estimated by changes in brightness and scale, but endoscope depth is typically inconstant and height only relative. A method we have developed to correlate laryngoscopic images with measurements of vertical laryngeal dimensions is to use simultaneous laryngeally positioned ultrasound, synchronizing the data with the audio signal, mapping parallel structures, and converting ultrasound pixels to millimetres of vertical change (see Section 3.2.3).

MRI and real-time MRI (rtMRI) (Lammert et al. 2010) are techniques that will likely prove pivotal in illuminating epilarynx behaviour in speech and its relation to the rest of the structures of the vocal tract. However, MRI research may still reflect the earlier tendency to neglect the epilarynx or conflate it with the laryngopharynx. Tiede's (1996) MRI study of tongue-root harmony in Akan and tense/lax vowels in English combines measurement of the epilarynx with that of the piriform fossae and groups the epilarynx together with the laryngopharynx. In Kröger et al. (2004), midsagittal traces of MRI neglect many details of epilarynx structure evident in the raw data, with the consequence that the epilarynx appears wider for the vowels they are documenting than it really is. A more recent study by Honda et al. (2010) of the hypopharyngeal/laryngopharyngeal cavities (the epilarynx and piriform fossae) shows the utility of MRI in studying how the epilarynx is configured during basic postures sustained over time (inspiration, humming, and whispering). With advances in rtMRI, new 3D visualization of time-dependent changes to epilarynx configuration are increasingly possible.

3.2.1   *Laryngoscopy: The Example of Aryepiglottic Trilling*

As described in Section 2.3.14, aryepiglottic trilling involves the vibration of the aryepiglottic folds at the top of the epilaryngeal tube. The production of voiceless and voiced pharyngeals in Iraqi Arabic is a good example. The classification of the vibration of this 'valve' of the larynx as trilling is analogous to how uvular vibration relates to uvular consonants (Edmondson and Esling 2006). The primary method for analysing and ultimately modelling the vibratory characteristics of the aryepiglottic folds (in Section 3.3.2) is high-speed laryngoscopy, in order to represent the relative periodicities of the two folds. Evaluating the images relies on epilaryngeal aperture estimation.

It is important to frame this discussion in the context of voice quality. Adding the laryngeal articulator to the vocal tract allows us to elaborate the interpretation of pharyngeal consonants to include aryepiglottic trilling. Since this trilling is located within the laryngeal mechanism, it has the potential to act as a source, much like glottal or ventricular vibration. Either voiceless or voiced trilling can act as a secondary or tertiary source, or as a primary source supplanting the glottal source. This has implications for the accurate description of voice quality, since states of the laryngeal articulator can generate multiple movements that contribute to the periodic (or aperiodic) characteristics of the signal.

Data and interpretation contributed by Zeki Majeed Hassan reveal the complex interplay of aspects of the laryngeal mechanism in producing pharyngeal consonants (Hassan et al. 2011). Although Arabic /ħ ʕ/ have often been labelled voiceless and voiced pharyngeal fricatives, the voiced pharyngeal is generally regarded as an approximant (Laufer 1996). They are identified generally in the pharynx for different varieties of Arabic, e.g. Tripoli Libyan (Laradi 1983), Sudanese (Adamson 1981), Qatari (Bukshaisha 1985), Iraqi (Laufer and Baer 1988), and Lebanese and Palestinian (El-Halees 1985, Pettorino and Giannini 1984). Heselwood (2007) notes the importance of epilaryngeal tube shape beneath the aryepiglottic folds and of larynx height variations. Aryepiglottic trilling in Arabic (or in Berber) is not widely attested in the literature, due initially to the absence of a model to explain the movement of laryngeal structures, but also perhaps because its incidence is limited to certain dialects or paralinguistic circumstances. In Basra Iraqi Arabic, the aryepiglottic folds are often heard to trill during /ħ/ or even /ʕ/, becoming trilled [ʜ] in /raħiil/ 'travelling' or trilled [ʢ] in /saʕad/ 'went up' or /saʕiid/ 'happy'. A medial geminate /-ħħ-/ becomes strongly trilled [ʜː], e.g. /raħħiil/ 'travel a lot', while the voiced counterpart geminate /-ʕʕ-/ is sometimes realized with voiced aryepiglottic trilling, but the auditory percept of rapid epilaryngeal tube compaction gives the impression of an epiglottal stop [ʕʔ], e.g. /faʕʕal/ 'made active', /saʕʕad/ 'made it go up', or /saʕʕiid/ 'make people happy'. This parallels the perception of a tight *'ayn* cross-dialectal allophonic variant of /ʕ/ – acoustically an approximant – as a stop (Heselwood 2007: 18, 24–25).

Video 3.1 demonstrates the vibratory pattern of the aryepiglottic folds using high-speed laryngoscopy. Table 3.1 enumerating the technical characteristics of the epilaryngeal vibrations that occur in Iraqi Arabic pharyngeals [raʕʜʕiːl], [raʕʜʜiːl], [saʕʕʕiːd], [saʕʕʔiːd] is in the media set, as are laryngoscopic videos of each Iraqi Arabic word cited.

Figure 3.2 displays the high-speed laryngoscopic images of a voiceless aryepiglottic trill (the [ʜː] in /raħħiːl/), aligned with acoustic, spectrographic, kymographic, and EGG signals. The analysis of aryepiglottic trilling indicates that the action of the aryepiglottic folds differs when combined with glottal voicing and with duration of the trilling. One important difference between voiceless and voiced trilling is the degree of epilaryngeal constriction, which increases in the order [ʜː, ʜ, ʕ, ʕʔ]. The geminates exhibit the greatest degree of aryepiglottic fold displacement, possibly because there is more time for the aryepiglottic folds to build up oscillatory momentum. The difference is partly reflected in trilling frequency, although [ʕ] is more rapid than in [ʕʔ], which may be due to the greater mucosal wave that occurs for the geminate.

Also relevant for the interpretation of aryepiglottic trilling is the EGG signal, which exhibits moments of interference while trilling is occurring. Changing laryngeal configuration, especially larynx raising, is the most probable cause of this effect. Once the larynx returns to a more neutral position, the signal often resumes (as in the latter parts of the /i/ vowels). Sometimes the EGG signal appears to register aryepiglottic vibration, as in Figure 3.2 (the moment between the two braces from approximately 0.25 to 0.35 s). In general (Figures 3.2a, b, c online), the speaker favours a single-channel, centro-lateral aperture because the cuneiform tubercles (c) do not come into contact with the epiglottic tubercle (et). Particular to the [ʜː] token (Figure 3.2), the posterior

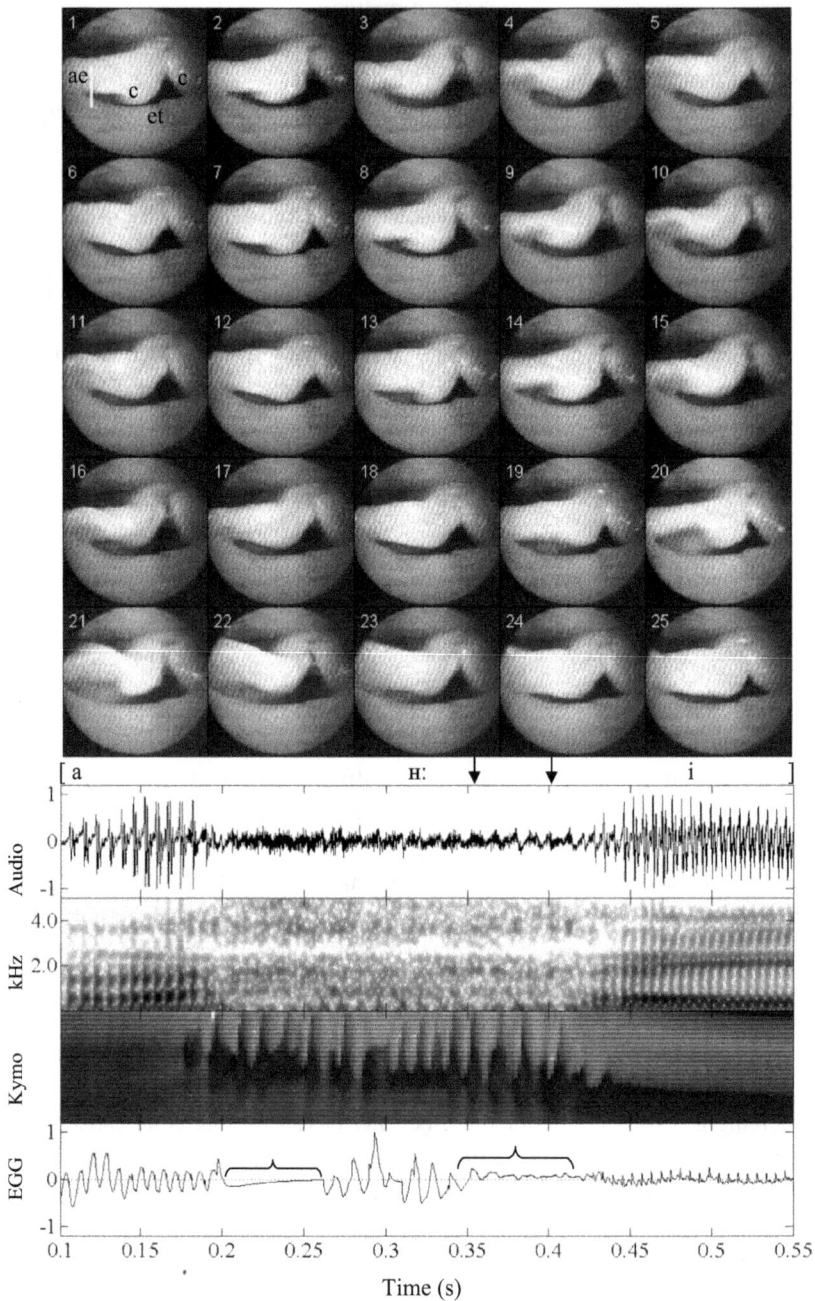

Figure 3.2 *High-speed laryngoscopic images and synchronized data for the geminate voiceless aryepiglottic trill [ʜ:] in Iraqi Arabic /raħħiːl/ 'to travel a lot' ae = aryepiglottic fold; c = cuneiform tubercles; et = epiglottic tubercle.*

arytenoid cartilage complex becomes engaged in oscillation, momentarily bifurcating the air channel during the trill.

In laryngoscopic videos, the laryngeal mechanism constricts more completely and for longer in /faʕʕal/ 'made active' (an epiglottal stop [ʔ]) than in /saʕʕiːd/ 'make people happy' in Iraqi Arabic, demonstrating that a precise target articulation is not replicated the same way each time a particular phonemic sequence (in this case, geminate /ʕʕ/) is realized. Figures 3.2a,b,c accompanying the videos show the comparative laryngoscopic, acoustic, kymographic, and EGG data for [ʜ, ʕ, ʕʔ] in Iraqi Arabic.

What is new in the Laryngeal Articulator Model is the view that the whole mechanism folds shut, so that all parts of the tube contribute to closing off the glottis and most parts above it (even when both aryepiglottic folds at the top of the tube might not be entirely adducted). The model defines how the supraglottic levels of articulation participate in what had always been considered to be just glottal voicing – that the whole mechanism can be responsible for different parts of the signal. The balancing of acoustic data against auditory judgements recalls Heselwood's discussion of the 'tight' version of Arabic *'ayn*:

> With low frequency and low amplitude, tokens [. . .of /ʕʕ/. . .] can sound like stops, a perceptual effect which is not unexpected in the light of results reported by Hillenbrand and Houde (1996: 1187–1189) who found that rapid decreases of F0 of about 10 Hz or more and sudden amplitude drops of at least 8 dB tend to give rise to the perception of a stop. This phenomenon raises an important question regarding how to categorise such tokens. If we class them according to instrumental data, they fall into the tight approximant category, but from an auditory-perceptual point of view they should perhaps be classed as stops if that is how people hear them.   (Heselwood 2007: 18)

We aim to detect the relevant articulatory elements in laryngeally articulated speech sounds and to weigh them proportionally as to how they contribute to the target. Assessing the components used by any particular speaker or speech community requires a significant corpus beyond the laboratory data we have assembled here.

3.2.2   Cineradiography

Cineradiography has been used in swallowing and speech research but fell out of favour because of risks associated with exposure to ionizing radiation in early equipment. We have used cineradiography to capture a small data set of intervocalic [ɑ]-context pharyngeal consonants [ʔ, ʜ, ʕ]. The benefit of cineradiography is the ability to obtain high-resolution images of the laryngeal-pharyngeal region at frame rates consistent with standard video. In articulating [ɑ], the pharynx becomes extremely narrow (Gauffin and Sundberg 1978), and adding 'pharyngealized' or 'raised-larynx-voice' quality [ɑˤ] adds epilaryngeal stricture. In discussions of pharyngeal stricture in the literature, the pharynx and larynx are often assumed to act in unison, as if the larynx were merely a downward extension of the pharynx. In modelling voice quality, it is therefore important to keep the action of the epilarynx conceptually separate from the pharyngeal space above it, particularly in analysing vowel quality.

Cineradiographic Video 3.2 (epiglottal stop [ɑˤʔːˤɑ]), Video 3.3 (voiceless aryepiglottic trilling [ɑˤʜːˤɑ]), and Video 3.4 (voiced aryepiglottic trilling [ɑˤʕːˤɑ]) were obtained by the first author with the assistance of Leonardo Fuks and Dr Milton Melciades Barbosa Costa at the Instituto de Ciências Biomédicas, Departamento de Anatomia, Universidade Federal do Rio de Janeiro. A PDF describes the technical details involved in capturing and analysing the data.

The cineradiographic frames in Figure 3.3 illustrate the states of the epilaryngeal tube from unconstricted to fully constricted. During forceful inhalation (a), the larynx is lowered and the tongue and epiglottis are advanced; the result is that the epilarynx is maximally expanded both in calibre and height to allow for unimpeded airflow into the lungs. The large separation between the hyoid bone and cricoid arch indicates vertical expansion of the epilarynx and concomitant vocal-ventricular fold separation. In the neutral configuration (b), associated with quiet breathing, the tongue is retracted so that the valleculae no longer appear in the image and the epilarynx is not as wide, but there is still vocal-ventricular fold separation and a large postero-anterior separation between the epiglottis and the arytenoid cartilage complex. During pharyngealization (c), the epilarynx is narrowed but remains open. To facilitate retraction, the hyoid bone lowers, implicating the thyrohyoid muscles, acting synergistically with the hyoglossus muscles. During [ʔ] (d), the epilarynx closes completely, but the pharynx does not close completely. While more pharyngeal narrowing occurs in [ʔ] than in [ɑˤ], it cannot account for epilaryngeal closure, which is driven primarily by the intrinsic laryngeal musculature. Additional tongue retraction aids in epilaryngeal closure and may facilitate lowering of the ventricular folds onto the vocal folds.

Figure 3.3a among the media files illustrates parameter extraction from the cineradiographic data using custom MATLAB (R2009a) GUIs (graphic user interfaces).

Figure 3.4 illustrates the relationships among estimated epilarynx area (solid line), estimated pharyngeal area (dashed line), and larynx height (dotted line)

(a) deep inspiration   (b) neutral   (c) [aˤ]   (d) [ʔ]

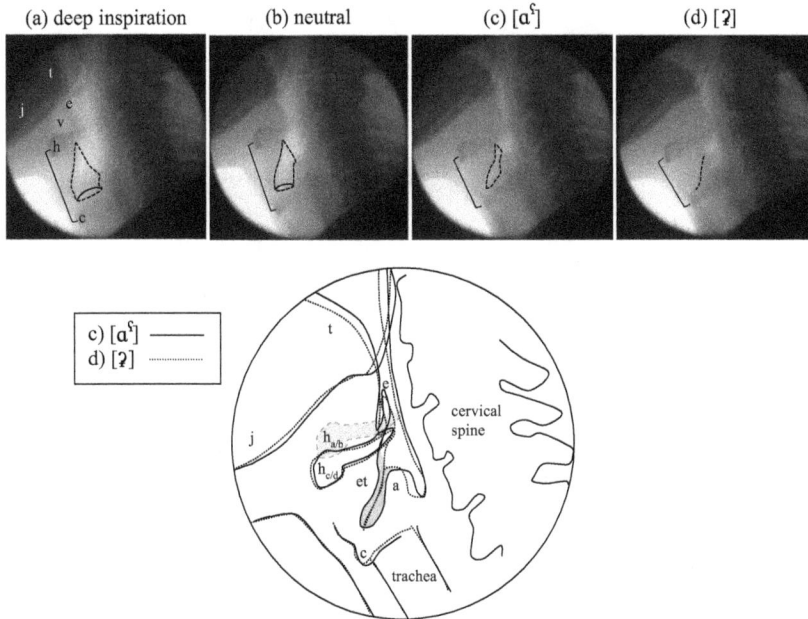

Figure 3.3 *Radiographic epilarynx images*
(a) fully unconstricted/open, (d) fully constricted/closed. States: (a) deep
inspiration, (b) neutral position, (c) [aˤ], (d) (aryepiglotto-)epiglottal stop
[ʔ]. Dotted line = approximate epilarynx sagittal area. Brace = hyoid-cricoid
gap. Arc (a) and (b) = ventricular fold edge. The diagram shows details of
frames (c) and (d): grey region = epilaryngeal tube; a = arytenoid complex
(arytenoid, cuneiform, and corniculate cartilages); c = cricoid cartilage; e =
epiglottis (apex); et = epiglottic tubercle; $h_{a/b}$ = hyoid bone location in (a)
and (b); $h_{c/d}$ = hyoid bone location in (c) and (d); j = jaw/mandible; t =
tongue; v = vallecula.

in the cineradiographic rendition of [ʔ]. After initial area expansion associated
with a quick inspiratory breath (a), epilaryngeal area diminishes at a much
faster rate than pharyngeal area in anticipation of the short-duration heavily
pharyngealized [aˤ] (b), then the epilarynx area closes entirely (c), while the
pharynx area slightly narrows. Finally, the second vowel (d) is less pharyngealized towards its offset than the first vowel, corresponding with a relaxation
of epilaryngeal stricture. The pharynx also relaxes, to roughly the same degree
as during (b). Larynx height has two peaks during the production: one in the
transition from (b) to (c), i.e. the onset of [ʔ], and one during the second vowel
(d), which probably reflects slightly increased fundamental frequency (f0)

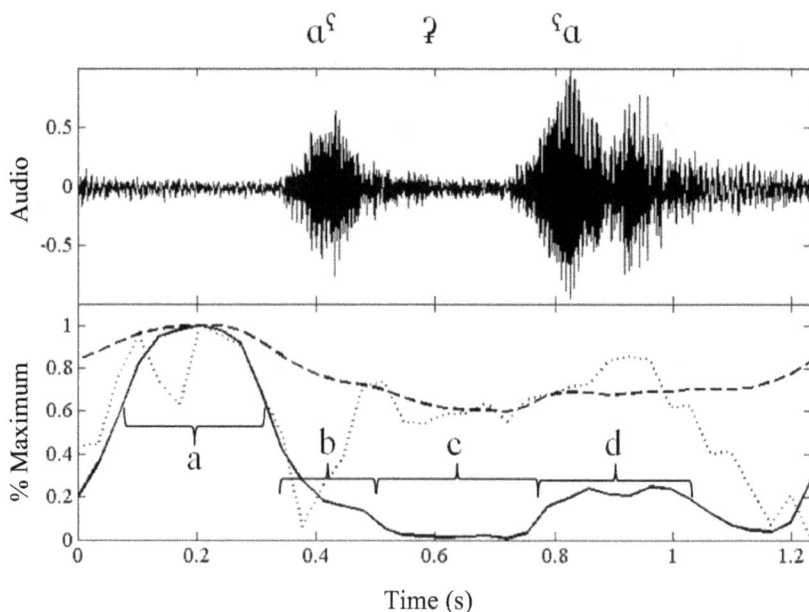

Figure 3.4 *Analysis of cineradiographic data for epiglottal stop [aʔa] Audio (top); Relative measures (bottom) as percentages of individual maxima of each time series: solid line = epilarynx area; dashed line = pharynx area; dotted line = larynx height. a = inspiratory breath; b = initial vowel; c = epilaryngeal closure; d = second vowel. Average f0: first vowel = 120 Hz; second vowel = 135 Hz.*

(~15 Hz higher than during the first vowel). Generally, epilaryngeal area relates to pharyngealization and stop production, while pharyngeal area corresponds to vowel production. The correlation between these two areas reflects the sharing of lingual retraction.

The analyses of cineradiographic data for [ʜ] (Figure 3.4a) and [ʕ] (Figure 3.4b) appear among the companion files.

The area measurements for [ʔ, ʜ, ʕ] reveal the aryepiglotto-epiglottal nature of the primary articulatory stricture. Narrowing of the pharyngeal cavity intrinsically accompanies the [ɑ] vowel, but it is intensified in the context of epiglottal/pharyngeal consonants. Enhanced [ɑˤ] or [ɑˤ] can be called 'epilaryngealization' in the sense of a secondary articulation, since changes in epilarynx area correlate most strongly with the performance of these closure or vibration gestures. The epilarynx-mediated nature of epiglottal/pharyngeal speech-sound production can explain previous observations that phonemic /ʕ/ in Arabic involves 'laryngealized' phonation or stop closure (Butcher and Ahmad 1987: 166). Once the vocal folds become compromised by ventricular fold contact, their dynamics can be biased towards creakiness or even harshness. The relationship is not so much between the pharynx and larynx, as sometimes suggested (Keyser and Stevens 1994: 213), but rather between the tongue, the larynx height mechanism, and the vocal folds, with the epilarynx acting as the 'conductor' of these activities.

3.2.3   *Laryngoscopy + Laryngeal Ultrasound*
Simultaneous laryngoscopy and laryngeal ultrasound (SLLUS) allows visual observations of changes in laryngeal state to be correlated with vertical movements of laryngeal structures and measurements of larynx height and its effect on the epilarynx. Laryngeal ultrasound is not ideal for characterizing internal laryngeal state but does provide clear information about changes in the vertical position of the larynx. The ultrasound transducer is placed onto the surface of the neck over the thyroid cartilage to obtain a (slightly oblique but roughly) coronal planar image. To perform the SLLUS technique, a standard laryngoscopic examination is conducted, with the attending physician seated in front of the participant, while the laryngeal ultrasound examination is performed simultaneously by approaching the participant from the side (photos in Moisik et al. 2014: 25, 27). With this technique, we are able to examine the interaction between larynx height and state during speech-sound production. In the case study presented here, we look at glottal stop and associated creaky voice, with and without laryngeal height suppression, produced in intervocalic [i] position. The focus is on larynx height, since it is an essential factor in setting the articulators of the lower vocal tract.

In the debate over the viability of the term 'constricted glottis', two critical issues emerge: whether glottal aperture reduction is a function of a more holistic constrictive action of the larynx, and to what extent there is vocal-ventricular fold contact. Larynx height is known to have several speech-related roles. Hardcastle (1976: 69) identifies two functions of larynx raising: swallowing-type closure (i.e. constriction) and glottalic initiation (as in ejectives). The correlation of larynx raising with pitch raising is also well known (Honda 2004). Closure in swallowing or in epiglottal consonants requires extreme epilaryngeal constriction, and our model predicts that larynx raising assists in such a gesture. It is less obvious that larynx raising should be important in a sound such as glottal stop. In standard phonetic and phonological theory, a 'constricted glottis' is assumed to be a vocal fold function and should be independent of larynx height. In this view, adductive force driven by the interarytenoid muscles maintains cartilaginous glottal closure while the lateral cricoarytenoid muscles manipulate medial compression or membranous compression of the vocal folds (Laver 1980: 109). A glottal stop should be sufficiently characterized by strong adductory force and medial compression. If the vocal folds are set into vibration in this strongly adducted state, then only the anterior, membranous portion of the vocal folds vibrate (the posterior, cartilaginous glottis being firmly closed by the adductive force). As Catford (1977a) pointed out, however, during this 'anterior voice' the 'whole upper part of the larynx may be constricted to some extent' (p. 102), and he inferred that 'it appears as if the arytenoidal constriction essential for anterior phonation is part of a general sphincteric constriction of the (upper) larynx' (pp. 102–103). This implies that 'glottal constriction' is necessarily a function of a more holistic action of the larynx, which must take into consideration the physiological nature of the epilarynx.

Quantifying larynx height during speech is not trivial (Honda 2004). Attempts have been made using thyroumbrometry (Ewan and Krones 1974, Sprouse et al. 2010), but this requires participants to have visible laryngeal prominences, and results can be confounded by rotational movements of the larynx. MRI can be used successfully on static postures (Honda et al. 1999), and real-time MRI is promising (Nissenbaum et al. 2002, Narayanan et al. 2011), but both techniques may be expensive or inaccessible. Our approach is to apply image-processing techniques to ultrasound data, such as optical flow, derived from the field of computer and robotic vision. We compute optical flow by breaking down each frame from the video sequence into an analysis grid and then looking for pixel correlations or minima of absolute difference convolutions performed between current and next frames. With an estimate of the optical flow, the vertical larynx velocity can be computed through a consensus approach (taking the mean of the vertical component of the velocities at or above a high percentile) and then converting from pixels to mm using the superimposed ultrasound depth indicator to obtain the pixel-to-mm scaling. Displacement over time can be obtained by integrating the velocity signal (but, because the constant of integration cannot be determined, the height changes must be interpreted relative to the starting point in the video).

Videos 3.5a and 3.5b demonstrate, respectively, the raw data and vector flow field used in validation of the optical flow algorithm, and Video 3.6 depicts laryngoscopy of epiglottal stop with optical flow in the ultrasound field. Accompanying Figure 3.5a provides a map of laryngeal structures to correlate with images in the text, and Figure 3.5b provides the results of the validation, showing accurate automatic measurement of displacement and velocity with reference to manual measurements of the same variables.

Here we present glottal stop (Figure 3.5) and creaky voice without height suppression (Figure 3.6) and with height suppression (Figure 3.7) in composite plots of the audio waveform, f0 trace, and larynx height (vertical larynx displacement), with key laryngoscopy frames beneath with temporal locations of these marked with vertical lines on the plots. In the SLLUS data for glottal stop in Figure 3.5, frame 20 shows modal phonation at the midpoint of the first vowel. (The audio signal has a high noise floor, due to the laryngoscopy and ultrasound equipment.) The larynx is unconstricted, the vocal folds (v) are adducted, and there is full glottal (membranous and cartilaginous) vibration – apparently unimpeded by the ventricular folds (f), which are laterally abducted. The apex of the epiglottis (e) is visible, but the epiglottic tubercle (et) is not. Frames 24, 28, and 32 then show the progressive adduction/ medialization of the ventricular folds during the glottal stop; some anticipatory ventricular fold adduction is evident at the very end of the first vowel (frame 24); and full adduction is attained early during the onset phase of the glottal stop (i.e. prior to the temporal midpoint). This adduction evidently continues to increase in degree of medial compression (frame 28) until offset occurs, where release of adduction must take place in anticipation of the upcoming vowel. Medial ventricular fold contact happens first at the anterior edges of the ventricular folds and progressively involves their posterior surfaces as constriction increases. During ventricular fold adduction, there is a reduction in the postero-anterior dimension of the epilarynx which correlates with a slight increase in larynx height. The observation of larynx raising is consistent with other reports in the literature. For example, Ewan reports larynx raising for Thai [?] (1979: 73–80), and Roach observes larynx raising and epilarynx closure in glottally reinforced stops in English (1979: 2). The change observed here is on the order of 1.24 mm and occurs in about 0.275 s. Somewhat surprisingly, raising continues to increase into the offset phase of the glottal stop, peaking at frame 32, then rapidly decreasing to its level during the following vowel and slowly continuing its descent. No obvious change in pitch occurs in relation to this vertical laryngeal displacement.

Videos 3.7, 3.8, 3.9, corresponding to Figures 3.5, 3.6, 3.7, are in the media set.

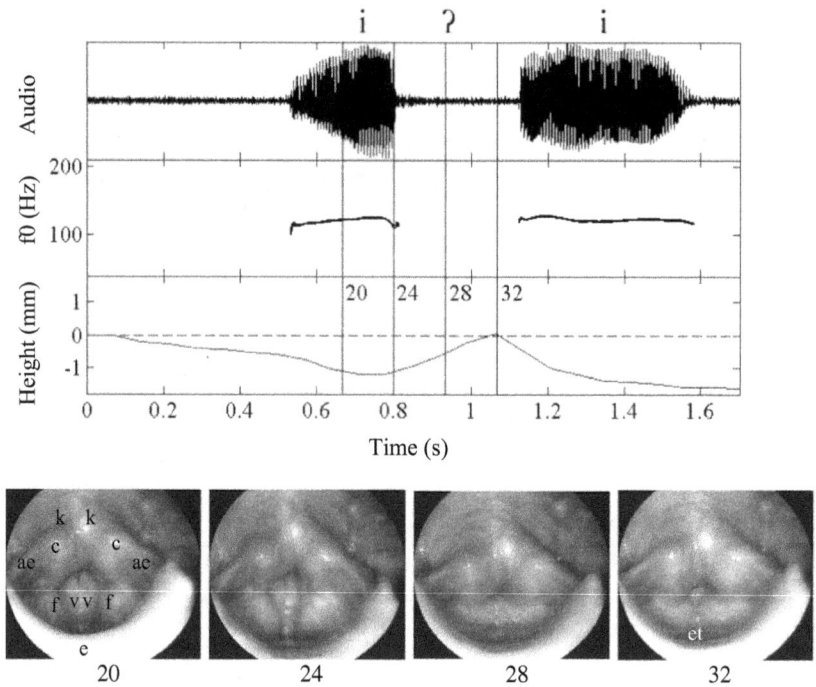

Figure 3.5 *SLLUS data for glottal stop*
ae = aryepiglottic fold; c = cuneiform tubercle; e = epiglottis (apex); et = epiglottic tubercle; f = ventricular (false) fold; k = corniculate tubercle; v = vocal fold.
Reprinted with permission from Esling and Moisik (2012).

Figure 3.6 illustrates the SLLUS data for creaky phonation, gradually being engaged during the midpoint of an extended [i] target. When larynx height is not deliberately suppressed (i.e. not actively lowered as it is in Figure 3.7), the larynx raises by 3.38 mm over the course of 1.1 s. A spectrogram is included in Figure 3.6 to show the impact of larynx raising on formant structure in the absence of tongue retraction: where both F1 and F2 (dashed-underline) exhibit arc-like increases. Raising can be discerned in the laryngoscopy frames by the relative enlargement in appearance of the structures. Ventricular fold medialization is again present, although unlike glottal stop, complete adduction of the ventricular folds does not occur; throughout the creaky section of [i] there is a posterior gap at the ventricular level. Postero-anterior narrowing of the epilaryngeal tube is comparable with glottal stop (Figure 3.5), but the degree of

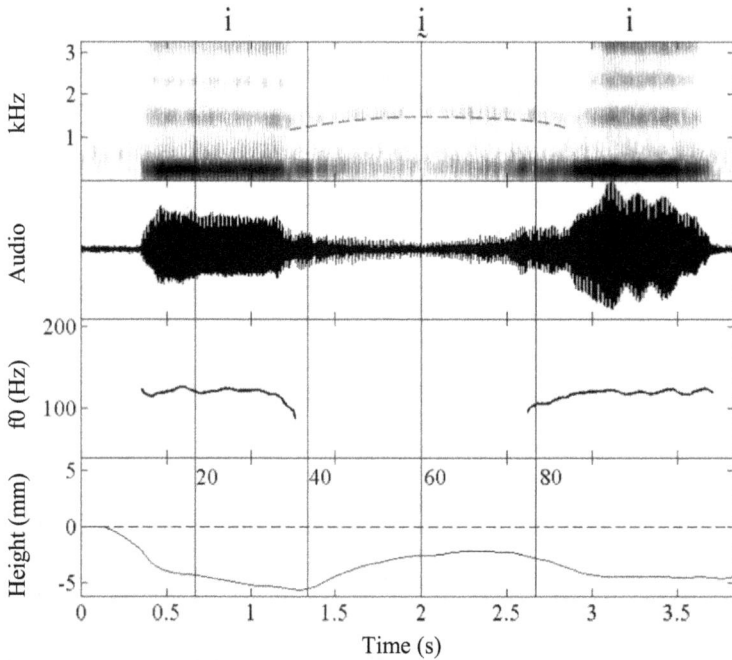

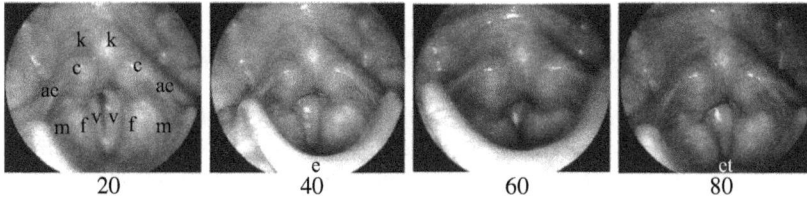

Figure 3.6 *SLLUS data for creaky voice without larynx height suppression ae = aryepiglottic fold; c = cuneiform tubercle; e = epiglottis (apex); et = epiglottic tubercle; f = ventricular (false) fold; k = corniculate tubercle; m = mucosa of inner aryepiglottic wall; v = vocal fold. Note: f0 is not detected (Kawahara et al. 1998) during creaky voice.*
Reprinted with permission from Esling and Moisik (2012).

arytenoidal adduction (as judged by the position of the cuneiform and corniculate tubercles) does not increase appreciably during production (the same is true of glottal stop production). Roughly maximal adductory displacement of the arytenoid complex (and vocal folds) is achieved even in the modal configuration (i.e. the adducted phonatory state) as in frame 20.

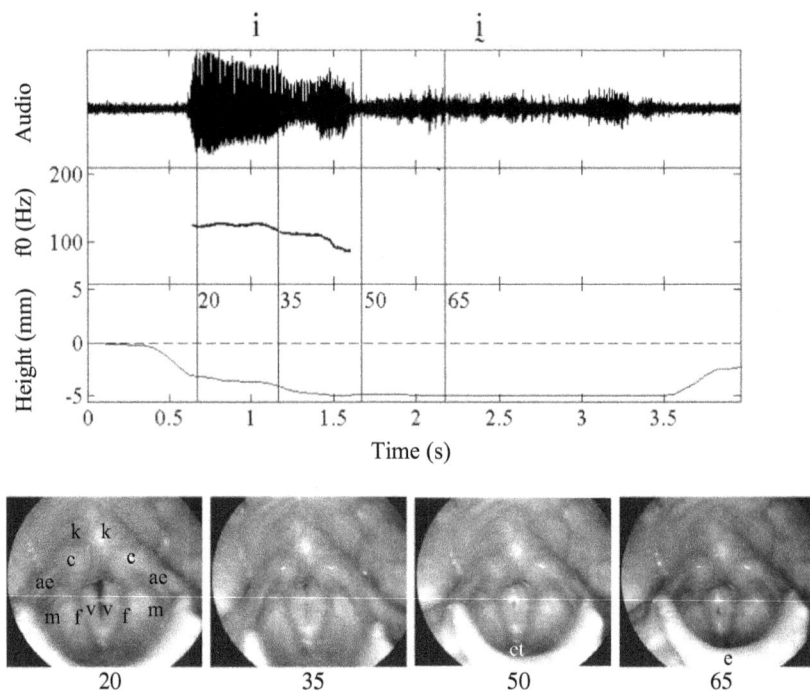

Figure 3.7 *SLLUS data for creaky voice with deliberate larynx height suppression (larynx lowering)*
ae = aryepiglottic fold; c = cuneiform tubercle; e = epiglottis (apex);
et = epiglottic tubercle; f = ventricular (false) fold; k = corniculate tubercle;
m = mucosa of inner aryepiglottic wall; v = vocal fold. Note: the pitch
extraction algorithm (STRAIGHT; Kawahara et al. 1998) does not detect f0
during the creaky portion of the vowel.
Reprinted with permission from Esling and Moisik (2012).

The production of creaky phonation while deliberately suppressing the height of the larynx (by forceful larynx lowering) is shown in Figure 3.7. While it is possible to produce creak in this lowered-larynx state without any obvious ventricular fold adduction, a state change occurs with the onset of creakiness at frame 50. There is a very slight elevation of the larynx at this point, accompanied by a substantial reduction of the postero-anterior dimension of the epilaryngeal tube, increasing in degree throughout the creaky region (frame 65). At the transitional point (frame 50), the vocal folds abruptly switch vibratory mode from one which allows for loose vibration along their entire longitudinal extent (frames 20 and 35) to one allowing only for limited lateral displacements confined to a short anterior (membranous) section along their longitudinal extent (frames 50 and 65). Adduction of the arytenoid complex does not change appreciably, and, somewhat surprisingly, the cuneiforms even separate slightly between frames 35 and 50, which, given that the larynx is lower in frame 50, is unexpected on the basis of camera perspective alone: they would be expected to appear even closer together. This may be due to increased aryepiglottic tension during constriction.

Glottal aperture was once thought to be the critical dimension of sounds involving a 'constricted glottis'. Figure 3.8 presents the axial-plane view of the forces acting to shape the longitudinal dimension of vocal fold vibration. The left column depicts forces thought to be shaping the glottis, and the right column illustrates the vibratory profile of the vocal folds depicted as a black region (a 'snapshot' of maximal glottal area during vibration). Modal voice (a) involves free vibration of the full glottis (membranous and cartilaginous). This state is essentially fully adducted and relies on activity of the lateral cricoarytenoid and transverse interarytenoid (tIA) muscles (Hillel 2001). The tissues manipulated by the arytenoids are in full contact. Further adductory engagement of the oblique interarytenoid (oIA) muscles will begin to engage epilaryngeal stricture in the ventricular and aryepiglottic planes according to the muscle-chain mechanisms described in Figures/Videos 2.7 and 2.8.

Creaky voice produced in raised-larynx in Figure 3.8(b) and lowered-larynx in Figure 3.8(c) conditions corresponds with Figures 3.6 and 3.7. Both qualify as 'anterior voice', i.e. only the membranous vocal folds vibrate. LCA activity must increase to hinder vibration of the cartilaginous vocal folds, but this does not account for the engagement of the epilarynx. We can infer further recruitment of the external TA and oIA muscles. The mechanism is engaged even with active height suppression (i.e. lowering the larynx by approximately 5 mm). Furthermore, whether raised or lowered, both states involve low-pitched creaky phonation, yet the entire larynx appears to be under considerable tension. The postero-anterior epilaryngeal narrowing is driven, in part, by the external and internal TA muscle branches (Moisik 2013: 27–47), with the effect of increasing vocal fold stiffness.

In order to resolve how low pitch is achieved, overall laryngeal articulation must be considered. In addition to glottal aperture control, there are two principal articulatory axes of the larynx: the axis of height and the axis of constriction. The former is causally associated with changing the volume of the pharyngeal cavity; the latter denotes action of the mechanism that induces stricture of the epilarynx. Both mechanisms have an impact on the pitch-control system. Larynx height positively correlates with pitch: larynx lowering

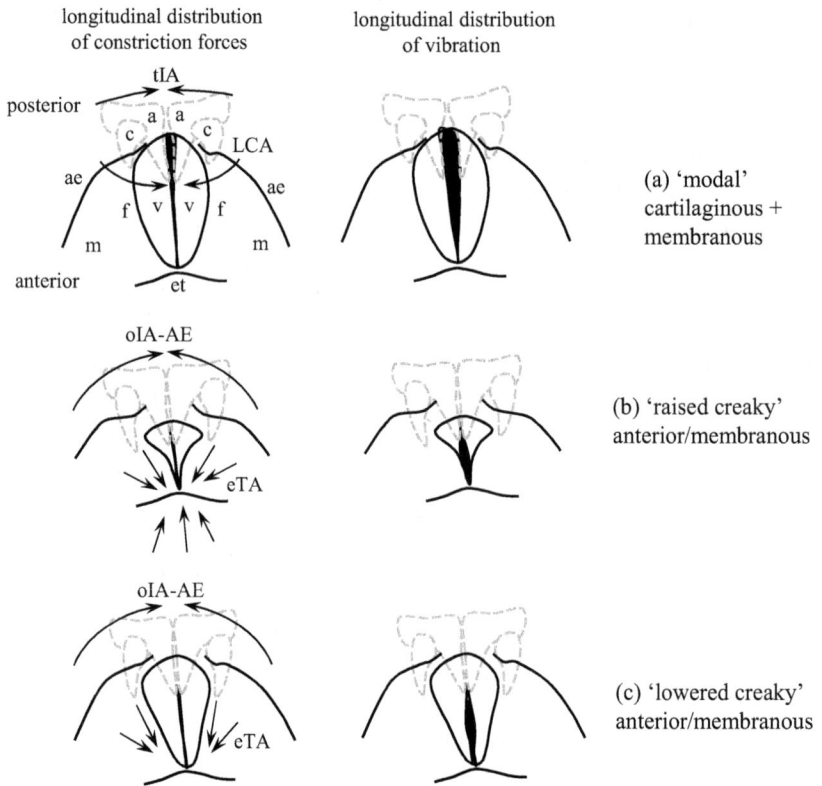

Figure 3.8 *Longitudinal nature of the effect of the epilarynx on the vocal folds*
Solid lines = structure edges visible in laryngoscopy; dashed outlines = cartilage structures; a = arytenoid cartilage; ae = aryepiglottic fold; c = cuneiform cartilage; e = epiglottis (apex); et = epiglottic tubercle; f = ventricular (false) fold; k = corniculate tubercle; m = mucosa of inner aryepiglottic wall; v = vocal fold; AE = aryepiglottic folds; eTA = external thyroarytenoid muscles; LCA = lateral cricoarytenoid muscles; oIA = oblique interarytenoid muscle; tIA = transverse interarytenoid muscle.

results in cricoid rotation favouring reduction of vocal fold tension (Ohala 1972, Honda et al. 1999); larynx raising increases vocal fold tension through anterior traction on the hyoid-thyroid complex and through thyrohyoid contraction in conjunction with contributions from other factors such as internal vertical tension and tracheal pull (Ohala 1972, Honda et al. 1995a, Vilkman et al. 1996). It is assumed that larynx height is relatively slow acting compared to the longitudinal pitch-control mechanism.

Laryngeal constriction is a function of three primary physiological compon-ents that act synergistically (Esling et al. 2007): tongue retraction (which is partly responsible for posterior displacement of the epiglottis), larynx raising, and contraction of the external TA muscle complex (Fink 1974a: 126, Rei-denbach 1998b: 367). Pitch is impacted by concomitant ventricular incursion through epilaryngeal stricture (Laver 1980, Moisik and Esling 2014); the ventricular folds impinge upon the upper surfaces of the vocal folds and mechanically couple with them. The increase in oscillating mass causes a lowered frequency response of vocal-fold vibration. Figure 3.9 provides a depiction of these relationships, the arrows indicating the direction of causal-ity. Larynx height plays a dual role in laryngeal control: it acts agonistically in the mechanisms for pitch control and for laryngeal constriction. The primary pitch-control mechanism stands in antagonistic relationship to the laryngeal constriction mechanism, because engagement of the laryngeal constrictor acts along the postero-anterior dimension to narrow the epilarynx – opposite to the antero-posterior lengthening of the glottal aperture and epilarynx caused by engagement of the cricothyroid muscles (Esling and Harris 2005). When unopposed by the pitch-raising mechanism, larynx raising has the effect of reducing the vertical dimension of the epilarynx. If all else is held constant, the vocal folds will approach the ventricular folds, which may be in descent because of active constriction forces (Reidenbach 1997, 1998b) and

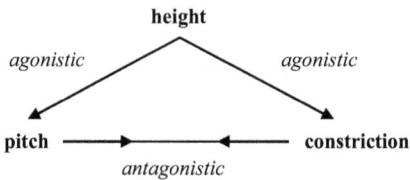

Figure 3.9 *The relationship amongst larynx height, constriction, and pitch control*
Raising larynx height helps the pitch mechanism to raise pitch; lowering the larynx assists in pitch lowering. Raising the larynx assists in compacting the larynx; lowering the larynx causes vertical expansion and separation of laryngeal tissues. The pitch mechanism expands the antero-posterior dimension of the larynx and diametrically opposes the constriction mechanism, which contracts the postero-anterior dimension. Engaging both at the same time results in the compromised configuration associated with harsh voice at high pitch (Esling and Harris 2005).
Reprinted with permission from Esling and Moisik (2012).

(a) lowered larynx   (b) neutral larynx   (c) raised larynx

traction from
supralaryngeal
linkage

compression from
supralaryngeal
linkage

f

v

raising force

lowering force

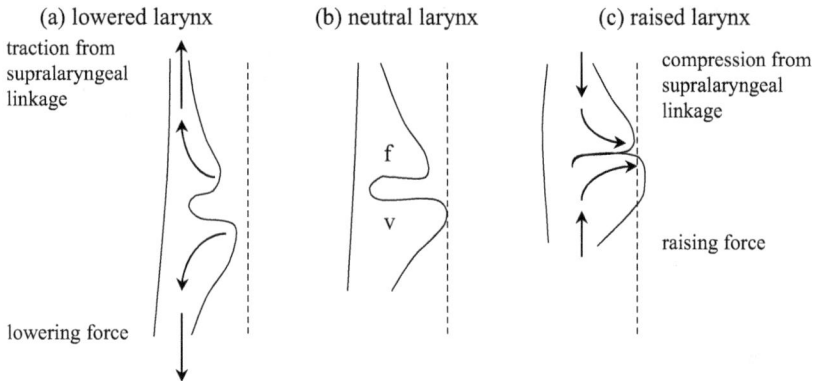

Figure 3.10 *The effect of larynx height on vocal-ventricular fold compression*
The relationship between the vocal folds (v) and ventricular (false) folds (f)
seen in a coronal half-section of the larynx. Dotted line = glottal midline.
Reprinted with permission from Moisik et al. (2014).

compaction from tissues above. The opposite effects are expected in the case
of larynx lowering, which Fink (1974a) described as driving anti-plication of
the larynx, i.e. laryngeal 'unfolding'.

The basic mechanical biases schematized in Figure 3.10 represent the vocal
and ventricular folds as half of the larynx in coronal section. Larynx lowering
(a) stretches and elongates the vertical dimension of the larynx – thereby
counteracting or reducing laryngeal constriction – biasing phonation towards
breathiness due to the lateral force on the vocal folds that draws them away
from the glottal midline. This lateral force results from the tendency for tissue
to thin as it is stretched along an axis, as described and illustrated by Fink
(1974a). Larynx raising (c) results in a collision between the two sets of folds,
which are forced to buckle towards the glottal midline as the laryngeal space
becomes more compacted in the vertical dimension – biasing phonation
towards harshness, tenseness, or creakiness depending on subglottal pressure
and other factors. These are tendencies or biases, not absolute relationships. It
is still possible to constrict the epilarynx in the lowered-larynx setting (Esling
1999), as larynx height is not the sole determinant of laryngeal constriction
(i.e. the intrinsic constriction mechanism and lingual/epiglottal retraction may
outweigh height). Even when larynx height is actively lowered, as in
Figure 3.7, laryngeal constriction appears to engage and still probably pro-
motes vocal-ventricular fold contact. However, the degree to which the epilarynx can narrow is hindered, in that ventricular fold medialization is slight by

comparison to the constricted phonation in Figure 3.6, where larynx height is not controlled and raises during the creaky voice phase.

Ultrasound allows us to document the relationship between narrowing of the epilarynx and larynx height. Sounds such as glottal stop and creaky phonation involve more than only the vocal fold mechanism. Combining laryngeal ultrasound with laryngoscopy allows us to quantify larynx height in relation to adductory or abductory manoeuvres, expanding on inferences drawn from laryngoscopic video (Esling 1999, Brunelle et al. 2010). While the case data presented here are limited to phonetic productions, the SLLUS technique can be readily applied to individual language studies (Moisik et al. 2014), and optical flow quantification of larynx height can be obtained using only laryngeal ultrasound. Larynx raising is an intrinsic part of epilaryngeal constriction in sounds that narrow the glottis and appears especially important in regulating the relationship between the vocal and ventricular folds, with dynamic consequences for the vibratory system. We believe that 'glottal' constriction has been overemphasized in previous phonetic models. Vocal fold adduction occurs in prephonation (Esling and Harris 2005), and medial compression is relevant to controlling which part of the vocal folds can vibrate. The creakiness and closure mechanisms rely critically on a general mechanism of laryngeal closure, and glottal closure is merely the first step in a larger, relatively slow-acting sequence involving narrowing, compression, and collapse of the epilaryngeal airway and associated tissues.

3.2.4   Magnetic Resonance Imaging

Magnetic resonance imaging (MRI) is a productive technique for examining lingual–laryngeal states because of its ability to capture rich information about the whole vocal tract in a safe way. Because MRI visualizes both the oral and laryngeal vocal tracts, long-term voice quality effects can be compared with changes in vowel postures. A familiar approach in examining voice quality is to perform contrasting settings on a text of phonemically balanced content (Harmegnies 1987, Harmegnies et al. 1989, 1994). A variation of this approach is to produce individual vowels with contrasting settings superimposed. To illustrate the changes that varying laryngeal articulatory posture makes to vowel targets, MRI data of peripheral vowels can be compared when influenced by the presence of glottal stop and of epiglottal stop. These comparisons are useful because of the often misunderstood status of glottal stop, its production and its scope as a laryngeal phenomenon, and because of the full-closure state of epiglottal stop, its relationship to pharyngealization, and its effect on the epilaryngeal tube. The vowels presented here are evenly spaced phonetic targets of [i e æ ɑ o u]. Sustained productions of each vowel were produced with modal voice, and then accompanied by glottal stop [V͡ʔ], holding both postures simultaneously, and by epiglottal stop [V͡ʡ], holding both postures simultaneously. 2D axial, coronal, and sagittal multi-slice and midsagittal MRI sequences were captured. MR analysis methods are described in Moisik et al. (2015), Dediu and Moisik (2019), and Moisik and Dediu (2019).

In addition to phonatory quality and tonal quality (interaction with pitch), larynx height also varies in relation to vowel quality (Ladefoged et al. 1972, Ewan and Krones 1974). Correlations have been inconsistent, dependent also on pitch, and some have suggested that the intrinsic f0 of vowels arises from lingual–laryngeal interactions (Ohala and Eukel 1987, Whalen and Levitt 1995, Whalen et al. 1998). Lingual–laryngeal interactions are central to the Laryngeal Articulatory Model, instigating a reshaping of vowel space organization to reflect the laryngeal component of vowel articulations (Section 1.2). Despite the evidence pointing to lingual–laryngeal interaction effects, uncertainty still remains about the nature of the articulatory changes involved, including pharyngeal resonator volumes and the internal configuration of laryngeal tissues in response to vowel articulation.

Near-midsagittal sections are shown in Figure 3.11, demonstrating the degree to which the coarticulatory laryngeal targets [ʔ] and [ʡ] produced by the first author alter the laryngeal cavity shaping and oral articulatory postures of otherwise identical target vowels. The MR images indicate that despite the laryngeal constriction in both [ʔ] and [ʡ], a very small ventricular space still exists. However, there are strong indications when examining slices on either side of the midsagittal plane that the vocal folds and ventricular folds are in contact in these states (Moisik et al. 2015). The epilaryngeal-tube space in [ʡ] context is fully reduced, paralleling the findings in Section 3.2.2. Figure 3.12 shows a similar set of vowels produced by the second author but with modal voice, creaky voice, and raised-larynx voice qualities. The creaky voice productions indicate more definitive contact between the vocal folds and ventricular folds than for the glottal stop configurations in Figure 3.11. Larynx height is variable between the modal and creaky states. Raised-larynx voice shows more laryngeal advancement than raising, for most vowels, although [i] does show clear larynx raising.

Technical specifications of MRI capture shown in Figures 3.11 and 3.12 are found in Moisik et al. (2015) and also provided in the media set.

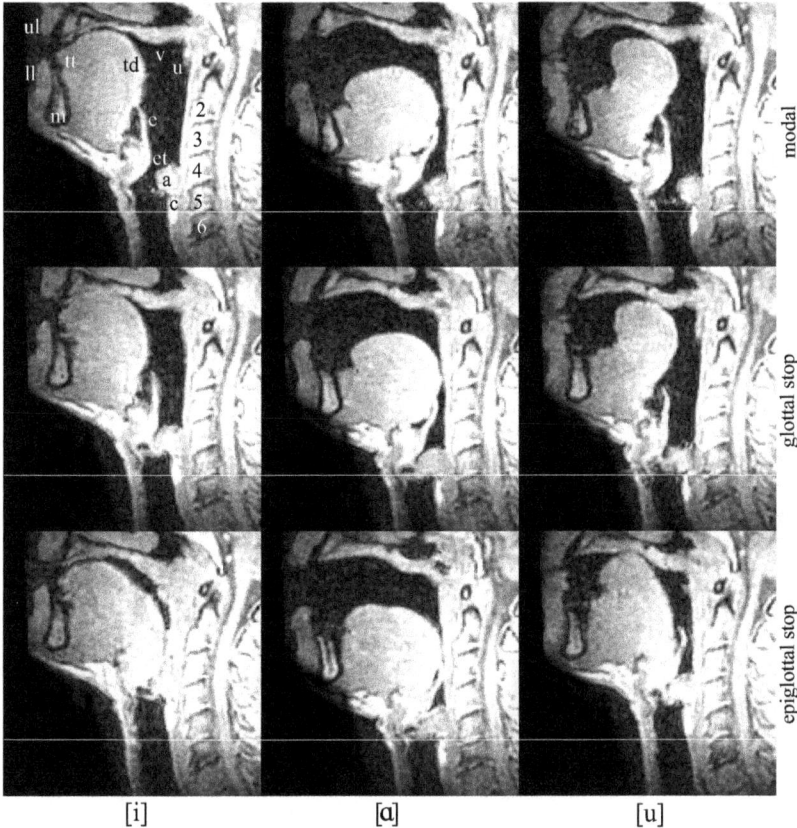

Figure 3.11 *MRI: three vowels in modal, glottal stop, and epiglottal stop conditions*
Near-midsagittal MRI sections of three vowel qualities (columns) in three laryngeal states (rows). The white bar positioned at the base of the fifth cervical vertebra provides a visual reference for comparing larynx height across the different productions. a = arytenoid complex (cuneiform + arytenoid + corniculate cartilages); c = cricoid (lamina); 2–6 = cervical vertebrae 2–6; e = epiglottis (apex); et = epiglottic tubercle; ll = lower lip; m = mandibular symphysis; td = tongue dorsum; tt = tongue tip; u = uvula; ul = upper lip; v = velum.

For the modal vowels, tongue position influences larynx height via epilaryngeal coupling. In both sets, [ɑ] is lower than [i], sometimes as low or lower than [u]. Retracted tongue positions characteristic of [ɑ] are predicted in the LAM to be especially susceptible to engaging laryngeal constriction on a

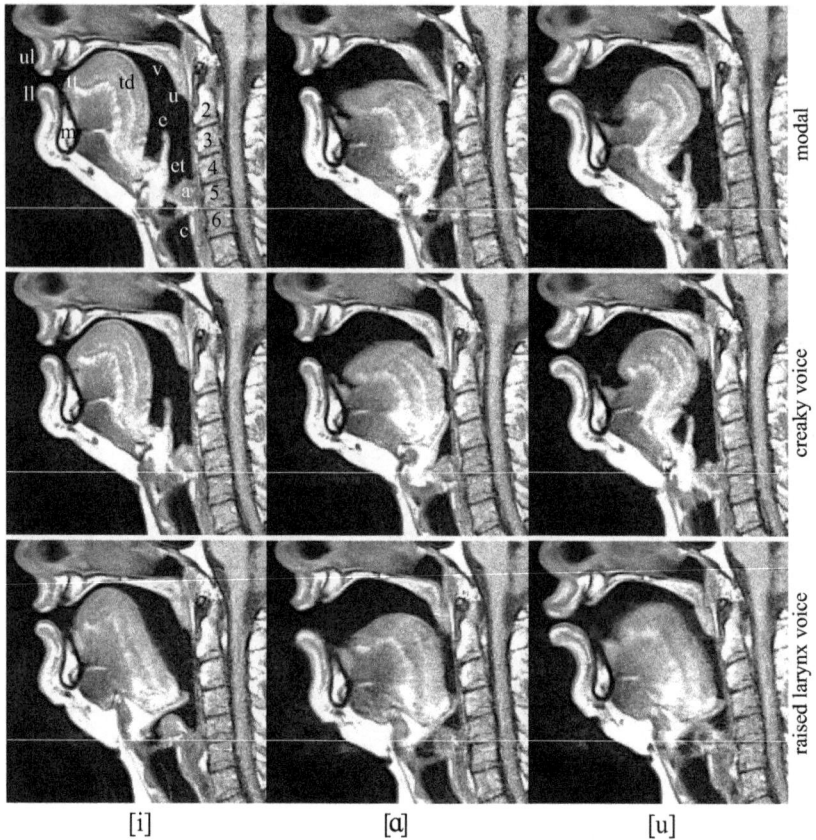

Figure 3.12 *MRI: three vowels in modal, creaky, and raised-larynx conditions*
Near-midsagittal MRI sections of three vowel qualities (columns) in three laryngeal states (rows). The white bar positioned at the base of the fifth cervical vertebra provides a visual reference for comparing larynx height across the different productions. a = arytenoid complex (cuneiform + arytenoid + corniculate cartilages); c = cricoid (lamina); 2–6 = cervical vertebrae 2–6; e = epiglottis (apex); et = epiglottic tubercle; ll = lower lip; m = mandibular symphysis; td = tongue dorsum; tt = tongue tip; u = uvula; ul = upper lip; v = velum.

passive basis, meaning that retracted and even open vowels in general might be more prone to the effects of constriction, such as spontaneous termination by glottal stops, creakiness, or effects arising from epilaryngeal vibration. A low-larynx position for these vowels helps to hinder this tendency. It may also

(a) Larynx height across three laryngeal
contexts produced by first author

(b) Larynx height across three laryngeal
contexts produced by second author

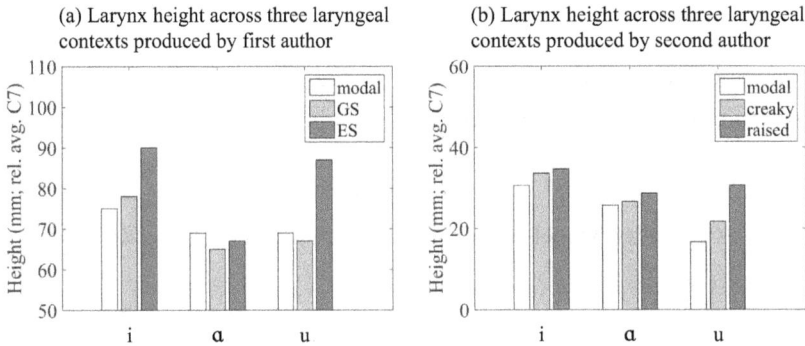

Figure 3.13 *Larynx height for three vowels in varying larynx-state conditions Produced by (a) the first and (b) second authors, measured as the distance between the inferior-most point on the cricoid lamina relative to the average location of the base of C7. The data in (a) relate to Figure 3.11. The data in (b) relate to Figure 3.12.*

simultaneously reflect jaw lowering (which is facilitated by lowering the hyoid bone and larynx complex). Conversely, laryngeal state can have unusual effects on tongue shape, especially noticeable for the less retracted vowels, such as [i]. The tongue appears to be 'cinched', or 'double-bunched' as Catford (1983: 349) noted for the pharyngealized vowels of certain Caucasian languages (Tsakhur and Udi), also attested in the South African Taa language, !Xóõ (Hess 1998: 340–364).

The MRI data reveal relationships between oral vocal tract and laryngeal vocal tract configurations when particular vowel targets are produced. Figure 3.13 demonstrates the shifts in larynx height that take place when a lower-vocal-tract condition accompanies a given vowel. Epiglottal stop has a strong effect on vocal tract space, as does a raised-larynx (pharyngealized) posture. The relationship of vowels to pitch must also take into account the role of the laryngeal vocal tract, although our results can only hint at the effects of vowel quality on f0 or of changing pitch on vowel quality. We can say, however, that articulatory targets for the tongue and the jaw, postures contributed by laryngeal (co)articulation, and pitch targets not only all codetermine the quality of a vowel, but they also constitute the phonetic groundwork for potential sound change when any one of those elements is altered. That is, one person's vowel may not be the same as another person's vowel, even though they are identified as the same on the basis of the auditory vowel quadrilateral. Secondary laryngeal 'colouring' (or pitch) may have influenced how the particular vowel is perceived. Perception is in turn influenced by the inherent normalization applied to vowels of a single speaker's vowel space or of the vowel repertory of a community of speakers. If the contribution of the laryngeal articulator is not taken into account, the primary description of the vowel itself risks being unreliable.

3.3   Computer Models of the Larynx and Laryngeal Constriction

3.3.1   A 3D Laryngeal Constrictor Model

The insights gained through various instrumental observation techniques have provided a basis for modelling the activity of the laryngeal articulator and incorporating an elaborated larynx into 3D models of speech production. An interactive 3D larynx model, intended primarily for visual illustration of laryngeal articulation (Moisik and Esling 2007, Moisik 2008), implements a biomechanical model of the aryepiglottic folds based on Titze's (1973) mathematical model of the vocal folds. Extending Titze's description, each aryepiglottic fold is modelled as a spring-mass lattice. Geometric configuration, determined by cuneiform positioning, is a manipulable parameter used to simulate the asymmetric modes observed in high-speed laryngoscopy data (Moisik et al. 2010). This 3D larynx model includes the original vocal folds from Titze's model, allowing for simulations of different combinations of vocal fold and aryepiglottic fold vibration (e.g. voiced vs. voiceless aryepiglottic trills). Based on Moisik's (2008) model, glottal stop [ʔ], glottal fricative [h], pharyngeal/epiglottal stop [ʡ], pharyngeal approximant [ʕ], pharyngeal fricative [ħ], and voiced pharyngeal (aryepiglottic) trill [ʕ] have been simulated.

Video 3.10 shows the 3D constrictor moving through a range of different postures (modal voice, breathy voice, pitch increase, and full vocal fold abduction) with simulated vocal fold vibration.

Video 3.11 shows the 3D constrictor engaging epilaryngeal constriction with simulated aryepiglottic fold vibration illustrating a left-right asymmetry (because of an anatomical difference in cuneiform configuration).

3.3.2   A Two-Trapdoor Model of Aryepiglottic Trilling

One complex action of larynx function is aryepiglottic fold trilling (Section 2.3.14). An important biomechanical feature visible in the high-speed frames of aryepiglottic trilling is a mucosal wave that radiates outwards across the surface of the aryepiglottic fold. The principles of vocal fold body-cover theory (Hirano 1974, Story and Titze 1995), which emphasize the importance of the vocal fold mucosal wave in self-sustaining oscillation, can be extrapolated and applied to mucosal wave action on the aryepiglottic folds. The two-trapdoor model of aryepiglottic trilling was designed to account for this possibility.

In terms of trilling biomechanics, we can infer that the aryepiglottic fold trilling frequency is correlated with the degree of laryngeal tension (or stiffness), and that the higher rate of vibration in the voiced trills is attributable to entrainment with the vocal folds, not just increased tissue stiffness. Sympathetic vibration of the aryepiglottic tissue with the vocal folds beneath during voiced trills occurs well before and after the trilling vibration proper in all cases. Once aryepiglottic vibration begins in earnest, however, the pulses are always highly irregular. All trills observed here involve the upper aryepiglottic mucosa, but the fact that the apices of the arytenoids also participate in the oscillation during the voiceless trill [ʜː], but not in the other trills, demonstrates possible variation in the nature of trilling. Despite such variation, auditory impressions do not vary markedly – both voiceless trills sound like 'raucous' pharyngeal fricatives.

Figure 3.14 diagrams the mechanical components of the model, which consists of the Story and Titze (1995) vocal folds surmounted by the aryepiglottic folds, each of which comprises a trapdoor component to represent the aryepiglottic fold body and a conventional (damped) spring-mass component to represent the mucosa of the fold, particularly at its upper free margin. The trapdoor formulation draws inspiration from McGowan (1992), in which the tongue tip is modelled as a trapdoor to better capture its geometric configuration. Each set of folds has adducted and abducted configurations, allowing for simulation of modal phonation (with no aryepiglottic vibration), voiceless aryepiglottic vibration (with no vocal fold vibration), and voiced aryepiglottic vibration (with both vocal fold and aryepiglottic fold vibration). Figure 3.15 illustrates the corresponding kinematic behaviour of the model's components for 100 ms of vibration. Details of modal voice and voiceless aryepiglottic trilling simulations can be found in Moisik (2013: 146–179).

Video 3.12 illustrates the trapdoor model of vocal fold vibration alone.
Video 3.13 illustrates the trapdoor model of aryepiglottic vibration alone.
Video 3.14 illustrates the trapdoor model of simultaneous oscillation of the vocal folds below and the aryepiglottic folds above.

A key insight arising from the model is that amplitude modulation of the glottal flow by the aryepiglottic pulses above creates an aero-mechanical

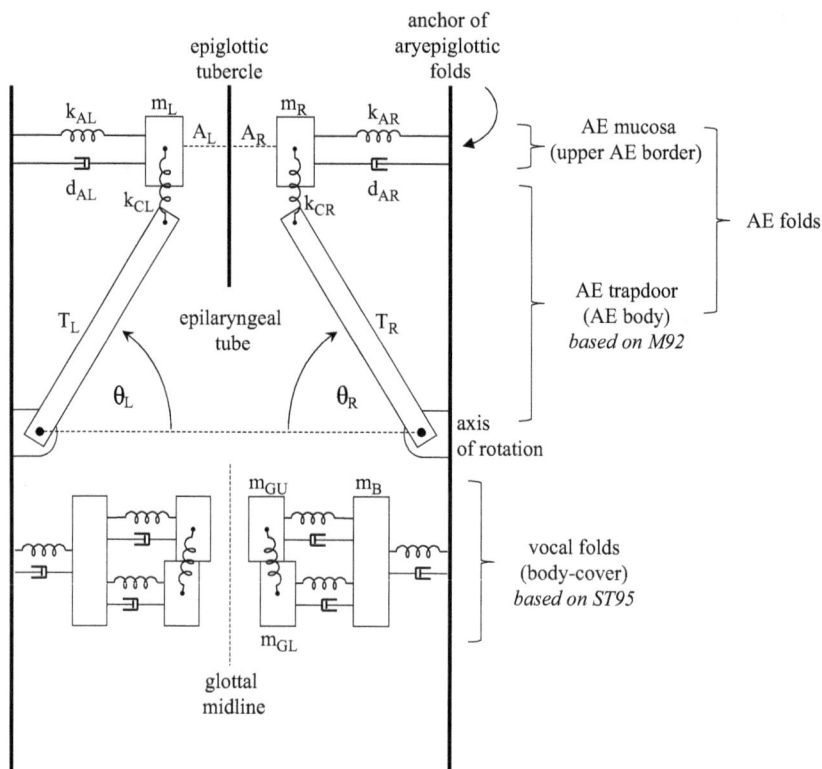

Figure 3.14 *Mechanical 'trapdoor' model of the aryepiglottic (AE) folds Parameters: A = aryepiglottic aperture area; d = damping; k = stiffness; m = mass; T = trapdoor; θ = trapdoor rotation angle. Subscripts: L = left; R = right; GL = lower glottis; GU = upper glottis; B = vocal fold body; AL = left AE fold; AR = right AE fold; CL = left AE trapdoor-mucosa coupling; CR = right AE trapdoor-mucosa coupling.*
Sources: *M92 = McGowan (1992); ST95 = Story and Titze (1995).*

interaction that generates subharmonic (s) structure in the glottal voice source spectrum: Figure 3.16(c). These subharmonics roughly correspond with the harmonics (h) generated by voiceless aryepiglottic vibration: Figure 3.16(b). The harmonics in Figure 3.16(c) roughly correspond with those produced in the case of modal vocal fold vibration without aryepiglottic oscillation in Figure 3.16(a). The subharmonics in Figure 3.16(c) are, therefore, due to the amplitude modulation of the glottal source by the aryepiglottic folds. The harmonics produced by voiceless aryepiglottic trilling in the model are much

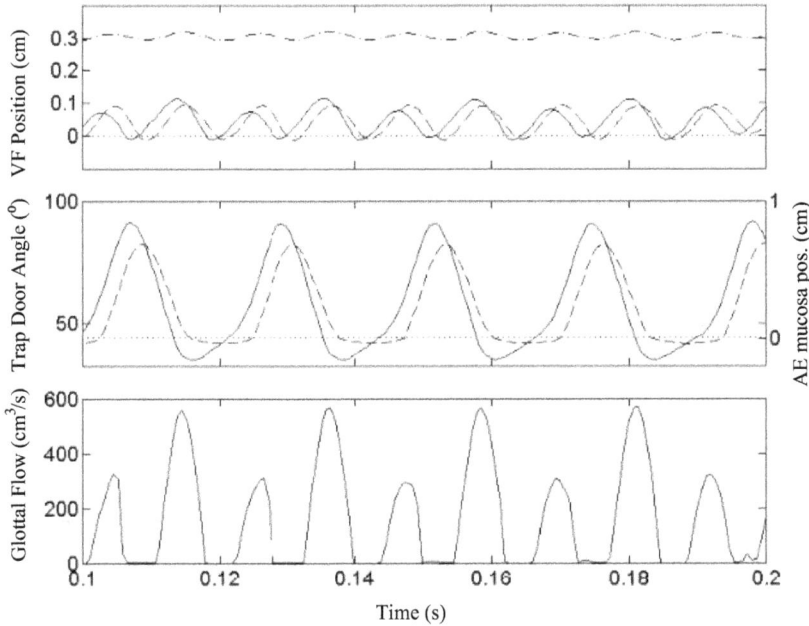

Figure 3.15 *Trapdoor model simulation of voiced aryepiglottic trilling Top plot: vocal fold mass displacements (solid line = lower glottal mass; dashed line = upper glottal mass; dash-dotted line = body mass); middle plot: angular displacement of the right side aryepiglottic trapdoor (left axis, solid line) and mucosa mass (right axis, dashed line) displacement; bottom plot: glottal flow.*

stronger than those that occur in reality, since the increased volume flow generates substantial turbulence and consequent noise in addition to general irregularity of AE vibration, which cannot be easily modelled with a lumped-element model (Moisik et al. 2010).

The model can simulate aryepiglottic trilling in the range of 40–60 Hz, with phase-lag values between the trapdoor and mucosa mass ranging from 24–64°. From experimentation, it is apparent that the major factor determining the frequency of the system is the stiffness of the trapdoor spring. While aryepiglottic vibration is typically reported at these frequency values, it is possible for rates as high as 90–100 Hz to occur, depending on the glottal frequency and the tightness of the configuration (Moisik et al. 2010). The higher frequency trilling likely involves far less effective mass than in the aryepiglottic model presented here. Specifically, as more postero-anterior narrowing occurs, a greater portion of the aryepiglottic fold body mass is prevented from

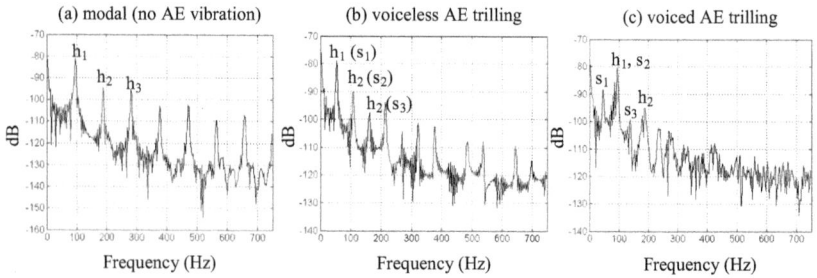

Figure 3.16 *Trapdoor model comparison of glottal source spectra*
Spectra (a) and (b) correspond with normal (modal) phonation and voiceless
aryepiglottic trilling, respectively (for corresponding time-series plots, see
Moisik 2013: 165–166). Spectrum (c) corresponds with voiced aryepiglottic
trilling shown in Figure 3.15. Harmonics = h; subharmonics = s.

oscillating due to contact and compression forces acting on the tissue. Gradually, only the upper mucosal border of the aryepiglottic fold oscillates. This is the case for the Iraqi Arabic data in Section 3.2.1. Evaluation of high-speed laryngoscopy with simultaneous EGG indicates that the changing aryepiglottic aperture during voiced aryepiglottic trills influences the dynamics of vocal fold vibration: the vocal folds oscillate in an alternating pattern of rapid and delayed closures depending on the state of the aryepiglottic aperture above the vocal folds.

Contrary to what is typically observed for aryepiglottic vibration, the model cannot simulate irregular motion very effectively, generally producing highly regular aryepiglottic motion. Consequently, harmonic/subharmonic structure, depending on whether the simulation is voiceless/voiced, is unrealistically strong and well defined. Sakakibara et al. (2004a) observe that the acoustic power of subharmonics in growl (vocal-aryepiglottic phonation, i.e. voiced aryepiglottic trilling) is weaker relative to kargyraa (vocal-ventricular phonation in Tuvan and Mongolian khöömei singing). This might be attributable to the oscillatory irregularity that characterizes aryepiglottic fold dynamics. In comparison to kargyraa, which exhibits surprisingly regular/periodic ventricular pulsing at typically half the glottal frequency, and vocal-ventricular vibration in general (Tsai et al. 2010: 210), aryepiglottic oscillation fluctuates between quasi-periodicity and aperiodicity (Edmondson et al. 2001, Moisik et al. 2010). One distinction between aryepiglottic and vocal-ventricular vibration is that aryepiglottic oscillation is characterized by topologically complex possibilities for airflow channels – the left and right aryepiglottic apertures, which can vary in time – which leads to greater complexity in the system in comparison to the vocal-ventricular mode. Strong periodicity in the flow signal corresponds with stronger harmonics in the frequency domain, since there are strong sinusoidal correlations with the signal. Irregularities or aperiodicities result in weak harmonic structure or harmonic smearing, since particular sinusoidal components are poorly correlated with the signal, and consequently the acoustic energy is dissipated over larger bands of sinusoids.

Ventricular oscillation has been observed to pass through a transient onset phase of irregular vibration, but it eventually locks into the oscillatory regime of the vocal folds (Fuks et al. 1998, Lindestad et al. 2001), vibrating at ½, ⅓, or equal to the glottal f0 (Sakakibara et al. 2004a). This frequency locking results from strong entrainment (synchronization tendency) of the two oscillating systems (the vocal folds and ventricular folds) coupled to a common aerodynamic source, i.e. the laryngeal airstream. The aryepiglottic folds have the potential to become entrained with the vocal folds, in the case of voiced aryepiglottic trilling, during which there is a degree of periodicity in the system. These instances, however, are relatively uncommon in comparison to the more irregular vibratory occurrences. Thus, the time evolution of the (real) system erratically shifts in and out of moments of vocal fold entrainment.

At the phonetic level, aryepiglottic trilling is often linked with the production of low-tone targets (Rose 1989, Edmondson and Esling 2006). This could stem from several factors (beyond the sphinctered laryngeal posture common to producing low pitch and constricted sounds), including the inherently low-frequency nature of epilaryngeal vibration and the presence of subharmonics in the case of voiced epilaryngeal vibration, both of which support the perception of voices with epilaryngeal vibration as low pitched (Teshigawara 2003). The model predicts that, through aerodynamically mediated entrainment, the vibratory frequency of the vocal folds will drop during aryepiglottic vibration. Even though this effect is small in the case of the model, if it occurs in real AE vibration, then this too could help explain the distribution of aryepiglottic trilling with low-tone productions. In general, this model provides a means to experiment with the vibratory mechanism of the extended phonatory function of the larynx. In voice quality analysis, this would apply to harsh voice with aryepiglottic vibration.

3.3.3   A Model of Vocal-Ventricular Fold Contact

During laryngeal constriction as in glottal stop, creaky voice, or epiglottal stop production, contact between the vocal folds and the ventricular folds – vocal-ventricular fold coupling (VVFC) – is evident (Section 3.2.3). A low-dimensional computational model to study the effects of this contact on the

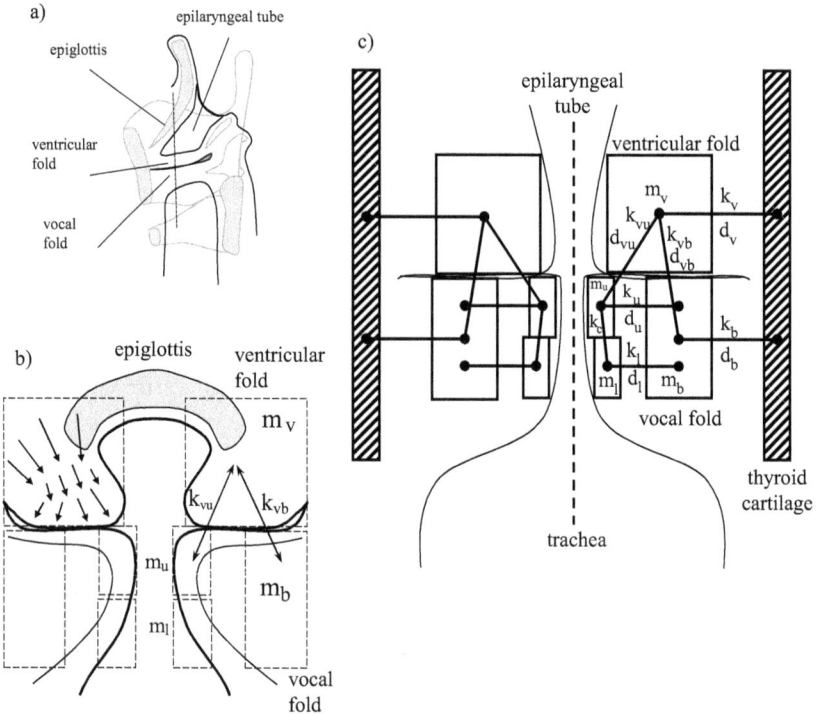

Figure 3.17 *Abstraction of VVFC into a low-dimensional model
(a) midsagittal profile of the larynx showing location (dashed line) of (b),
which is an anterior coronal section of the larynx showing the anatomical
distribution of model masses (dashed outlines) and an illustration of the
compressive forces of ventricular incursion as a vector field (left side; single-
headed arrows) and the representation of these forces as coupling springs
acting on the upper (m_u) and body (m_b) masses of the vocal folds (right side;
double headed arrows). (c) schematic of the model. In (b) the vocal folds are
depicted as partly abducted (following the anatomical photo of the dissected
larynx used to create the diagram), but they are more adducted in constricted
states.*
From Moisik and Esling (2014), reprinted with permission.

vibratory behaviour of the vocal folds (Moisik and Esling 2014) adds additional ventricular fold masses and coupling springs to the Story and Titze
(1995) model of the vocal folds, as depicted in Figure 3.17. The anatomical
distribution of the lumped masses represented in Figure 3.17(b) illustrates the
configuration of the VVFC springs (right side) and the compressive forces

acting on the vocal-ventricular-epiglottal complex (left side). Three forces are responsible for driving the adduction and descent of the ventricular folds and their consequent compression into the vocal folds: a downwards force from the epiglottis, likely driven by the aryepiglottic and thyroepiglottic muscles (Kimura et al. 2002), a downwards force from the anteromedial component of the craniolateral extension of the thyroarytenoid (TA) muscle, and an adductory force from the postero-lateral component of the TA muscle system (Reidenbach 1998b). Additionally, postero-anterior action of the epilaryngeal stricture mechanism should result in compression of the ventricular folds, effectively contributing to their medial and downwards motion into the vocal folds.

Video 3.15: The operation of a VVFC low-dimensional model of modal voice.
Video 3.16: The operation of a VVFC low-dimensional model of creaky voice.

In speech, the force exerted on the vocal folds by the ventricular folds has a vertical component; however, all VVFC-model masses are limited to a single, latero-medial, degree of freedom: no motion in the vertical (inferosuperior) dimension is considered. This abstraction is due to simplifying choices made in representing the vocal folds with a lumped-element approach and the aero-acoustic simulation of the vocal tract; introducing a vertical degree of freedom would complicate the calculation of glottal flow. As a first attempt at repre-senting VVFC, the goal is to maintain simplicity, so the coupling acts exclu-sively in the latero-medial dimension. Similar to Story and Titze's (1995) abstraction in its representation of the body and cover masses of the vocal folds, in the VVFC model, upper-cover mass m_u and body mass m_b move in the same dimension; but, in reality, the 'cover' mass is spatially distributed medially and superiorly around the 'body' as in Figure 3.17(b). The mucosal wave travels across the vocal fold upwards and laterally, as depicted in Figure 3.18(a). Thus, the cover has vertical and latero-medial influences as the mass is redistributed throughout the glottal cycle. Figure 3.18(b) adds to this VVFC and illustrates how collision (col) between the mass in the mucosal wave and the ventricular fold mass above drives the horizontal component of the coupling force.

Modelling VVFC using a low-dimensional, lumped-element computational model of laryngeal biomechanics can reproduce the anticipated effects of VVFC (Allen and Hollien 1973, Laver 1975, 1980, Moisik and Esling 2011). Increased effective mass and damping of the laryngeal system and the introduction of new modes of oscillation cause f0 lowering, inhibit oscillation,

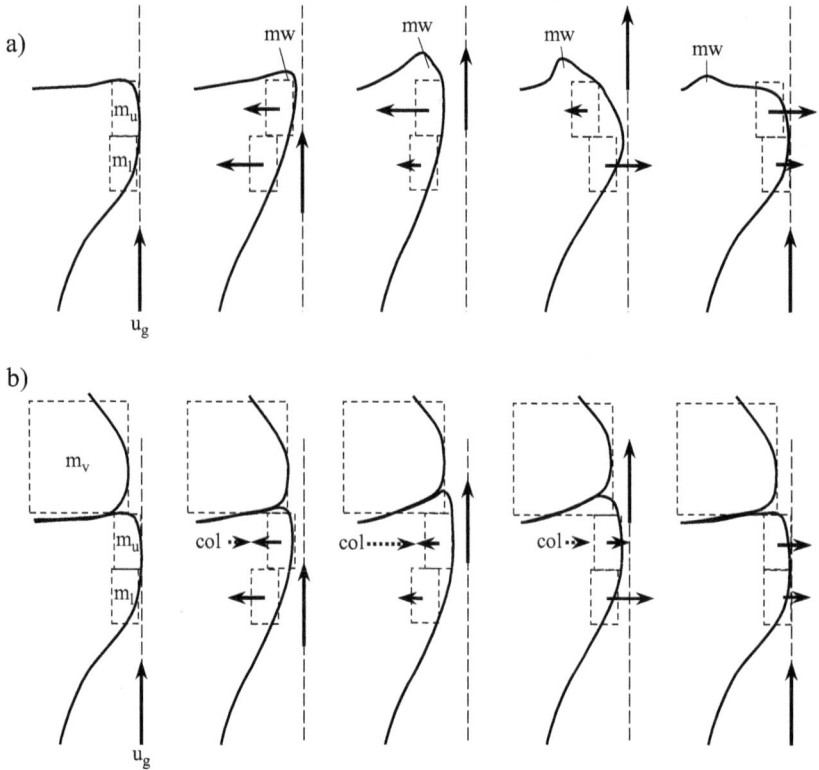

Figure 3.18 *Spatial abstraction and mass movement during the glottal cycle (a) without VVFC and (b) with VVFC. Dashed vertical line: glottal midline; Dashed outlines: model masses; horizontal arrows: velocities of the masses; mw = mucosal wave; col = force due to 'collision' between the ventricular fold mass and the upper-cover mass; m_u = upper-cover mass; m_l = lower-cover mass; m_v = ventricular fold mass; u_g = glottal flow.*
From Moisik and Esling (2014), reprinted with permission.

and can change vocal fold dynamics to result in constricted phonation. Figure 3.19 shows the effects of an incremental, percentage-wise increase of VVFC (10% increments starting at 10%). The increase of coupling strength coincides with the expected effect along each of the measures: f0 decreases and cover-mass phase difference (ϕ) increases. The products of simulation with coupling are auditorily classifiable as creaky-like or harsh-like. Other effects not mentioned in previous literature include mucosal wave interference, reinforcement of irregular patterns of vibration ('irregularity reinforcement'), a form of (2:1) amplitude modulation ('period-alternation') consistent with

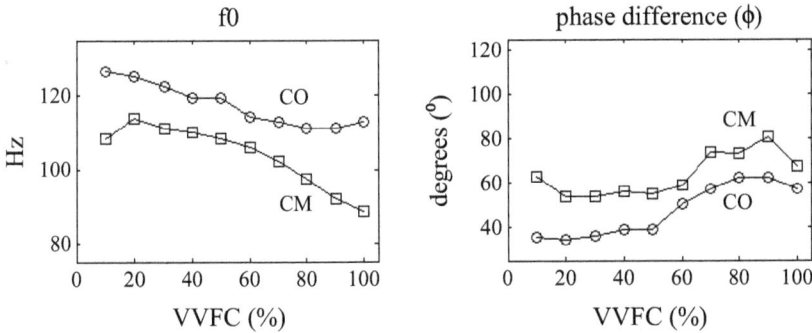

Figure 3.19 *Model performance as a function of percentage-wise increasing VVFC ([a] context)*
Squares: CM-VVFC; circles: CO-VVFC. (Note: CM = collision-and-mucous-type springs (push-pull); CO = collision-only-type springs (push only).)
Regardless of coupling type, f0 tends to decrease and φ (phase difference between upper and lower cover masses) tends to increase with VVFC.
From Moisik and Esling (2014), reprinted with permission.

previous observations of constricted forms of non-modal phonation (Gerratt and Kreiman 2001), and enhancement of laryngeal closure in glottal stop articulation. The model supports the view that vocal-ventricular fold coupling and epilaryngeal stricture in general are essential in explaining the nature of constricted phonation and laryngeal closure in vocalization and speech. The significance for phonetics and phonology, particularly in relation to the physiological basis of sounds such as glottal stop and creaky voice, is that both were long considered to be primarily attributable to action of the vocal folds rather than to the action of the laryngeal constrictor mechanism. The work also has significance for speech simulation, where it is desirable to use computationally inexpensive models (such as the lumped-element formulation presented here) to simulate natural-sounding voices (Birkholz 2005, 2011).

3.3.4   The ArtiSynth Model of the Larynx
The experimental phonetic techniques that we have employed to evaluate and quantify the articulatory function of the lower vocal tract have contributed to the elaboration of ArtiSynth, a 3D software platform primarily intended for (but not limited to) biomechanical simulation of vocal tract function (Fels et al. 2003, Stavness et al. 2011, Lloyd et al. 2012). An ArtiSynth model (called QL2) of the laryngeal articulator is described and diagrammed in Moisik and Gick (2017). Our intention is to demonstrate how the laryngeal constrictor

mechanism operates by illustrating its progressive degrees of closure and elucidating the most extreme strictures that the mechanism performs. By focusing on the stricture points, we are calling attention to the consonantal (or 'contoid') elements of speech, around which 'vocoid' elements and other continuants carry the majority of voice quality information, including the transitions between strictures and more open articulations.

Video 3.17 ArtiSynth model of plain glottal stop.
Video 3.18 ArtiSynth model of vocal-ventricular (reinforced) glottal stop.
Video 3.19 ArtiSynth model of (aryepiglotto-)epiglottal stop.

The ArtiSynth model reveals the 3D interplay amongst the folds of the larynx under constriction, which progressively increases through a simulated series of laryngeal stops: plain glottal stop, vocal-ventricular ('reinforced') glottal stop, and (aryepiglotto-)epiglottal stop. We observe in these models that, with the progressively greater aryepiglottic narrowing required for reinforced glottal stop, vocal-ventricular fold contact occurs. The results also demonstrate the articulatory-biomechanical instability of plain glottal stop relative to reinforced glottal stop and aryepiglotto-epiglottal stop, which predicts that plain glottal stop might be less common. While there is some endoscopic evidence for plain glottal stop (Iwata et al. 1979, Edmondson et al. 2011, Garellek 2013), glottal stop with ventricular reinforcement is more commonly encountered (Esling and Harris 2003, Edmondson et al. 2004, Esling et al. 2005, Edmondson and Esling 2006). Even in apparent cases of plain glottal stops, it is still possible that the ventricular folds come into contact with the vocal folds, even if the ventricular folds do not completely adduct (Moisik et al. 2015).

The aryepiglotto-epiglottal stop state represents a culmination of biomechanical stabilization events beginning with corniculate tubercle contact and leading to extensive compression and contact of most of the vocal fold and epilaryngeal surfaces. The simulation results indicate that this configuration is highly stable (for details, see Moisik and Gick 2017). Tongue retraction tends to accompany this state (Edmondson and Esling 2006) but has not been included in this simulation. The quality of phonation surrounding an epiglottal/pharyngeal stop is inevitably influenced by the extreme degree of stricture, the raising of the larynx, and the compression of the epilaryngeal tube, also producing key resonance effects in any surrounding vocalizations. Since tongue position can influence the position of the epiglottis, and displacement of the epiglottis impacts aryepiglottic stricture and the positioning of the ventricular folds, the model implies that the vocal folds can be perturbed by lingual position. Related to voice quality, this might characterize what occurs in many Germanic languages which exhibit a tendency for glottal stop insertion in vowel-initial syllables, particularly on open and retracted vowels (Brunner and Żygis 2011, Pompino-Marschall and Żygis 2011).

ArtiSynth modelling offers a sophisticated means of examining how laryngeal action operates to form the basic configurations underlying different voice quality settings. Future models are intended to allow for exploration of its interactions with other vocal tract structures, including the tongue and pharynx, as in the context of the FRANK model (Anderson et al. 2017). It may also be possible to study how voice quality interacts locally with segmental-level structure, which will be important in understanding the articulatory mechanisms underlying sound change.

4 Linguistic, Paralinguistic, and Extralinguistic Illustrations of Voice Quality

Chapter 4 presents examples of speakers whose voices illustrate the voice quality taxonomy outlined in Chapters 1 and 2. The aim of the chapter is to provide the reader with search terms to assist in locating individual speakers and languages that typify each voice quality category. As in Chapter 2, categories are organized from the lower to the upper vocal tract, paying specific attention to laryngeal categories as defined by the Laryngeal Articulator Model. Examples of well-known actors, singers, and media or political personalities, whose performances, speeches, or interviews are readily found online, are cited to illustrate extralinguistic long-term articulatory settings. Citations of specific works are found in the Multimedia References listing, following the academic References. Examples of paralinguistic instances of voice quality 'registers' are also provided, where categories are used in stylistic or shifting sociophonetic contexts. Examples of the linguistic (phonemic) incidence of each voice quality category are also given, where the short-term presence of the target sound quality signals contrastive meaning in the language.

Media files, organized by section, are found on the companion website to illustrate numerous instances of the articulatory postures that generate specific qualities. A PDF of the Multimedia References section is posted online, in the Chapter 4 set, for the reader's convenience in searching for examples.

We begin the illustrations with voice quality categories originating in the laryngeal articulator, starting with glottal phonation. We present examples of long-term settings, where each voice is characterized by one predominant voice quality category. These are exemplifications of voice quality in the broader sense – habitual or preponderant articulatory settings that impart a characteristic auditory quality to the voice. We also identify examples of stylistic registers or paralinguistic uses of voice qualities. Each individual category can potentially occur on all three strands of accent – segmental, voice dynamic, and voice quality – differing only in the length of time the quality lasts. Many linguistic sound systems use the lower vocal tract in particular to signal contrasts, applying properties to vowel nuclei or syllables to create register differences, as in languages that have tonal register – pitch and quality contrasts that distinguish lexical items. Linguistic realizations of laryngeal voice qualities are intertwined with the identification of pharyngeals. While pharyngeal consonants are rapidly fluctuating segments, they exhibit the same characteristics of the laryngeal articulator mechanism as in more sustained production. That is, a voiceless pharyngeal fricative parallels whispery voice; a voiced pharyngeal approximant parallels pharyngealized voice or raised-larynx voice; and a voiceless or voiced pharyngeal trill parallels aryepiglottic trilling as a long-term phonatory setting. Following the examples of laryngeal phonation and articulation, we illustrate voice quality settings of the oral vocal tract: the velopharyngeal port, tongue, jaw, and lips. Our aim is to highlight the auditory similarity of each quality across the range of speech functions.

4.1   Laryngeal Categories

4.1.1   *Glottal Phonation Types*
4.1.1.1   Breath

Pure breath as sustained phonation occurs in the 'whispered singing' techniques of Burundi (Ocora 1968, 1988). When the whispered singing is very soft, the phonation type is phonetically breath. When the whispered singing becomes louder and more forceful, the phonation type becomes phonetic whisper. If voicing is added, the phonation type is whispery voice or slightly harsh whispery voice.

Voice quality schemata rarely specify the aerodynamic flow of breath through the vocal tract as an independent parameter. When the airway is constricted by the laryngeal constrictor mechanism, airflow is impeded and can be assumed to be reduced (e.g. in harsh voice). The higher rate of airflow combined with the narrowing of the airway produces greater turbulence and/or aperiodicity (e.g. in laryngeal constriction at high pitch, pressed voice). Conversely, when the airway is not constricted and the flow of breath is relatively unimpeded, greater aerodynamic flow can act as a quality modulator, introducing characteristics of breath at susceptible points during the stream of speech. This occurs in the case of pre-aspiration in some Scandinavian and Celtic language varieties. Theoretically, the habitual presence of sustained, greater-than-usual airflow can be detected as a quasi-permanent property of an accent, especially during segments that favour breathy flow (e.g. [h], other voiceless fricatives, some voiceless consonants such as /t/) and lengthened flow (e.g.

vowels). In this way, duration interacts with positioning of the articulators (in this case, of the glottal abductors) to add an aerodynamic element to the articulatory description of the voice quality. This characteristic marks Southern Irish accents, such as Jim Beglin's TV football commentary (2007–12) and also O'Malley (1993–2006), Donnelly (1996–2001), and Kirwan (1996–2001). The propensity for fricativized coda [t] to occur in the context of persistent breathy flow in accents such as Irish English, although a subject for further research, can be hypothesized to link voice quality to segmental production.

4.1.1.2 Modal Voice

Laver (1980: 109–111) uses the term 'modal', after Hollien (1974), for the neutral setting of the larynx for voicing. This implies that modal voices are commonly found in the general population. Many fine singing voices that make optimal use of regular unimpeded vocal fold vibration exemplify modal voice (Reynolds 1970). However, professional singing voices with extensive training, e.g. in the operatic tradition, may fall outside the scope of phonetic taxonomies for describing voices in normal speech. The professional speaking voices of newsreaders (Mansbridge 1988–2017) and other radio/television announcers are likely to include more modal than non-modal voicing, as a reflection of aesthetics (geopolitical preferences), although elements of salient local (regional or social) articulatory settings may appear in such contexts.

4.1.1.3 Breathy Voice

The speaking and singing voice of Marilyn Monroe (1959) often typifies breathy voice. Many songs by Julio Iglesias (1978) are sung with breathy voice. These classic productions of sustained breathiness on voiced segments are typically associated with 'sexy voice'. From the perspective of physiological competence, they differ from many cases of 'breathy voice' encountered in clinical contexts, which are often dysphonically non-continuous, alternating between breath, voicing, breathy voicing, and glottal arrest. Sociolinguistically, breathiness has been reported as a marker of Welsh women's voices (Hejná 2015) and of Panjabi voices in the UK (Wormald 2016). Evidence suggests that breathiness is not only physiologically opposite to constricted phonation, such as harshness, but that it is also functionally opposite to constricted phonation in human social interaction. Xu et al. (2013) report that certain male listeners may show a preference for female voices that are higher pitched and breathy, and that female listeners, while finding male voices more attractive if they are lower pitched, may also prefer slightly breathy male voices, presumably to counteract acoustic cues of large body size, which may also signal aggressiveness.

4.1.1.4 Falsetto

Falsetto is used as an honorific register in Tzeltal (Brown and Levinson 1987). Falsetto in singing has a long history, especially since Renaissance Italy, and usually refers to a low-range male singer, singing in a high range. The history of the countertenor revolves around finding an ethereal quality (disembodied and therefore divine) in church music, a hint of sexual ambiguity, and an air of social confusion (Bidisha 2011). There are many famous examples of twentieth-century rock and pop singers using falsetto: Frankie Valli, the highest-pitched singer in The Four Seasons' four-part harmony (1962, 1963), Lou Christie (1966), and the Bee Gees (1977a,b). In some harmonies, breathy falsetto can be found along with falsetto (Bee Gees 1977c), as in the singing of the title line 'How Deep Is Your Love'. Jimmy Somerville usually sings in breathy falsetto (1990).

4.1.2   *Phonation Types with Laryngeal Constrictor Effects*
4.1.2.1   Whisper

Whisper as a discourse style of speaking quietly or secretively can be realized by phonetic breath or phonetic whisper. Degrees of harshness can be added to the latter, as these are compatible with the laryngeally constricted state of whisper. As noted above, whispered singing from Burundi (Ocora 1968, 1988) moves beyond soft breath and demonstrates phonetic whisper or harsh whisper when more constriction is involved, or slightly harsh whispery voice when voiced.

4.1.2.2   Whispery Voice

Whispery voice is often known as 'stage whisper', as the addition of voicing helps the voice to carry over a distance while preserving its quiet or secretive implication. Like whisper, it is a laryngeally constricted state, with potential for other constricted states to occur. Jeremy Irons' character Rodrigo Borgia (2011–13) uses whispery voice when speaking quietly or secretively, becoming harsh whispery voice when speaking more forcefully, and harsh voice when speaking most forcefully. In contrast to the Bee Gees' preference for breathy falsetto (1977c), Lou Christie's falsetto takes on a momentary harsh (irregular) component, in the style of Frankie Valli (1962a), leading into slightly whispery falsetto, viz. 'yai-yai-yai-yai-ya'a-ai' (1963). It is whispery rather than breathy, since whisper is a function of the constrictor mechanism, even though pitch remains high.

4.1.2.3 Creaky Voice (Creak)

Creak and creaky voice are identified by the low frequency of bursts in the glottal cycle, from a few occasional or irregular bursts for creak to a regular slowing of periodicity for sustained creaky voice. The Standard Edinburgh English of upper-middle-class speakers is known for its use of creaky phonation (Esling 1978). Even where most voicing is creaky, a speaker's voice can descend to even lower-frequency creakiness phrase-finally. As a Germanic language, English generally favours laryngeal constriction towards the ends of intonational phrases, sometimes only on the final syllable of a long phrase. Many newsreaders with otherwise modal voices employ this strategy of phrase-final creak. This is also the sociolinguistic usage of many young English-speaking women, referred to in the media as 'vocal fry speaking' (Salie 2013, Podesva 2013). The creaky voice of Kim Kardashian (2007–16), especially phrase-finally, is a good example of low creakiness for attitudinal effect. Many songs by Kenny Rogers are sung with creaky voice when his register is in the low pitch range (1978). His quality often becomes harsh creaky voice, although when his register is higher in pitch, his voice is modal.

Files illustrating creaky voice can be found in the media set for this section.

As a constricted setting, creakiness can be combined with other constricted traits, such as whisperiness or harshness, but pure creaky voice reflects only the shortening of the vocal folds due to constriction and its regular very-low-pitched periodicity. Anthony Hopkins uses whispery creaky voice in his portrayal of Dr Hannibal Lecter in *Silence of the Lambs* (1991). Judi Dench's Queen Elizabeth (1998) varies between modal and slightly breathy phonation, with the breathy component becoming slightly whispery as pitch drops (with gravitas) to creaky phonation. Both creak and whisper are functions of constriction. Vincent Price often performs whispery creaky voice in intonational phrase codas in *Thriller* (1983). The 'broken pitch' aspects of the voice of Slow Mobius (Romano 2014) give it the quality of creaky falsetto. Chris Diamantopoulos uses falsetto as Mickey Mouse (2013), which becomes creaky falsetto when Mickey is excited and speaking quickly. Frankie Valli alternates between falsetto, creaky falsetto, and harsh falsetto in 'Sherry' (1962a). Craig Ferguson (2014) uses whispery creaky falsetto when he imitates David Beckham. Pitch is high, airflow increased, and the 'squawky' arresting of phonation gives the impression of creak.

4.1.2.4   Harsh Voice (Mid Pitch)

Irregular, aperiodic voicing and noise as a function of narrowing of the laryngeal constrictor can be found in many speaking voices and singing styles, with quite broad variation in the exact quality of the harshness. Harshness also interacts with pitch in many varied ways. Even in examples at mid-range pitch, harshness may become harsh creakiness in phrase-final contexts. Norman Goodland's renditions of Hampshire dialect, as performed on BBC Radio Solent, exemplify harsh phonation (1981). The singing of The Kinks (Davies 1964a,b) provides a contrast, with modal voice becoming harsh voice in the louder chorus lines. Rod Stewart demonstrates harsh voice in all of his songs (1970a,b,c). There is an exceptionally clear contrast towards the end of 'Country Comforts' (1970c) between his harsh voice quality and the modal voice vibrato backing vocals of Jack Reynolds. In some later performances, and where pitch is higher, Stewart's harsh quality has more isometric longitudinal+constricted 'pressed' tightness (see Section 4.1.2.7). His singing-voice quality is reminiscent of the traditional singing of central Italy (Bravi 2017), which may engage multiple levels of vibrating folds or pressed voice. A good example of harsh voice singing is the Mongolian rap-style group, Fish Symboled Stamp (2013). Battogtokh Odsaikhan, the rapper wearing cap and furs, has consistently harsh voice quality, in contrast to his partner, who uses primarily ventricular voice (see Section 4.1.2.5).

Kenny Rogers' creaky singing style (1978) often acquires an aperiodic mode, becoming slightly harsh creaky voice. Slightly harsh moderately creaky voice predominates in Rogers (1969). Pitch is mid to low, which facilitates the production of creak, and the final verse changes to slightly harsh whispery voice. Moderately harsh slightly whispery phonation is characteristic of Glaswegian phonation (Connolly 1982, Ferguson 2014). Dr Claw from *Inspector Gadget* (Welker 1983) has extremely harsh whispery voice with slight aryepiglottic trilling. These components also comprise Yoda's voice (Oz 1980). Mimicking the harsh to harsh creaky voices of boxing announcers (Meriman 1979), the announcer voice on *Timmy Turner vs Mac - Cartoon Showdown #2* (2016) combines harshness and whisperiness with high pitch to effect a cartoon voice. Although the voice is not yet falsetto, longitudinal tension combined with tension of the laryngeal constrictor creates a third dimension that distinguishes it from lower-pitched productions of harshness and whisperiness. Because of maintained tight constriction, falling pitch introduces an intermittent periodicity that emulates creakiness (harsh whispery creaky voice). Frankie Valli's falsetto becomes harsh falsetto in 'Sherry' (1962a), viz. 'make-a you mi-i-i-ine'. His performance in 'Big Girls Don't Cry' (1962b) also reaches into harsh falsetto, viz. 'cry-y-y'. James Brown's high-pitched squealing screaming mode (1966) produces a quality that alternates between harsh creaky falsetto and harsh whispery creaky falsetto, with falsetto shifting to the isometric tightness of longitudinal stretching plus aryepiglottic compression (as in Section 4.1.2.7). Marge Simpson's usual harsh whispery voice becomes harsh whispery falsetto when she is emotional, screams, or is represented as a child (Kavner 1989–2016).

4.1.2.5 Ventricular Voice

Given the high degree of airflow necessary to drive the ventricular folds into self-sustaining oscillation and the requisite adduction of the vocal folds to medialize the ventricular folds, vocal fold vibration is virtually guaranteed to occur. Ventricular voice is therefore always voiced (accompanied by vocal fold vibration below). In some instances, the vibration ripples up through the lower portion of the epilaryngeal mucosa (just above the ventricular folds). This may be the more typical mode of 'dist' tones in the singing style of hard rock, metal, and similar genres (Zangger Borch et al. 2004). An example of ventricular voice as primary phonation type is the cartoon voice of Popeye the Sailor Man, as performed by Jack Mercer (1935–45, 1947–84). The voice-over performance is the speaking-voice equivalent of the 'deep' chant of a Tibetan monk chant master. Tibetan chanting illustrates virtuosity in the use of the instrument of the human voice – a practised form where the vocal folds, ventricular folds, supraventricular mucosa, and mucosal ring are shaped in the cylindrical tube above the glottis to produce sustained oscillation. Sanjjav Baatar, the sleeveless Mongolian singer in Fish Symboled Stamp (2013), employs ventricular phonation in his deepest pitch range, alternating with a number of other throat-singing techniques (such as overtone singing). The linguistically contrastive tense low-tonal register of the Tibeto-Burman language Bai may couple some ventricular vibration with (glottal) vocal fold vibration for some speakers, or exploit the inner mucosa of the epilarynx, as in /tɕi̤²¹/ 'flag', but primarily recruits aryepiglottic fold vibration, as aryepiglottic trilling is more commonly observed in general populations whereas ventricular voice is more restricted to clinical populations or specialized performances. We use a version of the Chao (1930, 1968: 25) system to mark tone, from 1 low to 5 high. Two or more numbers written together represent a pitch contour. Vowels are often marked with a diacritic to emphasize the difference in phonatory quality.

A laryngoscopic video example of 'deep' chanting by a Tibetan Buddhist chant master is in the media set. We hypothesize that vertical separation is optimal, isolating the ventricular folds, up through the level of the mucosal ring circling the top of the epilaryngeal tube.

4.1.2.6   Harsh Voice (Low Pitch, with Aryepiglottic Fold Trilling)

Sakakibara et al. (2004a) point out that growl phonation is a common effect in some of the music of the Xhosa people in South Africa, the beginning of Kakegoe used by Noh percussionists, and pop styles (e.g. jazz, blues, gospel, Enka in Japan, samba in Brazil). Some singers use growl extensively through a song, while others use it as a vocal effect for expressive emphasis. Some of the best examples of aryepiglottic-trilled phonation occur in blues, rhythm and blues, and jazz singing. Bobby 'Blue' Bland (1961) and Koko Taylor (1969) sang many songs with very pure modal voice, embellishing certain lines or sections of the performance with pronounced aryepiglottic fold trilling. In a different context, this quality could be called growling. It typically occurs in a lower pitch range, hence the association of harshness at low pitch. It can also occur paralinguistically, in a Germanic language like English for example, as an intensifying quality in heated conversation or on stressed items marked by anger or emphasis. In *Atanarjuat: The Fast Runner*, one scene portrays shamanistic embodiments of a polar bear (Ulayuruluk 2001) and a walrus (Kotierk 2001). The polar bear is realized with ventricular voice, while the walrus uses aryepiglottic trilling. Canadian country music singers Paul Brandt (2001) and George Canyon (2008) use, in addition to their modal and low creaky voice, evocative aryepiglottic-trilled (growled) onsets that echo, inversely, the prevalent female coda creak reported in the sociolinguistic literature (Podesva 2013). A paralinguistic use of aryepiglottic trilling even occurs in Japanese, to denote surprise. Louis Armstrong (1967) used aryepiglottic-trilled phonation as a norm throughout most of his singing, notably in his later years. In the 1920s and 1930s, his improvisational vocalizing (1926) and the lower-pitched portions of his scat singing (1931) were performed with aryepiglottic trilling, in contrast to more melodic modal portions, but some of his singing was already dominantly aryepiglottic (1929). A raised-larynx quality can also be heard in his singing. In later years, his speaking voice was also dominated by aryepiglottic-trilled phonation, which can be heard as one African-American speaking style, which is employed in stereotype voices (Moisik 2012). Many of Chris Rock's stand-up comedy routines adopt this sociolinguistic style of speech (1996). Rock frequently exhibits aryepiglottic trilling (or other enhanced epilaryngeal vibration) at very high pitches – glottal f0s of ~300–400 Hz (Moisik 2012: 204). As a linguistically contrastive trait, aryepiglottic fold vibration can be heard in the lowest-pitched Bai syllables, /tɕi̱ ²¹/ 'flag' or /tɕḭ̃ ²¹/ 'bracelet', possibly involving some vertical coupling of all laryngeal folds but primarily vibration of the inner mucosa of the epilaryngeal tube and the aryepiglottic folds. There is no reason that aryepiglottic trilling cannot be combined with falsetto (e.g. Henley 1964), since the vibrations are produced at separate locations; because the trilling is low pitched, its effect is very different from the tight high-pitched phonation described in Section 4.1.2.7.

An illustration of the paralinguistic incidence of aryepiglottic trilling in Japanese can be found in the media for Section 4.1.2.6, as well as the examples of Bai 21 register tones.

4.1.2.7 Laryngeal Constriction at High Pitch (Pressed Voice)

When the sphincteric closing of the laryngeal mechanism combines with longitudinal stretching of the vocal folds for increasing pitch, the isometric tightness that results produces a high-frequency quality with slow airflow release. Force is applied in two opposing directions: antero-posteriorly (longitudinally), resulting in stretched vocal folds; and postero-anteriorly (aryepiglottically), resulting in medial and vertical compression. The air is held in the lungs to stabilize the chest, so this quality can be heard in cases of physical exertion as in straining to lift a heavy load. It would not be unusual for laryngeal constriction at high pitch (pressed voice) to alternate with aryepiglottic fold trilling as a result of vertical compaction, especially if air is suddenly expelled more forcefully from the lungs. The harsh phonatory quality of the young Gipsy Kings approaches this pressed quality when pitch and amplitude increase, as on the stressed syllable of 'bamboléo' (Reyes 1987), and as stretching for high pitch strains against the tightened laryngeal constrictor. A heavy-lifting vocalization realizing pressed quality can be heard from Polish weightlifter Paweł Najdek (2001) on a clean and jerk. Russian Andrei Chemerkin, when he vocalizes (2000 Olympics), also produces pressed voice (harsh constriction at high pitch). Hossein Rezazadeh's version is tight enough to be pressed, but considerable aryepiglottic vibration flows through, as pitch is not as high. Although auditorily identifiable in these contexts and distinct from other constricted qualities, this quality requires further analysis of its detailed components.

4.1.3   Laryngeal Constrictor and Larynx Height Settings
4.1.3.1   Constricted (Aryepiglottic Sphinctering, Retracted Lingual Setting, Raised Larynx Height)

4.1.3.1.1   Raised-Larynx Voice   Raised-larynx voice is a resonance effect rather than a vibration and is therefore not classified with phonation types. It is nevertheless a setting of the laryngeal constrictor, which is responsible for pharyngeal sounds, predisposing vibratory actions to occur. When the laryngeal articulator is constricted, the larynx is normally raised; hence the co-occurring relationship of a narrowed passageway and a vertically shortened pharynx (complemented by retraction of the tongue). As a long-term setting, raised larynx is associated with Jim Henson's muppet character Kermit the Frog (1955–90). Many well-known voices are permeated with raised-larynx resonance (shortened pharynx and narrowed epilaryngeal tube), such as influential blues artist, Robert Johnson (1937). Many singers follow this tradition, including Canadians Roy Forbes (1975) and Steven Page, whose lead vocals with the Barenaked Ladies (1992) are distinguished by higher pitch and raised-larynx quality. Related to aryepiglottic trilling (through pharyngeal constriction), raised-larynx voice is also an African-American speaking style with associated stereotypes (Moisik 2012). The Schmenge Brothers (Candy and Levy 1982–83) used pronounced raised-larynx voice as a comedic parody of foreign accent. Rowan Atkinson's Mr Bean tends towards raised-larynx voice when he speaks (1992). Inuit katajjaq or katajjait describe traditional throat-singing vocal games where one singer often adopts a raised-larynx-voice rhythmic pattern while the second singer adopts various laryngeal vibrations in counterpoint (CBC Northern Service 1984). Many times, however, the rhythmic pattern is breathy, while the counterpoint is laryngeally constricted and/or epilaryngeally vibrated. The sound of raised-larynx (narrowed-laryngeal-constrictor) vocalization is remarkably replicated by the sound of the jaw harp, which can accompany traditional Inuit music. The short distance between the source jaw harp vibrations and the tongue replicates the resonance properties of the compressed space between glottal vibration and the top of the epilaryngeal tube in raised-larynx voice. The contribution of the shape of the performers' vocal tract cavities to the sound of their musical instruments is a fruitful line of research, e.g. the techniques of virtuoso performance on trumpet (Antonsen 1997) and ultrasound of didgeridoo (Zolotas and Bird 2010) and of trombone (Heyne and Derrick 2015).

4.1.3.1.2   Pharyngealized Voice   When pitch is lowered (inducing downward tilting of the thyroid), a raised-larynx setting (due to laryngeal constriction) produces pharyngealized voice quality (maintaining laryngeal constriction). These qualities are directly implicated in linguistically contrastive realizations of laryngeal constriction, including pharyngeal segments and pharyngealized syllables (Section 4.3). Similar to the phonemic occurrence of constricted quality in Tibeto-Burman languages, the 'high' chant of a Tibetan monk chant master illustrates how narrowing through the epilaryngeal tube and pharyngeal channels combines with a relatively low-pitched voice to produce pharyngealized voice. The voices introduced by Jim Henson (1955–90) and his muppeteers exploited larynx raising as a setting, varying in pitch to create different characters – a style contrasting with the earlier Warner Bros. voices of Mel Blanc (1937–89) that often introduced a secondary periodic source generated in the oral cavity. A classic example of the low pitch of pharyngealized voice as a marker of 'serious' personality is Frank Oz's muppet character Sam the Eagle (1975–2000). Günter Grünwald's (2009) comedic impressions of an Arabic accent in German could also be called pharyngealized voice quality because of the repetitive accumulation of pharyngeal stricture articulations.

Pharyngealized voice in a Tibetan 'high' chant is illustrated in a video file (about halfway into the chant, where the laryngeal structures elevate to approximate the retracting tongue).

4.1.3.2 Unconstricted
4.1.3.2.1 Lowered-Larynx Voice   Lowering the larynx without laryngeal constriction is the setting for lowered-larynx voice. Low pitch is the default with lowered larynx. Gary Cooper's character Robert Jordan and Akim Tamiroff's character Pablo in *For Whom the Bell Tolls* (1943) often employ a lowered-larynx posture in their authoritative personae. Interestingly, Cooper's dubbed voice in German is non-modal and constricted, e.g. *Zwölf Uhr mittags* (Lukschy 1952). Downward expansion of the pharynx characterizes some Russian voices and singing styles. Leonid Kharitonov (1965) adopts lowered larynx at low pitch and even in higher ranges, reflecting an Eastern Orthodox Church singing style and conceivably Russian speech, giving the voice what is recognized even impressionistically as an 'open' resonance. Lowered larynx was a 'serious' posture for American radio and public address announcements in the mid twentieth century (Clapper 2011). The *Talking to Americans* announcer voice from *This Hour Has 22 Minutes* on CBC TV (Mercer 2001) parodies this style. Jean-Yves Le Borgne (2014) illustrates how lowered-larynx voice can occur in standard French – a language favouring openness and breathiness (both enabled

by larynx lowering) rather than constriction. Lowering of the larynx can occur as a paralinguistic effect in some varieties of Southern British English, marking an attitudinal comment or rhetorical enhancement on select phrases (Bruce 2011). The *Monty Python* Gumby voices, notably Michael Palin's (1969), have lowered larynx, an excessive amount of airflow (which is correlated with lowered larynx), but with slight constriction, adding harshness (not normally correlated with lowered larynx). When pitch rises in their performance, auditory perception shifts to the quality of faucalized voice, although with unexpected harshness. These counterintuitive combinations of qualities give the voices their bizarre character.

4.1.3.2.2 Faucalized Voice   When the larynx is lowered and pitch is increased, faucalized voice results. This is best illustrated by the advertising voice of Tony the Tiger (Ravenscroft 1953–2004), starting off with lowered-larynx voice and then crescendoing rapidly to high pitch at the end of 'grrreat!' yielding faucalized quality. This voice quality setting is often associated with New York City or Boston dialect speech. It is slightly present in John Ratzenberger's character Cliff Claven (1982–93) in his New England accent when he raises his voice. Ben Affleck sometimes affects a broad Boston accent in this way. It can also be found as drill sergeant voice in some US Army ads (2012). Joe Pesci portrays the faucalized larynx setting of a New York/ New Jersey accent in his character Tommy DeVito (1990). Marlon Brando's character Don Corleone (1972) has elements of larynx height control, possibly with a slightly lowered setting with counterintuitively higher pitch (slight faucalization), even though his voice is dominated by moderately harsh phonation, which is a function of constriction, modulated by slight nasality (not to mention creative oral settings). The Godpigeon voice (LaMarche 1993) explicitly exploits the faucalized potential of the Godfather voice, dominating over slight harshness, as a parody. We suspect that stage/screen roles will not display the extreme versions of single qualities that parodies do. The parody may also exploit traits of underlying regional and social accents that a stage/ screen actor moderates but which the comedian or voice-over actor recruits.

4.2   Supralaryngeal (Oral) Categories

4.2.1   *Velopharyngeal Port Settings*
4.2.1.1   Nasal Voice
Nasality is a component of many accents, e.g. British English of higher social status (Esling 1978), American English, particularly of the South Midland

region, or Brazilian Portuguese. Bluegrass music imports local regional accent into song with pronounced nasal voice (Osborne Brothers 1967, Soggy Bottom Boys 2000, Foggy Hogtown Boys 2010). In the American folk music tradition, nasal voice is endemic, as revived by Bob Dylan (1963, 1965). If a hint of nasality contributed to Don Corleone's voice (Brando 1972), then considerably more nasality characterizes accents of European French. Nasal vowels occur plentifully in French, but nasal voice quality is also a function of sustained velopharyngeal opening. This can be heard in prosodic embellishments, along with larynx lowering and breathiness. Audrey Tautou (2010) exemplifies this combination of qualities, along with other distinctive oral settings.

4.2.1.2 Denasal Voice

Related to nasality and to velarization as an articulatory setting, the cold-in-the-nose quality of denasal voice is exemplified by Gilda Radner's character Lisa Loopner (1978a). The requirement of tongue raising (velarization) for denasal quality is exemplified by the presence of both elements in the voice of Lucy Worsley (2013, 2014).

4.2.2 Tongue-Body Lingual Settings
4.2.2.1 Fronted Lingual Settings
4.2.2.1.1 Dentalized Voice   Advancing the tongue body so that it habitually impinges on the teeth or partially protrudes through the teeth produces the quality of dentalized voice. It would be surprising for a speaker with dentalized voice not to have dentalized consonants. Bricio Segovia (2012) demonstrates this auditorily and visually. Section 4.2.5.4 explores further the relationship of tongue-front consonants and long-term setting in standard Castilian Spanish, in particular the facilitation of consonant production by adopting compatible settings. Idiosyncratically, Harry Kane's lingual setting is dentalized, favouring dental stops and nasals (2015). Since a dentalized front-lingual setting does not preclude the back of the tongue from assuming a raised or retracted posture at the same time, it is not impossible to find a voice where the tongue is displaced in two directions at once.

4.2.2.1.2 Alveolarized Voice   Italian offers an example of the tongue operating primarily in the alveolar region. Bertinetto and Loporcaro (2005) cite six dental phonemes, three alveolar phonemes, and three postalveolar phonemes. Theoretically, a setting with a locus of articulatory activity around the alveolar ridge can be hypothesized to facilitate the production of several consonants. Personalities Benedetta Rinaldi and Andrea Cavalieri illustrate the alveolarized locus (Rinaldi 2013). The pre-alveolarized lingual consonants of German also fit with a generally alveolarized tongue-body setting, illustrated by Deutsche Welle presenter Ariane de Hoog (2012). In her case, English bilingualism is also a factor, and therefore a potential reinforcement, as much English speech can also be characterized as front-lingual.

4.2.2.1.3 Palato-Alveolarized Voice A more mid-tongue-body-oriented posture can be heard in Greek (E.R.T. 2013), as palato-alveolarized voice. The same locus of postural preference characterizes a Greek accent in English (Tsipras 2015). Our premise is that auditory phonetic identification, as in these selected illustrations, can serve as a guide in experimental studies of individual speakers' segmental production in conjunction with their centre-of-gravity locus over time.

4.2.2.1.4 Palatalized Voice Russian president Vladimir Putin demonstrates recurrent palatalized sequences in his formal speeches (2012). The cumulative effect of palatalized consonants and palatalization in morphophonemic alternation in Russian can create the context for palatalized voice as a setting. Russian also has productive velarization (Yanushevskaya and Bunčić 2015), which can occur as a dominant background setting. We posit that a habitual velarized posture might serve as the voice quality 'ground' to enhance the distinctiveness of palatalized consonants in the language. The research challenge is to demonstrate a relationship between phonemic or morphophonemic tendencies and an identifiable 'centre' of movement or postural locus. A case where palatal segments predominate, for example, a children's jeering taunt ['ɲaː⁴ ɲa³ɲa⁵ 'ɲaː⁴ɲaː³] (on the notes sol-mi-la sol-mi), demonstrates a palatalized tongue-body setting, with allowance made for jaw opening for [a]. In a Japanese animation (Fujimoto 2011), persistent reiteration of [ɲ] (along with [n] and reduced vowels) lends a predominantly palatalized quality, reinforced with nasalization. An intense version of baby talk in English uses palatalized voice (tongue tip down, tongue body up) as well as close rounding, nasal voice, and lowered larynx. This setting may emulate the tongue in a small infant vocal tract.

4.2.2.2 Raised Lingual Settings
4.2.2.2.1 Velarized Voice In velarized voice, the body of the tongue is raised up and back, giving a secondary colouring to consonants produced with the front of the tongue and altering vowel quality by superimposing the

auditory/acoustic characteristics of an [ʊ] or [u] vowel. Harold Wilson, British Prime Minister, 1964–70, 1974–76, had distinctively velarized voice quality (1970), characteristic of some Huddersfield accents and other parts of the north of England, notably Liverpool (Gerry Marsden 1963, see Knowles 1974). Cristina Serban Ionda in the New Zealand TV drama *The Brokenwood Mysteries* (2014–17) uses a velarized setting to embody her Russian character, pathologist Gina Kadinsky. Velarization can be heard in Jill Barber's singing (2008), most noticeably on vowels further away from /u/. Lucy Worsley's (2013, 2014) presentations illustrate velarized lingual quality as well as the affinity of a raised (velarized) tongue-body position with denasal quality (Section 4.2.1.2). Her sustained velarized/denasalized quality influences not only the front /i/ but also the raised /kw/ of a word such as 'queen'. The lingually raised setting may also restrict the way tongue-front segments, such as /r/, are pronounced. It can be hypothesized that lifting the tongue body up and back interferes with the front of the tongue adopting a retroflex posture, favouring a tip-down variety of /r/ (cf. Lindau 1985). Velar stricture may also facilitate trilling (labial in Worsley's case), due to the effect of channelled airflow on downstream strictures (Solé 2002).

4.2.2.2.2 *Uvularized Voice*

Another lingually raised voice quality of the north of England is uvularized voice. It can be heard throughout Yorkshire in many broad accents. It is a prominent element of Tony Capstick's performance of broad Rotherham dialect (1981). It also enters into footballer Michael Dawson's Leyburn accent (2013). The example of Richmond Yorkshire dialect on the classic BBC (1971) recording of regional dialects is moderately uvularized. Many of Sacha Baron Cohen's Israeli characters use uvularized voice (Cohen 2018). The attempts of the crew of *Red Dwarf* (1997) to speak the GELF language could also be called uvularized voice quality (with harsh phonation) because of the recurrence of only [χ] and neutral vowels.

4.2.3 Tongue-Front Lingual Settings

4.2.3.1 Tongue Tip Articulation (Apical)

A refinement of habitual lingual activity is the posture of the tip of the tongue. Many accents of English are described as apical. The (Canadian) English and German accents of Ariane de Hoog have apical quality (2012). In theory, the more frequent the incidence of apical pre-alveolars, the more their spectral characteristics contribute to overall voice quality. One research challenge is to isolate what those characteristics are and how they affect perception.

4.2.3.2   Tongue Blade Articulation (Laminal)

In contrast to apicality, when the apex of the tongue is lowered and the blade articulates consonantal strictures, the gestures are laminal. In contrast to English, the French accent of Audrey Tautou (2010) demonstrates generalized tongue blade articulation.

4.2.3.3   Retroflex Articulation

While the tongue tip and blade affect primarily the quality of transitions between strictures and vowels, retroflexion of the tongue has a pronounced effect on the resonance of the oral vocal tract as a whole. Curling the tongue tip rearwards not only affects how individual consonantal strictures are heard but also influences spectral frequency globally, playing a role in throat singing (Section 4.3.4). Many local accents of the south coast of England exhibit retroflex articulation (Sussex, Hampshire, Dorset, Somerset, Devon, Cornwall). The BBC (1971) recording of regional dialects illustrates the degree to which each is retroflexed. Robert Newton's (1954) character Long John Silver represents archetypal pirate voice with retroflex oral quality and harsh phonatory quality. Norman Goodland's (1981) presentations on BBC Radio Solent represent a Hampshire accent, with retroflex effects and harsh phonation resembling Robert Newton's Dorset rendition. The degree to which intermittent /r/ phonemes contribute to voice quality perception is an issue, but the interaction of retroflexion and harshness on an /a/ vowel extends beyond just consonantal influence. In a Johnny Carson interview (1989) of Jimmy Stewart, both have slightly retroflexed sibilants, which may contribute to retroflexion in the perception of their voice qualities if frequent enough. The classic Jimmy Stewart accent is famously retroflexed, focusing on sibilants and approximants /r/ and /l/ but also on lengthened vowels (1946).

4.2.4   *Jaw Settings*

4.2.4.1   Close Jaw

A close jaw setting is one marker that distinguishes Standard Southern English from General American accents. Bill Nighy's character Johnny Worricker in *Salting the Battlefield* (2014) and most of the other English actors in that series (Ralph Fiennes, Saskia Reeves, Rupert Graves, Felicity Jones) use slight to moderate close jaw settings, especially in neutral conversation. Naturally, in more heated conversation, jaw movements become more dynamic. Not all American accents have an open jaw setting. Labov (1963, 1972: 40) identified the 'close-mouthed' setting of 'old Yankee' islanders on Martha's Vineyard as a favoured articulatory posture, lending a characteristic auditory quality to their 'up-island' speaking style and giving a number of phonological variables a closer, more centralized pronunciation in juxtaposition to the more standard open jaw setting of down-island and mainland speakers. Some accents of the Northern US dialect region, across New York State, Michigan, Wisconsin, Minnesota, and parts of the Dakotas have a preference for a closer jaw (with labial spreading), e.g. Rod Serling (1959–64). French and Polish are examples of European languages that use close jaw. Audrey Tautou (2010) demonstrates this along with distinctive lingual and labial settings. Professor Jan Miodek (2012) and *TV Polonia* presenter Piotr Kraśko (2009) speak Polish with an extremely close jaw setting.

4.2.4.2   Open Jaw

Many American accents have an open jaw setting. Jimmy Stewart (1946) uses slightly open jaw in a classic style. The New York comedic styles of Henny Youngman and Milton Berle (1966) have slight or moderate open jaw settings. In the comedic style of Jerry Lewis (1961), jaw opening is more extreme. Frank Sutton's character Sgt. Vince Carter (1965) exaggerates jaw opening, as do Gilda Radner's *Saturday Night Live* character Roseanne Rosannadanna (1978b) and Bradley Cooper's *SNL* character Craig Kristofferson, parodying a California accent so that even close vowels have open jaw (2015). Such parodies often have a basis in accents that reflect familiar stereotypes and changing sociolinguistic patterns. Pratt and D'Onofrio (2017) explore this intertwining of language semiotics and embodied stereotypes in performance. Just as not all American accents have open jaw, not all accents of England have close jaw, but there are dialect affinities. The retroflex accents of the south coast of England (Newton 1954, Goodland 1981) tend to jaw opening – a plausible historical source for many North American speech settings.

4.2.4.3   Protruded Jaw

Many Scots adopt protruded jaw posture, particularly in broader accents. Sean Connery exemplifies protruded jaw in his portrayal of James Bond (1962, 1983) and in his everyday speech. Alex Salmond also demonstrates the lower lip position that results from protruded jaw posture (2014). Jim Nabors' character Gomer Pyle (1965) moves his jaw quite a bit, including protrusion (jutting). We have not discussed range of motion, but extreme excursions of the articulators exert a potentially strong effect on the perception of voice quality.

4.2.4.4   Labiodentalization

June Brown's character Dot and Gretchen Franklin's character Ethel in *East-Enders* (1985) mirror the old Cockney accent of London's East End. Retracting the jaw leaves the upper teeth to overbite the lower lip in a labiodentalized setting. Helen Morse's character Jean Paget in *A Town Like Alice* (1981) is slightly labiodentalized, in juxtaposition to the slightly protruded jaw (and lower lip) of Gordon Jackson's Scottish persona Noel Strachan and to the slightly unilateral upper lip raising of Bryan Brown's Australian archetype Joe Harman (see Section 4.2.5.4). Robert Glenister's character Ash Morgan in *Hustle* (2004), and to a lesser extent Marc Warren's character Danny Blue, portray London accents with slight labiodentalization. *Monty Python* 'Upper Class Twit of the Year' sketches parody the labiodentalized articulatory posture in an acrolectal English accent (1970). Although the characters hardly speak, the mere visual representation of this articulatory trait suffices to reference the social class accent. Footballer Luis Suárez (2014) demonstrates a distinctly labiodentalized posture, if not an explicitly retracted jaw. It is the task of sociophonetic research to separate idiosyncratic anatomical traits of accent from socially acquired dialect commonalities and to identify the prevalence of specific voice quality settings within a language community.

4.2.4.5   Laterally Offset Jaw

Extremely laterally offset jaw imbues Jim Carrey's character The Grinch with uniquely coloured vowels and enhanced sibilants (2000). Carrey's Grinch jaw setting is usually laterally offset to the right, but it often switches effortlessly to the left. The effect on vowels and consonants is similar, whichever side is selected. Jim Nabors (1965) also experiments with lateral jaw movement to good effect in prosodic/paralinguistic expression. Laterally offset jaw is a difficult articulatory posture to maintain, especially switching sides, as it interferes more than other postures with the function of the temporomandibular joint and therefore with mandibular, dental, and lingual alignment for chewing and speech. Overarticulated behaviour in any setting may be interpreted as disordered speech, where key diagnostic criteria apply (see Chapter 7).

4.2.5   Labial Settings

4.2.5.1   Close Rounding

Audrey Tautou (2010) illustrates an articulatory predisposition towards close rounding of the lips. Her constellation of postures characterizes one archetypal French accent (lowered larynx, nasality, dentalization, blade articulation, close jaw, lip rounding). Even front unrounded vowels such as /i/ undergo a type of rounding in this accent, enforcing the perception of long-term roundedness, even though the /i/ of French is traditionally described as unrounded. In this case, the rounding of /i/ differs in degree and character from the rounding on /y/, from which it must remain distinct. Although back rounded vowels are already rounded (technically not susceptible to roundedness), the close rounded setting can enhance rounding on homorganic segments, making them in effect hyper-rounded. In our example, initially unrounded segments may increase marginal lip-muscle contraction, while rounded vowels may acquire greater peripheral lip-muscle contraction as well as marginal sphinctering (see Honda et al. 1995b, Section 1.5.4). However, other complex labial adjustments may be required to keep a 'rounded /i/' auditorily distinct from /y/.

4.2.5.2 Open Rounding

Open rounding of the lips can be heard in some Norwegian accents. Jim Henson's Swedish Chef exaggerates this characteristic as an indexical token for comic effect (1975–90). Introducing a trademark singing style, Mick Jagger intersperses an open-rounded quality in his performance (1966, 1978), so that front unrounded vowels in particular are influenced by the open and protruded labial posture. This stylistic effect is applied effectively to the maximally susceptible /eɪ/ vowel in the pronunciation of 'name' and 'game' (Jagger 1968), lending a front-rounded quality. The change brought about by the superimposed setting replaces the usual quality of the vowels with different vowels altogether.

Files illustrating Norwegian open rounding (one in English read by a Norwegian who does not speak English) can be found in the media examples.

4.2.5.3 Labial Spreading (Spread Lips)

Howie Mandel's early comedic style (1981), characterized by extreme labial spreading, probably helped induce smiles from the audience. Rod Serling (1959–64) complements close jaw with spread lips. Bricio Segovia (2012) uses labial spreading in Spanish together with upper-lip raising. Michael Dawson's North Yorkshire accent is also spread lipped (2013). Sean Bean often adopts labial spreading for his character Richard Sharpe (1993–97), which mirrors his own South Yorkshire accent. It is noteworthy that his labial setting has both horizontal and vertical expansion (see Laver 1980: 36–37).

Labial spreading (shortening the front vocal tract) contrasts acoustically with close rounding (lengthening the front vocal tract) by raising formant frequencies. Unlike laryngeal settings, we suspect that the auditory and visual correlates of spreading vs. rounding are commonly identified because of their familiar role in vowel production and in describing vowel quality phonetically.

4.2.5.4   Upper-Lip Effects

The upper lip can adopt symmetrical or asymmetrical vertical expansion as a habitual posture. We observe that many Castilian Spanish speakers raise both sides of the upper lip. In the standard Castilian Spanish of Bricio Segovia (2012), dentalized lingual advancement and horizontal lip expansion are accompanied by an upper-lip posture that exposes the upper teeth. Spanish television presenters Marta Jaumandreu and Francisco José Caro (2013) illustrate the same setting. Mónica Esgueva (2014) articulates her Castilian consonants by raising the upper lip and expanding the lips horizontally. It is fundamental in voice quality theory to ask whether this elevated superior labial setting facilitates the production of segmental articulations in the consonantal and vocalic inventory of Iberian Spanish, with dental stops [t̪ d̪], a dental fricative [θ], and a fricative with distinctive sibilance that could be represented as [s̠] or as [s̺] (an apical postalveolar fricative). In theory, it is hypothesized that a habitual articulatory posture facilitates or predisposes the production of the rapidly fluctuating segments (Honikman 1964), or at least that it should not hinder their production by imposing a contrary basis for reaching the segmental target. As a research question, it could be hypothesized that the raising of the upper lip facilitates the rapid production of the distinction between /θ/ and /s/ in Castilian Spanish (Martínez-Celdrán et al. 2003), as opposed to the labial setting of other varieties of Spanish that have only /s/. To stimulate research, we observe that the setting and these tongue-front targets co-occur.

Unilateral raising of the upper lip can be found in some Australian English accents. Australian accent expert Alanna (2012) demonstrates this online. Slightly unilateral upper-lip raising appears in the speech of Bob Katter (2013), Bryan Brown (1981), and Hugh Jackman (2008). Edward G. Robinson (1948) was noted for unilateral horizontal and vertical expansion, usually to the right, aided or even induced by habitual cigar smoking. A theoretical question posed here is whether modifying long-term lip position asymmetrically facilitates the articulation of some consonants or vowels in those accents. One functional element of the observed Australian setting is that it accompanies diphthongized pronunciations of close vowels /i/ and /u/. Such modifications have been hypothesized to be facilitative in peripheral vowel shifting (Labov and Kim 2015).

4.3 Other Realizations of Laryngeal Constriction

4.3.1 Glottalization and Laryngealization

A sound sequence is glottalized when its coarticulatory gesture involves a glottal stop, i.e. closing the glottis (Esling et al. 2005). By extension, a sound sequence is epiglottalized when its coarticulatory gesture involves an epiglottal stop (completely closing the airway). A sound sequence is laryngealized when its coarticulatory gesture involves narrowing the laryngeal constrictor mechanism to produce a continuant with one of a number of constricted qualities. These can include creakiness, harshness, ventricular voice, or aryepiglottic trilling. The term pharyngealized is applied when the secondary quality is a resonance rather than a vibratory pattern. One low falling tone in Hanoi Vietnamese illustrates glottalization (Kirby 2011). It is low in pitch and short, tone 21, with a slightly pharyngealized (raised-larynx) component finishing in a glottal stop 21-ʔ, contrasting with a longer, breathier (lowered-larynx) 21 tone. The so-called 'broken tone' or 'interrupted tone' is also glottalized. It is a mid-rise interrupted by a glottal stop 2-ʔ-4. With glottalization, laryngealization can also occur before or after the glottal stop component, while the glottis is closing or opening.

Mpi, a Tibeto-Burman language investigated by Jimmy G. Harris, also in the UCLA database (Ladefoged and Maddieson 1996: 315–317), has a laryngealized series, marked by greater constriction of the laryngeal articulator. The laryngealized quality is generally creaky voice; however, even in the same speaker, the quality can change with tone. Because creak is 'cleaner' at lower pitch, lower tones have purer creaky voice, while higher tones have a tighter or harsher quality. Some speakers may use harsh creak or harsh voice in general, but the constricted series is always tighter than the laryngeally open series. In its resonance quality, the laryngealized/creaky series is articulated with raised-larynx voice or pharyngealized voice, depending on pitch height, as a product of the aryepiglottic constriction that is also responsible for laryngealized phonation. Glottal squeaks sometimes occur after glottalized obstruents (Redi and Shattuck-Hufnagel 2001, Hejná et al. 2016), adding complexity to the association between laryngeal constriction and pitch, perhaps revealing dual possibilities arising from the tense vocal fold body (in contrast to its increased mass per unit length and slackened cover) needed for glottalization.

The Jimmy G. Harris files illustrating the phonemic contrasts in Mpi are among the media illustrations:

[si] 33 open (a colour)	[si̱] 33 constricted (a classifier)
[si] 45 open 'four'	[si̱] 45 constricted (a name)
[si] 35 open 'to roll a rope'	[si̱] 35 constricted 'to smoke'
[si] 13 open 'to be putrid'	[si̱] 13 constricted 'to be dried up'
[si] 52 open 'to die'	[si̱] 52 constricted (a name)
[si] 21 open 'blood'	[si̱] 21 constricted 'seven'

Two low-tonal pairs in Hanoi Vietnamese illustrate contrasting laryngeal articulator options. Two higher long tones are included for comparison. One low falling tone is breathy with a lower larynx, i.e. signalling an open laryngeal mechanism; the second is glottalized, i.e. constricted, with a closing epilaryngeal tube and rising larynx. One low rising tone is open, i.e. unconstricted; the second is glottalized, but word internally instead of finally. At the constricted end of the continuum, any of the possibilities concomitant with a constricted laryngeal articulator can occur, here primarily laryngealization through an increasingly compressed lower-vocal-tract mechanism:

> [dɔ̌ː] high rising 'accordingly'
> [dɔ̄ː] (high) mid level 'measure'
> [dɔ̰̀ː] low falling (lowered larynx, breathy) 'small river ferry'
> [dɔ̀ˀʔ] low falling, checked (raised larynx, constricted) 'to compare, (boxing) bout'
> [dɔ̌ː] low rising (open, modal) 'red'
> [dɔ̌ʔɔ̰] low rising, broken (glottal interrupted, laryngealized) 'apiary'

4.3.2   *Laryngeal Constriction in Segmental Contrast*

Languages described as having a pharyngeal place of articulation in their phonology use the laryngeal articulator to produce short-term sounds. The segments /ħ ʕ/ in Semitic are a function of the aryepiglottic constrictor. They may contrast with /h/, with no constriction, and /ʔ/, with slight constriction. In Moroccan Arabic, /ħ ʕ/ are produced with supraglottic constriction stronger than whispered or creaky [i] (Zeroual et al. 2008). In Iraqi Arabic, trilling sometimes occurs on /ħ/ and /ʕ/; prevalently in the case of geminates /ħħ/ and /ʕʕ/, which become trilled [ʜː] and [ˤʔ] where the [ʔ] stop effect dominates due to a dramatic decrease in amplitude of vibratory pulses and of noise as the epilaryngeal tube reduces in volume (Hassan et al. 2011; see analyses in Chapter 3). In Tigrinya, there is also a four-way contrast between /h ʔ ħ ʕ/. The prevalence of pharyngeals in Semitic languages can be enough to lend an utterance a long-term pharyngealized voice quality. The Austronesian language Amis also has epiglottal stop [ʔ] and aryepiglottic trilling [ʜ] (Edmondson et al. 2005). A Saudi Arabian tap reflex of /r/ has been reported with aryepiglottic trilling (Heselwood and Maghrabi 2016) and could be transcribed as [r̝ˤ]. Languages of the northwest coast of North America also contain pharyngeals. The Wakashan language Nuuchahnulth of Ahousaht is documented as having /ħ ʕ/ phonologically (Jacobsen 1969), but phonetically they are [ħ ʔ] (Carlson et al. 2001). In the 'Story of Sea Lion', narrated by George Louie in the Department of Linguistics at the University of Victoria, the pronunciation of /ħ ʕ/ in the speech of a young man transformed into a sea lion may be realized as trilled [ʜ ʢ], with repeated interjection of sustained [ʜʢ͡e:] or [ʜʢ͡a:] (Esling 1996), giving the altered voice the harsh long-term quality of aryepiglottic trilling. Interior Salish languages of British Columbia, Spokane/Kalispel (Npoqínišcn/Qalispé) (Carlson and Flett 1989), Nxaʔamxčín (Czaykowska-Higgins 1998) and Nlaka'pamuxcín (Carlson et al. 2004), illustrate what have been described as voiced pharyngeals /ʕ ʕʷ/ and 'glottalized pharyngeals' /ʕ' ʕʷ'/. The latter are more accurately described phonetically as epiglottal stops [ʡ ʡʷ] (Carlson and Esling 2000). Some pharyngeals may be rendered with uvulars, and even many of the uvulars in Nlaka'pamuxcín are likely to be produced with secondary pharyngealization, signalling the potential for a sound shift (Carlson and Esling 2003). That these articulations are in fact different manners performed by the laryngeal articulator is an important basis for determining the voice quality of the language, since the laryngeal constrictor mechanism explains how the pharynx is related to the glottis. It is also important to observe that, despite similar transcriptions, different languages render the sounds differently, because the options for combining with the laryngeal articulator are so broad. Consequently, although these are segmental articulations, secondary modifications that accompany each sound may constitute part of the voice quality component of accent. These simultaneous gestures can interact to function as a vehicle for sound change (see Chapter 8).

The four-way glottal and pharyngeal/epiglottal contrast in Tigrinya /h ʔ ħ ʡ/ is illustrated with media files. The videos of Tigrinya [hi:] and [ʔi:] illustrate particularly well how the aryepiglottic constrictor compacts the epilaryngeal tube, then the tongue retracts as the larynx elevates. The contrasts in Nuuchahnulth include:

[ha:] 'yes'
[wi:ʔu:] 'nephew'
[ħu:w] 'over there'
[ʔɪħu:] 'to cry after'

Instances of paralinguistic aryepiglottic trilling from the Sea Lion story are also illustrated.

The contrast between the production of glottal stop and epiglottal stop in Nlaka'pamuxcín is also illustrated:

[ʔimˀnmˀ] 'make a noise' (initial glottal stop /ʔ/ and two glottalized /mˀ/ in the word)

[nː -paˤʔʷ] 'ice' (This stop is labialized /ʔʷ/, as opposed to plain /ʔ/.)

In Spokane (Npoqíniščn), a language that contrasts plain and labialized velars, uvulars, and pharyngeals (including some ejectives), it is not surprising that there should be a four-way distinction between /ʕ ʕʷ ʔ ʔʷ/. It is also possible that there is some ambiguity in the phonetic realization of all occurrences, given the scope for sound change in such a system.

/pʔiʧ/ [pʰə̣ʔˈiʧ] 'bear grass, skunk cabbage'
/ʕaw-n/ [ˤawən] 'to name someone, to read'
/ʕʷos-n/ [ʕʷːɔ·sn̩] 'I lost it'
/hi-ˈʕʷił/ [hiəˈʕʷɨɬ] 'it is one piece'
/tsaʔʔ/ [tsˤa̰ʔə̣] 'crow'
/maʔʷ-t/ [maˑʷʔʷə̣tʰə̰] 'broken'

Iraqi Arabic items illustrate /h ʔ ħ ʕ/ and the phonetic realizations [ʕ ʕ ħ ʔ]. The versatility of the laryngeal mechanism allows it to move quickly (for a pharyngeal tap [ʕ]), to supplement glottal voicing with aryepiglottic periodicity [ʕ], to use only aryepiglottic vibration [ħ], and to close the airway entirely with epiglottal stop [ʔ]:

/hiib/ [hiːb̤] 'digging tool'
/ʔiid/ [ʔiːd̥] 'hand'
/hanna/ [ħɐnːa] 'Hanna (name)'
/ʕiid/ [ʕiːd̥] 'festival'
/saʕiid/ [saʕiːd̥] 'happy'
/ʕanna/ [ˤʕɑnːə] 'on his behalf'
/saħħar/ [sɑħːar] 'made magic'
/saʕʕiid/ [sɑ̰ʔiːd̥] 'make people happy'

The Caucasian language Agul, described in Ladefoged and Maddieson (1996: 38, 167–170) and archived in (2009), offers a clear example of an epiglottal stop /ʔ/. Agul is also represented as contrasting two voiceless pharyngeal continuants. The one symbolized as pharyngeal /ħ/ can be described using the terminology proposed here as a voiceless pharyngeal fricative with lowered larynx, i.e. expanded lower cavity resonance. The one sounding more constricted and symbolized as epiglottal /ʜ/ can be described as a voiceless pharyngeal (aryepiglottic) fricative with raised larynx, potentially a voiceless pharyngeal trill. The voiced pharyngeal approximant /ʕ/ of Agul sounds slightly trilled in one example, but the purported /ʕ/ is not represented in the database. These contrasts are analysed in Moisik (2013: 410–415).

Catford's auditory evaluation that /ʜ/ and /ʢ/ are more 'genuinely fricative' than /ħ/ and /ʕ/ (1990: 26) is supported by our interpretation that they are fricatives with the addition of aryepiglottic trilling. Since trilling mimics glottal phonation as a vibratory source, the contrast between these two pairs of sounds could be framed as the overlay of a phonatory quality.

Many Germanic varieties demonstrate a relationship between approximant consonants, specifically /r/ in many cases, and vowel quality. A pharyngeal component has been identified in American English [-ɹ] (Redi and Shattuck-Hufnagel 2001). In Standard Southern English, three of the vocalic coda /-r/ realizations [ɪə ɛə ɑː ɔː ʊə ɜː] are monophthongal, without the schwa reflex (Roach 2004). The [ɔː] in particular reflects retracted vowel quality and the potential for laryngeal constriction to occur. This potentiality even affects Jones's production of Cardinal Vowel 6 (1956). Australian unstressed coda /-ər/ can have an open vocalic quality, described as [ɐ] by Harrington et al. (1997) as in 'here' [hɪːɐ]. Its quality can move towards the retracted corner of the vowel space, with the potential to engage the laryngeal articulator (viz. Alanna (2012) or New Zealand actor Sara Wiseman).

Northern British varieties may have a more pharyngealized variant of the final-/r/ schwa reflex. Some Lancashire dialects realize /-r/ as a pharyngealized vowel. John Henshaw's character Wilf Bradshaw (2002–05) often performs the schwa coda as [ɔˤ], viz 'here, year'. Stuart-Smith (2007) describes Glasgow working-class adolescents' coda /-r/ realizations as laryngeally constricted gestures, i.e. as [ʢ], retracted vowel qualities, laryngealization, or as pharyngeal frication [ħ]. Lennon et al. (2015) present evidence that only pharyngealization in the /-r/ context distinguishes pairs such as 'hut/hurt', 'bust/burst'. The same phonetic realization has been observed in working-class Edinburgh adolescents' accents, with only a pharyngealized quality being audible, although a silent lingual consonantal gesture may still be detected, using ultrasound, after the sound has finished (Lawson et al. 2015). Upper Saxon German is the archetype of coda [oˤ] for /-ər/, in addition to pharyngealized long vowels in the /r/ environment [ʊˤː oˤː ɔˤː ʌˤː aˤː] (Khan and Weise 2013). Wolfgang Stumph (1989) and Uwe Steimle (2015) illustrate the Dresden variants of these sounds. The Chemnitz renditions in the Khan and Weise (2013) *Journal of the International Phonetic Association* illustration are clearly pharyngeal. Günter Grünwald's character Danilo aus Sachsen (2013) parodies these regional indicators, in juxtaposition with Bavarian dialect. In another sketch (2011), although the imitation of the pharyngealized sounds of Upper Saxon is not as strong as other vocalic, consonantal, and prosodic aspects, Grünwald's comedic switch into his Bavarian accent embodies lowered-larynx voice, contrasting dramatically with the pharyngealized (raised-larynx) Saxon setting. The /-r/ of older Parisian French dialect, as in northern Picard dialects, can be realized as [ʕ], which also occurs as a paralinguistic marker independently of the /r/ environment. Guy Lecluyse's character Yann Vandernoout (2008) performs /-r/ as a pharyngeal in his 'ch'timi' dialect representations. A preponderance of such pharyngealized items in a stretch of speech in this dialect lends a generalized auditory character of pharyngealization to the speaker's voice quality.

From the perspective of the Laryngeal Articulator Model, these segmental adaptations engage the laryngeal constrictor, establishing a link between the oral vocal tract and the laryngeal vocal tract. Any such link creates a potential for parallel effects to lend new qualities to utterances of varying duration. The frequency or persistence of these effects can contribute to the perception of voice quality. Because of the complexity of the laryngeal articulator, the variety of possible concomitant effects goes far beyond the familiar link between oral stops and the timing of glottal opening and closing or glottal phonation type, which usually do not persist beyond segmental duration. The laryngeal articulator allows creakiness, harshness, aryepiglottic trilling, or other vibratory effects, as well as pharyngealization or other resonances due to epilaryngeal-tube constriction or larynx height, to enter multiple levels of the sound stream.

4.3.3   *Laryngeal Constriction in Syllabic Contrast*

It has been pointed out (viz. Delattre 1971) that pharyngeals may occur in European languages, mostly as subtle vowel-quality effects. More overtly, Danish stød is largely predictable by syllable structure, there are numerous minimal pairs, and it is generally regarded as 'a laryngeal syllable rhyme prosody' (Basbøll 2014). Considering its attributed descriptive referents, such as 'creaky voice', 'laryngealization', glottal stop, compressed character, intensity drop, and pitch effects (Grønnum 1998, Grønnum et al. 2013, Hansen 2015), stød is consistent with our description of laryngeal constrictor action. That 'the stød/non-stød distinction is a difference in laryngealized versus modal voice' (Grønnum et al. 2013: 70) is accounted for globally by laryngeal constriction and its co-related effects. Fischer-Jørgensen (1989) offers a comprehensive instrumental account of stød effects, as does Hansen (2015), corresponding elegantly with our LAM interpretation. Both also observe that the stops /t, k/ affricate when they occur initially in syllables containing stød – perhaps an enhancement in force across the syllable, as we have found where labial trilling increases in tense-register syllables in Nuosu Yi (see below). Lindqvist-Gauffin (1972) speculated on the historical relationship between low tone, laryngealization, and glottal stop, citing the instance of the development of stød (see Lindblom 2009).

Laryngoscopic videos of Danish illustrate how degrees of laryngeal constriction produce the phonetic effects that accompany instances of stød – a suprasegmental effect on certain syllables in Danish with various possible phonetic realizations, all consistent with narrowing/tightening of the laryngeal constrictor mechanism. Despite deficiencies in the representativeness of the recorded data, the performance of items with stød reflects categories of sounds that we expect to observe in a constricted context, such as laryngealization in general, creaky voice in particular, glottal stop, larynx raising, and degrees of pharyngeal resonance. The performance of items without stød involves sounds consistent with an open laryngeal mechanism (modal voice, lack of glottal stop or of larynx raising or of pharyngeal resonance). The falling pitch in these citation-context performances of words with stød, contrasting with rising pitch on words without stød, although not obligatory, is consistent with the presence of laryngeal constriction as a vehicle for lowering pitch. The presence of any one of these attributes of laryngeal constriction would be enough to signal stød. Videos 1–5 contain two instances of each item in a minimal pair, the first with stød, the second without. In Video 6, the order is reversed (stød second). The Danish words are spoken by a female speaker and a male speaker. Stød is represented by superscript glottal stop [$^{?}$] in the phonemic notation:

1 væsen /ˈvɛːˀsn̩/ 'creature'   hvæsen /ˈvɛːsn̩/ 'hiss'
2 hvalen /ˈvæːˀln̩/ 'the whale'   valen /ˈvæːln̩/ 'half-hearted'
3 musen /ˈmuːˀsn̩/ 'the mouse'   musen /ˈmuːsn̩/ 'the Muse'
4 moden /ˈmoːˀðn̩/ 'ripe'   moden /ˈmoːðn̩/ 'the fashion'
5 skal /sɡ̊alˀ/ 'shell'   skal /sɡ̊al/ 'must'
6 man /man/ 'one, you'   mand /manˀ/ 'man'

Languages that use the laryngeal articulator to contrast resonances over the duration of a syllable take advantage of constriction (for pharyngealization) vs. a neutral or modal setting, or larynx lowering, which in turn may be low pitched or higher pitched (faucalized). Some languages add vibratory contrasts (constricted vs. non-constricted). These 'register' differences have often been termed (narrowly) differences in voice quality. Even at the syllabic level, the laryngeal articulator effect introduces interactions between vowel quality and voice quality, often supplemented in these languages with tonal quality. Thurgood (2017) reports that speakers of Iu-Mien exploit the phonetic interplay between pitch and register by alternating laryngealized quality variably with modal quality (between the first and last tone-2 pitch) to differentiate a low 232 tone over the duration of a vowel.

The Tibeto-Burman language Nuosu Yi of Sichuan contrasts a 'lax' series with a 'tense' series (Edmondson et al. 2017). Lax syllables have modal voice (as a baseline, since individual speakers will always vary). The predominant resonance quality of the tense series is raised-larynx voice (Lama 1991). Tense vowels of the five syllabic pairs have a distinctly laryngeally constricted posture, with a more retracted oral vowel quality, while the lax vowels are unconstricted (Lama 2012). The constricted acoustic signature of the tense vowels makes their quality more retracted in vocalic terms, or pharyngealized (elevated F1, slightly reduced F2), than their lax counterparts. Most minimal pairs occur at mid tone, since constriction favours low tone and laxness high tone. It is significant that bilabial trilling [ʙ̥ ʙ] accompanying front consonants is enhanced in the tense/constricted vowel series, ostensibly a function of increased force, as postulated for Danish (above). In Bruu, a Mon-Khmer language (UCLA 2009), we interpret tones described as having 'stiff vocal cords' and 'tense vocal tract walls' as the result of aryepiglottic constriction and larynx raising, judging by their auditory contrast to the 'non-stiff' series. The Tibeto-Burman language Bai of Jianchuan, Yunnan, contrasts a lax series with a tense series over five tones (Edmondson et al. 2001). Eight syllables are oral, and seven can be nasalized. At mid 33 tone, the lax register is modal, but the tense register is harsh. Lax syllables become breathy voiced at 31 tone, and harsh tense syllables become harsher, with vibrations (trilling) occurring at the inner mucosa of the epilarynx or at the aryepiglottic folds at low 21 tone. At 55 tone, lax syllables are modal, but tense counterparts add constriction, which results in a quality similar to pressed voice (constriction at high pitch) and elevating pitch to 55+. Bai provides a key to the interpretation of voice quality. Viewed as a register, voice quality differs on each of fifteen syllables in Bai; viewed as a long-term setting, voice quality in Bai could be an amalgamation of all of these elements; but that would require a sociophonetic analysis of speakers within the community. High-pitched constriction (55+) is one realization of harshness; harsh constriction in the middle pitch range (33+, 31+) assumes a massed vibratory character; and harsh vibration at low pitch (21) is compatible with adding vibration from the ventricular or aryepiglottic levels. It may be that voice quality setting in such a language is more a question of proportionate fluctuation across competing forms than of permanently maintained postures (in this case, of the laryngeal articulator).

Figure 4.1 in the companion material enumerates the fifteen-way syllabic tonal register contrast in Jianchuan Bai. A laryngoscopic video illustrates each syllable, demonstrating the mix of phonological register contrasts that combine to generate long-term laryngeal settings. We are grateful to Li Shaoni and Jerry Edmondson for this analysis and to Li Shaoni for the recorded items.

Somali has two series, or registers, contrasting laryngeally constricted syllables with lowered-larynx syllables that may be termed faucalized if tone is high, lowered-larynx voice if tone is low. The Nilotic language Dinka of Bor, South Sudan, has a four-way register distinction – modal vs. breathy vs. pharyngealized vs. faucalized (Edmondson and Esling 2006). The latter has been called 'hollow' in the literature. Modal voicing contrasts with a lowered-larynx posture that maximizes openness (breathy register), similar to the way that lax register behaves in Bai. Constriction with larynx raising (pharyngealized register) contrasts with a lowered-larynx posture that lacks open breathiness (faucalized register).

The two registers in Somali are illustrated: /dʕ̰d/ 'to faint' has a constricted laryngeal articulator setting (moderately narrowed epilaryngeal tube, larynx slightly raised); /dʕ̥d/ 'to refuse' has an open laryngeal articulator setting (not constricted, larynx lowered). The tongue fronts for the [iː] in both cases. Several diacritics could indicate a contrast in the posture of the laryngeal constrictor. The raising and lowering diacritics used here emphasize the raising and lowering of the larynx differentiating the two series, even though larynx height is not explicitly mentioned in the chart of the IPA. The retracting and advancing diacritics [i̱ i̟] could be recruited to refer to the constrictor mechanism, but the 'ATR' emphasis on the tongue's role in constriction is not sufficient here. Reducing the vowel *and* adding the retraction symbol [ɪ] is the practice in Padayodi (2008) where both vowel quality and phonatory quality are symbolized. Narrowing the constrictor produces similar effects and transcription preferences ([ɛ]) in Nuosu Yi (Edmondson et al. 2017). Other retracted and advanced diacritics [ˍ ˎ] could be used, although these are usually applied to vowels. A retracted subscript [i̠] is an acceptable phonemic marker. If phonation is involved in the distinction, as in Bai, a subscript tilde, or two in the case of 21 tone, can convey degrees of harshness, although that does not apply to Somali.

Languages exhibiting the [–ATR] (not advanced, or possibly retracted tongue root) vocalic phenomenon are another case of a constricted ([–ATR]) posture contrasting with an unconstricted ([+ATR]) aryepiglottic posture. Lindau's x-rays (1979) identify pharynx width and larynx height as the key elements that distinguish the 'expanded pharynx' vowel set and the 'constricted pharynx' vowel set in Akan (Twi). Lindau's observation that [+ATR] is independent of raising of the tongue body is crucial, because it signals that [+ATR] is not primarily a lingual distinction. Tiede's MRI data confirm that overall pharyngeal volumes, beyond movements of the tongue root alone, define the contrast in Akan (1996). From the perspective of the LAM, both the x-ray and MRI data need to be interpreted through the functioning of the aryepiglottic constrictor mechanism, which is challenging because its actions cross a number of diagonal planes that do not all appear in a single image. Constriction tightens the aryepiglottic constrictor while raising the larynx and retracting the tongue in the [–ATR] set, with the consequence that vowels sound more open/retracted than the vowels in the corresponding [+ATR] set, in which the laryngeal constrictor opens while lowering the larynx and advancing the tongue to expand the pharynx. The vowel-quality effect in the constricted set is acoustically similar to producing an open vowel such as [ɑ]: raising F1 and lowering F2, as in pharyngealization. This interpretation accounts for the vowel-quality distinctions in experimental observations of Igbo and Akan (Ladefoged and Maddieson 1996: 300–302). In her illustration of Igbo, Ikekeonwu (1999) associates the four vowels in the more fronted harmony set [i e o u] with Lindau's 'expanded pharynx' category. The four vowels in the more retracted harmony set [ɪ a ɔ ʊ] are auditorily constricted through the epilaryngeal tube, giving them the acoustic characteristics of vowel openness. In her illustration of Kabiye, Padayodi (2008) describes the constricted ([–ATR] = [+RTR]) syllables as a function of aryepiglottic constriction, so that [ɪ ɛ ɔ ʊ] are marked for both vowel quality and laryngeal register vs. unconstricted [i e o u], with an [a] vowel that varies allophonically. The variety of Akan described by Lindau has this same vowel system, while some varieties of Akan, such as the one we illustrate here, contrasts a fifth pair [a ɑ] (Edmondson et al. 2007). It is important to remember that the more open vowel set is retracted lingually but is also laryngeally constricted, predisposing the larynx to elevate towards the tongue. The tendency of vowels to have increased F1, decreased F2, and also decreased F3 in some dialects in the retracted set is consistent with the effects of laryngeal constriction, as in pharyngealization. Moisik (2013: 293–308) confirms the F3 lowering effect of larynx raising. Increased F1 for all [–ATR] vowels and decreased F2 for most [–ATR] vowels – consistent with aryepiglottic constriction and larynx raising – is also reported in the Nilotic language Lopit (Billington 2017). Similar acoustic results are found for the Tungusic language Even (Aralova et al. 2011), suggesting a system that also patterns along laryngeal constriction lines.

The laryngeal constrictor in Nuosu Yi is observed to behave as in 'ATR' languages. Notwithstanding the global folding action of the aryepiglottic mechanism, each language may organize its phonological space on the basis of different components of constrictor action, and different vowels within a given system may respond variably to those effects. In the nine Nuosu Yi minimal pairs, the second (tense) counterpart illustrates the tubular narrowing of the laryngeal articulator that affects resonance to shift register and alter vowel quality towards openness. Fieldwork and analyses were carried out by Jerold Edmondson and Ziwo Lama. Detailed transcriptions and illustrations of the sound system can be found in Edmondson et al. (2017).

The four registers of Bor Dinka differentiate modal voice [tʰik] 'woman' (neutral setting), breathy voice [tʰe̤e̤k] 'action' (more open phonation), harsh voice [tʰɪ̰ˤk] 'divide' (more constricted tube *and* phonation, elevated larynx), and faucalized [tʰi*k] 'chin' (open tube but *lowered larynx *without lowering pitch*) (Edmondson and Esling 2006: 185–188). The distinctions exploit 'cardinal corners' of laryngeal contrast: phonatory quality, sphincteric tightening, and larynx height (with concomitant effects on vowel quality).

Minimal pairs in 'ATR' languages Akan and Kabiye demonstrate the role of laryngeal constriction in the register contrast. Akan files /tú/ 'pull out by the roots' and /tʊ̠́/ 'to throw' show how reducing vowel quality parallels tightening of the constrictor with larynx raising, as do /midí/ 'I eat' and /mɪ̠dɪ̠̀/ 'I am called'. The configurational shift in Kabiye from /tú/ 'elephant' to /tʊ̠́/ 'bee' and from /lò/ 'cut at (imper)' to /lɔ̠̀/ 'thatch (imper)' also illustrates the effects of laryngeal constriction. Analyses of Kabiye were carried out by Cécile Padayodi.

In a role similar to register tone, 'strident' vowels in !Xóõ (Traill 1986) are produced by a tightened laryngeal constrictor, causing the aryepiglottic folds to vibrate (see Figure 1.4). The quality is similar to a number of singing-voice qualities recognized by Yanagisawa et al. (1989) and Honda et al. (1995a) (see examples in Section 4.1.2.6). Secondarily epiglottalized vowels in N|uu (Miller et al. 2009) and Ju|'hoansi (Miller-Ockhuizen 2003, Miller 2007) are reported to have non-modal phonation due to laryngeal constriction, and acoustic analysis confirms the presence of epilaryngeal vibration in N|uu (Moisik 2013: 119–131).

4.3.4 *Throat Singing*

The multifaceted art of throat singing exploits articulatory movements and airflow through the entire vocal tract as well as the interspersed timing of productions by the oral articulators and the laryngeal articulator. The singing instructions accompanying *Deep in the Heart of Tuva* (Leighton 1996) implicate the laryngeal articulator as primary, comparing different styles to Kermit the Frog (sygyt), Howlin' Wolf or Wolfman Jack (khöömei), or Popeye (kargyraa) voice qualities. The instructions to produce sygyt include: making a Kermit voice (establishing a narrowed epilaryngeal tube and reduced pharyngeal volume), curling the tongue back (adding rear-oral-tract resonances), protruding the lips (adding front-oral-tract resonances), and making the voice nasal (coupling nasal resonances) (Ondar 1996). Tuning a harmonic to align with the narrowly peaked resonance this produces in the mid-frequency range (similar to the typical F3 of a North American English /r/) will generate the overtone effect. Vibratory effects linked to laryngeal constriction, such as aryepiglottic trilling or vocal-ventricular coupling, are characteristic of kargyraa. Tanya Tagaq's Inuit throat singing (2014) illustrates exceptional timing alternations between a range of laryngeal articulations and rapid oral articulations, fricatives and different degrees of closure of the airway, and varying egressive and ingressive airflow.

The laryngeal articulator, as observed and described here, is also the likely source of the so-called 'glottal whistle' which David Abercrombie taught his students at the University of Edinburgh. Moolenaar-Bijl (1957) described it as a 'laryngeal whistle', and Catford characterized the glottal whistle as 'voiceless falsetto... partly due to a kind of wake turbulence – in this case, periodic vortex-formation in the turbulent wake of airflow past the thinned edges of the vocal folds' (1977a: 38). A sound originating in the throat, it could reportedly be produced by some as a true whistle, even during labial closure. This implies that the sound is postuvular, but it is unclear how the whistle could be solely glottal. Optimal narrowing of the immediate supraglottal space, between the ventricular folds and continuing between the angled aryepiglottic folds and the base of the epiglottis, could provide the channelling necessary to effect a whistle. This manner of constriction is essentially the same as for a pharyngeal fricative but with the correct angle and aim to produce a sine wave, just as the fricative [s] may be channelled between the tongue front, teeth, and lips into a whistle. This interpretation conforms with Moolenaar-Bijl's description of an 'inclination of the epiglottis, together with a narrowing of the pharynx' (1957: 166). The most reasonable hypothesis at this stage, consistent with the LAM, is that the whistle is a fine adjustment of the laryngeal constrictor and vertical larynx positioning.

5 Phonological Implications of Voice Quality Theory

Chapter 5 explores the implications of the Laryngeal Articulator Model for phonology and the place of voice quality in phonological analysis. The chapter begins with a brief consideration of previous theoretical treatments that neglect to posit a direct connection between the laryngeal and supralaryngeal systems – a gap that parallels the linear source-filter dichotomization of the lower and upper vocal tracts. The Laryngeal Articulator Model has implications for linguistic theory, providing deeper phonetic grounding at numerous levels of phonological argument. The LAM provides the possibility of a laryngeal phonetic approach to phonological theory, implemented as the Phonological Potentials Model (PPM) introduced by Moisik et al. (2019), that formalizes the essential intersection between phonation, tone, vowel quality, and global vocal tract states that underlie the concept of voice quality. Several illustrative cases demonstrate the analysis of both synchronic and diachronic phonological processes.

Voice quality is not an explicit part of phonological theory; however, voice quality is unavoidably a strand of accent and a component of phonetic theory. In Laver's notion of 'figure to ground' (1980: 5), segments are the figures that appear against the background of articulatory settings, signifying a link between the voice quality level and phonology. Labov expressed the relationship of articulatory setting to segmental phonology elegantly in his sociolinguistic analysis of 'old Yankee' speech on Martha's Vineyard.

> There are no less than fourteen phonological variables which follow the general rule that the higher, or more constricted variants are characteristic of the up-island, 'native' speakers, while the lower, more open variants are characteristic of down-island speakers under mainland influence. We can reasonably assume that this 'close-mouthed' articulatory style is the object of social affect. It may well be that social evaluation interacts with linguistic structures at this point, through the constriction of several dimensions of phonological space. Particular linguistic variables would then be variously affected by the overall tendency towards a favored articulatory posture, under the influence of the social forces which we have been studying. (Labov 1963: 307, 1972: 40)

Labov's observation encapsulates what a closer jaw setting imparts to various segmental articulatory preferences. Settings of the laryngeal articulator can also have a profound effect on segmental articulations, and reconstructing the vocal tract as a composite two-part articulator implies changing existing phonological assumptions and constructs. The descriptive terminology used in the literature for laryngeal events and for vowel systems that contrast in their laryngeal settings has left a confused array of phonological interpretations (with sometimes conflicting conclusions). The Phonological Potentials Model (PPM) outlined in this chapter takes all of these descriptive traditions into account and provides a more phonetically coherent approach by unifying these phonological tendencies as realizations of voice quality potentials.

Sounds of the lower vocal tract (LVT), which involve articulatory activity of the larynx and pharynx, have posed challenges for traditional phonological analysis (Clements and Hume 1995, Rice 2011). Unlike sounds made in the upper vocal tract (UVT), many LVT sounds intertwine phonation and articulation together, and their production often entails broad changes to vocal tract shape, not just localized articulatory movements. These aspects are not well represented by current theoretical models of phonology. Revising phonological constructs from the perspective of how the UVT and LVT function together phonetically, specifying the potentials for interaction, gives us an opportunity to relate prevailing phonological processes in a language to the language's long-term speech postures – to begin to build a relationship between the phonology of a language and its voice quality settings.

5.1   Voice Quality in Phonological Theory: Previous Approaches

The general contemporary approach to the phonology of LVT sounds derives from, on the one hand, the arguments of Halle and Stevens (1971) concerning the features relevant for describing laryngeal state, and on the other, those of Hayward and Hayward (1989) and McCarthy (1994) for a guttural (or post-velar) natural class formed by laryngeal, pharyngeal, and uvular sounds. The difficulty these proposals face is in accounting for the (phonological) coupling between the laryngeal and supralaryngeal systems. A few researchers, however, have identified a relationship between gutturals and other sounds or sound classes which exhibit a link between the larynx and pharynx (Colarusso 1985, Czaykowska-Higgins 1987, Trigo 1991, Halle 1995). These include 'tense', 'head', or 'harsh' vocal registers in Tibeto-Burman and Mon-Khmer languages and in cross-height or so-called 'ATR' harmony languages of Niger-Congo and Nilo-Saharan families, pharyngealized vowels found in Caucasian and some Tungusic languages, and 'sphincteric' vowels found in Khoisan-group languages. These phenomena present the necessity of connecting phonatory quality and vowel quality: what is required is a model that incorporates voice quality as a means to logically connect these (and other) properties.

Many formal phonological models assume lingual–laryngeal independence, as in the laryngeal–supralaryngeal dichotomization of distinctive features (Steriade 1987) and their organization (Clements 1985, Sagey 1986, McCarthy 1988: 89). This has become the established *de facto* view of the phonological function of the larynx. As Montler puts it, 'it is well known that glottals are not supposed to affect vowels... since laryngeal articulation is physically independent of tongue articulations' (1998: 371). This separation is so firmly held by phonologists that Uffmann is able to observe that 'the general existence of a LARYNGEAL class node is undisputed' (2011: 648). However, some phonologists have argued that phonological models must address the lingual–laryngeal–pharyngeal interactions that characterize LVT sounds (Czaykowska-Higgins 1987, Trigo 1991). The LVT effects on vowel quality and tonal quality documented instrumentally in Chapter 3 demonstrate an intricate LVT–UVT dependency that is especially relevant in languages that exploit tonal register or 'ATR' in their phonologies (e.g. Tibeto-Burman, West African, Nilotic) or that make extensive use of pharyngeal articulations (Semitic, Wakashan, Salishan), as illustrated in Chapter 4. These LVT–UVT interactions cannot be excluded from phonological description; indeed, LVT-rich phonologies provide a crucial link between how these phonetic phenomena perform linguistic contrasts and at the same time relate to long-term voice quality setting.

Chomsky and Halle (1968) proposed the feature [covered] for sounds 'produced with a pharynx in which the walls are narrowed and tense and the larynx raised; uncovered sounds are produced without a special narrowing and tensing in the pharynx' (pp. 314–315). Painter (1973: 97–98) evaluated [covered] in an x-ray study of Twi/Akan vowel harmony, which is based on what he called 'tense' [i e æ o u] vs. 'lax' [ɪ ɛ a ɔ ʊ] vowel sets. While pharynx volume distinguishes the Twi/Akan vowel sets, Painter argued that tense–lax was sufficient to characterize the phonemic system. He noted the entanglement of vowel, voice, and phonatory quality intrinsic to the Twi/Akan contrast (Painter 1973: 117).

The feature [covered] faded into obscurity, along with short-lived proposals by Lindau (1975, 1978) for [expanded] (cf. Keyser and Stevens 1994, Davis 1995), both being eclipsed by the feature [Advanced Tongue Root] or [ATR], originally proposed by Stewart (1967, cf. Halle and Stevens 1969) for the Akan harmony system and extended to tonal register in Mon-Khmer by Gregerson (1976). By denotation, [ATR] gives primacy to movement of the tongue root in the production of these contrasts, which usually cross-cut entire vowel systems, and, thus, it does not capture the more holistic nature of voice quality.

Czaykowska-Higgins (1987: 7) proposed a tongue-root articulator with two different types of behaviour: Type I, a 'mutual cooperative relationship between tongue root position and laryngeal behaviour'; Type II, an independent action of the tongue root constricting the pharynx. These correspond, respectively, to the features [±lower pharynx] (or [±LP]) and [±upper pharynx] (or [±UP]). In justification of this cooperative but independent analysis of the tongue root, she argues that languages with Type II tongue-root behaviour may exhibit phonatory correlates in the retracted group but not in the non-retracted group (e.g. retracted vowels in Nxaʔamxčín are creaky, but non-retracted vowels are not breathy); however, Type I always involves phonatory effects in both tongue-root states (advanced and retracted).

Czaykowska-Higgins's approach established that correlated or cooperative lingual–laryngeal activity needs to be accommodated in phonological analysis. Trigo (1991) takes this notion one step further by exploring the hypothesis that tongue-root position and larynx height are independent phonetic parameters, with corresponding phonological features [ATR/RTR] and [lowered larynx/raised larynx] (or [LL/RL]). Her survey spans 'voice quality or register' contrast in African and Southeast Asian languages, laryngeal, pharyngeal, and uvular consonants, and the association between voiced stops and enlarged pharyngeal volume. In her conclusion, she concedes that the evidence for orthogonality of the features [ATR/RTR] and [LL/RL] is weak and that the 'co-occurrence of pharyngeal and laryngeal effects is attributed to a mechanical link between pharynx and larynx' (p. 132). Thus, Trigo (1991: 116–119) posits a mechanical relationship between larynx height and vocal fold functioning that operates independently of vocal fold abduction/adduction (phonologically expressed by [±spread glottis] and [±constricted glottis] features). This premise is used to explain the occurrence of breathy phonation with larynx lowering and 'squeezed'/'pressed' (p. 117) phonation with larynx raising. Concomitant with this is a peripheralization–centralization of the vowels – moving away from or towards [ə] in the vowel space (Trigo 1991: fn. 5) – which, in the case of Caucasian languages, she claims is caused by 'a peculiar distortion of the tongue' (fn. 7) similar to a bunched-r in North American English.

Trigo's analysis represents a concerted effort to address the phonological relevance of lingual–laryngeal connection in forming register contrasts.

(a) Herzallah (1990: 61–62)   (b) McCarthy (1994: 223)

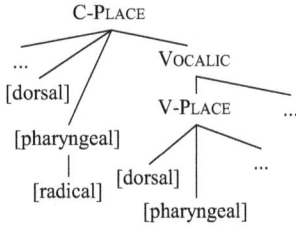
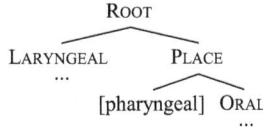

(c) Davis (1995: 471)   (d) Rose (1996: 80)   (e) Halle et al. (2000: 389)

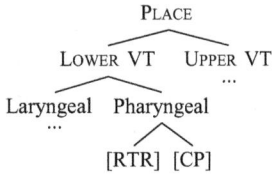
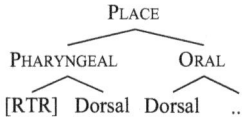
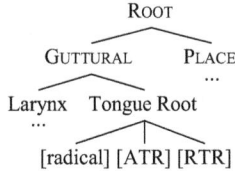

Figure 5.1 *Five variations on guttural/post-velar feature geometry*
RTR = retracted tongue root; CP = constricted pharynx.

The lack of impact of Trigo's findings may be attributed to its timing, as it came at the time when Feature Geometry (FG) was in ascent as a popular formalism for phonological analysis. The requirement in FG of strict dominance – a feature may be dominated by one, and only one, feature (McCarthy 1988, cf. Ohala 2005) – may have caused reinforcement of the already well-established view that laryngeal and supralaryngeal activity were separate in phonological terms.

The number of different proposals for feature geometric representation in general is considerably large, and the 'guttural' part of the tree is no exception. Bessell (1992: ch. 2) provides a survey of some prior models; summaries of the 'guttural' section of the tree are also provided by Clements and Hume (1995: 274) and more recently by Uffmann (2011: 648). Here we briefly examine five proposals depicted in Figure 5.1.

All models posit a representational unit (node or feature) associated with guttural/post-velar classhood: [pharyngeal], PHARYNGEAL, GUTTURAL, LOWER VT. All of these suggest the idea of the pharynx or pharyngeal part of the vocal tract. For example, in Herzallah's (1990) model in Figure 5.1 (a), which is framed in Unified Feature Theory (UFT, Clements 1989, Clements and Hume 1995; for a review see Halle et al. 2000: 399–412), gutturals/post-velars and the /a/ vowel are argued to be specified with the [pharyngeal] feature; in McCarthy's model in Figure 5.1(b), [pharyngeal] is tantamount to a region of articulation rather than a specific articulator, hence its status as sister to the ORAL node (also a region of articulation). This regional status of [pharyngeal] is later emphasized in the proposals by (c) Davis (1995: 471), (d) Rose (1996), and (e) Halle et al. (2000, cf. Halle 1995), though it has nodal status rather than being a feature (and is variably named and organized into subnodes and features). Halle (1995: 18) and Halle et al. (2000) claim that lingual–laryngeal interaction is a corollary of the structure of their vision of FG, in which the GUTTURAL node exclusively dominates the TONGUE ROOT and LARYNGEAL articulator nodes, implying a phonological lingual–laryngeal affinity for segments specified with TONGUE ROOT features such as [±ATR] (advanced/non-advanced tongue root). The problem with this approach is one of causality. The FG formulated by Halle does not intrinsically express the direction of correlation amongst the phonetic properties character-izing all of the registers. There is no reason for the articulatory configuration entailed by [±ATR] to correlate with any particular laryngeal state.

Attempts to account for guttural/post-velar patterning resulted in a shifting perspective on the nature of phonological place of articulation. Prior to these accounts, there were Place and Laryngeal categories of features (Clements 1985, Sagey 1986). The vocal tract was roughly split into laryngeal and supralaryngeal zones for phonological purposes, and laryngeals were viewed as being 'placeless'. With the advent of guttural/post-velar phonology (e.g. Hayward and Hayward 1989, Herzallah 1990, McCarthy 1991), phonologists were forced to reconcile the relationship of laryngeal features to place features. The introduction of a pharyngeal zone of articulation undermined the logical unity of the PLACE category. This is reflected in the change in nomenclature seen in the Davis, Rose, and Halle et al. models: what was formerly PLACE becomes associated with the oral or upper vocal tract, and the pharyngeal part of the vocal tract is then given place status (although the Halle et al. model resisted the renaming trend – but GUTTURAL vs. PLACE is basically the same division). The status of the laryngeal node was also called into question, leading to the following split in approach: Rose's (1996) model follows McCarthy's proposal by keeping LARYNGEAL external to PLACE; Davis's model (1995) and Halle et al.'s model (2000) admit LARYNGEAL/LARYNX into the domain of the other articulators.

This split in the treatment of laryngeal features reflects conflicting beliefs about how the organization of feature geometry should be defined and the deeper metatheoretical tension found in the debate about the phonetics–phonology interface: should definition proceed by patterning or by anatomical organization? Feature geometries are phonological, so they are assumed to be categorically organized on the basis of observed phonological patterns; however, at the time, there was a notion that FG is a mapping of the physical organization of the vocal tract (Keyser and Stevens 1994, Davis 1995, Halle 1995, Halle et al. 2000). Thus, many of these models constitute, more or less, a schematization of the physical layout and operation of the vocal tract (e.g. Ohala 2005).

Although much of the discussion relates to the larynx, generally the larynx is conceptually reduced to just the 'glottis' constituting what we call a 'flat' view of the larynx. Only recently has it become apparent to researchers that the vocal folds might interact with the structures above (e.g. Borroff 2007, Shahin 2011). The fact remains that despite this 'flat' viewpoint, there are still early, prominent observations of the lingual–pharyngeal–laryngeal interaction (Trigo 1991, McCarthy 1994, Keyser and Stevens 1994, Halle 1995) and awareness of the supraglottal structures of the larynx and their involvement in 'glottal' sounds (Halle and Stevens 1971).

The rest of this chapter will argue that when anatomo-physiological and phonetic understanding of the epilarynx is admitted into the domain of 'phonological' explanation, many issues raised in LVT phonological analyses can be attributed to the articulatory interaction between the epilarynx, vocal folds, and the rest of the vocal tract.

5.2   Phonological Potentials, the Laryngeal Articulator, and Voice Quality

Our model concerns the factors governing 'potential' phonemic organization at the physical/physiological level (possible divisions and patterning of the system), and compares this to 'realized' systems. The idea of potentials (metaphorically borrowed from the notion of potentials in physics) is useful because it is not absolute or deterministic: it does not describe the way phonological systems must be; it describes the way they tend to be and the factors that go into determining these tendencies. Unlike traditional or current phonological formalisms (such as Feature Geometry or Optimality Theory), the model we develop here, following the theoretical stance of Ohala (1990, 2005, 2011), is not a model of mental representations. We are focused on 'articulatory' factors, but potentials are not limited in this way. Phonological potentials can also be aerodynamic, acoustic, perceptual, and even cognitive in nature (and the alignment and interaction of these factors). The focus is on how voice quality, as mediated extensively (but not exclusively) by actions of the

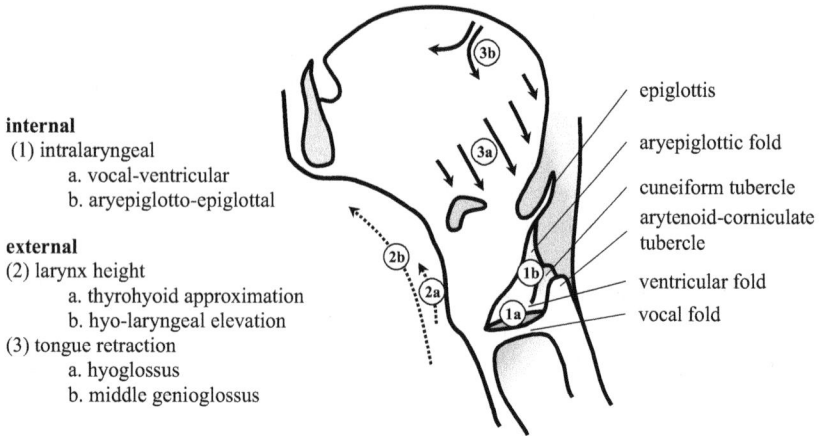

internal
(1) intralaryngeal
   a. vocal-ventricular
   b. aryepiglotto-epiglottal

external
(2) larynx height
   a. thyrohyoid approximation
   b. hyo-laryngeal elevation
(3) tongue retraction
   a. hyoglossus
   b. middle genioglossus

epiglottis

aryepiglottic fold

cuneiform tubercle
arytenoid-corniculate tubercle

ventricular fold

vocal fold

Figure 5.2 *Key components of epilarynx operations (sagittal schematic)*

laryngeal articulator, plays a role in shaping speech-sound systems and patterns. The model is thus discussed in terms of laryngeal physiology and its interrelations to other articulatory components of the vocal tract.

We begin with a brief summary of some of the key elements of the laryngeal articulator, focusing on the epilaryngeal level. This system is characterized by internal and external physiological control mechanisms which aid in its constriction: (1) the intralaryngeal musculature, (2) the larynx height mechanism, and (3) tongue retraction. Mechanism (1) is an epilarynx-internal mechanism; (2) and (3) are epilarynx-external mechanisms. Each component can be further broken down into subcomponents, as illustrated in Figure 5.2. Detailed definitions of these components are provided in Table 5.1.

Component (1), the intralaryngeal musculature, is the most important in driving epilaryngeal constriction. The lower epilaryngeal subcomponent (1a) pertains to the musculature acting primarily in the ventricular plane to cause downward and medial motion of the ventricular folds; the relevant musculature comprises the external thyroarytenoid and its projections into the transverse interarytenoid muscle. Vocal fold adduction (as in prephonatory or phonatory postures) enables constriction in this plane. The upper-epilaryngeal subcomponent (1b) involves the musculature driving motion in the aryepiglottic plane – the thyroepiglottic muscles and the sphincteric chain formed by the lateral cricoarytenoid, oblique interarytenoid, and aryepiglottic muscles. The vocal folds do not need to be adducted for constriction to occur in this plane.

Table 5.1 *Definitions of the components of epilaryngeal control*

	Component		Subcomponents	Description
1	intralaryngeal	a.	vocal-ventricular	lower epilaryngeal
		b.	aryepiglotto-epiglottal	upper epilaryngeal
2	larynx height	a.	thyrohyoid approximation	'local' larynx raising
		b.	hyo-laryngeal elevation	'global' larynx raising
3	tongue retraction	a.	hyoglossus	primary retraction
		b.	middle genioglossus	'double-bunching' retraction

Dashed line separates epilarynx-internal [above] from epilarynx-external [below] components.

Component (2) involves larynx height, which plays a key role in changing the vertical dimension of epilaryngeal constriction. The 'local' subcomponent (2a) involves approximation of the thyroid cartilage and hyoid bone driven by the thyrohyoid muscles. This can occur regardless of the 'global' position of the hyo-laryngeal complex – subcomponent (2b), which involves the suprahyoid and pharyngo-laryngeal musculature to lift the larynx upwards. Epilaryngeal constriction is more efficiently accomplished when both subcomponents are engaged. Because of the muscular linkage through the hyoid bone, component (2) can cause the tongue to retract/lower, but this will depend on the activation level of the suprahyoid muscles and other forces acting on the tongue.

Component (3) is the tongue retraction component. Primary retraction (3a) involves a hyoglossus-driven motion that is obliquely oriented downwards towards the larynx (as Figure 5.2 depicts). Secondary retraction (3b) involves displacement of the posterior body of the tongue under the influence of middle genioglossus (GGM) action (the extreme contraction of which produces the 'double-bunching' state seen in a canonical variant of American English /r/: Type 4 in Delattre and Freeman's 1968 taxonomy). The GGM has been shown to contract in the production of front vowels (Takano and Honda 2007: 56). An important effect of general tongue retraction (3) is to push the epiglottis posteriorly and to distort the pre-epiglottic (fat) body, the stresses of which are transferred to the level of the lower epilarynx and probably assist posterior displacement of the epiglottic tubercle. Tongue retraction does not entail active epilaryngeal stricture, which depends on the contribution of components (1)

Table 5.2 *Typical concomitant phonetic properties of epilaryngeal states*

Property	Anti-constriction	Constriction
C1: intralaryngeal	relaxed	contracted
C2: larynx height	lowered	raised
C3: tongue position	advanced	retracted
phonatory quality	breathy or modal	creaky or harsh
voice quality	lowered-larynx voice	raised-larynx voice
vowel quality	peripheralized	condensed

C# = component #; see Figure 5.2.

and (2). If retraction is strong, and the larynx is not lowered, then the epilaryngeal space will narrow, but this is passive – not active – epilarynx engagement. Thus, tongue retraction biases but is not sufficient for active epilarynx stricture. Broadly speaking, the epilarynx has two basic states: constricted and unconstricted. Table 5.2 lists general physiological and auditory descriptors applied to these polar opposite configurations.

5.3   Synergistic Relations Network

Underlying each sound is a neuromuscular module (NMM), a concept discussed in Gick and Stavness (2013), Gick (2016), which engages certain states of the vocal tract, such as tongue retraction, larynx raising, vocal fold adduction. These NMMs are associated with particular speech sounds and denoted using ⟦ ⟧ (for instance, the neuromuscular basis for a plain glottal stop with no ventricular fold reinforcement would be ⟦ʔ⟧). NMMs are discussed in detail in Moisik et al. (2019). Phonological potentials of the LVT can be expressed as the tendencies for interaction amongst various physiological states of the vocal tract when placed in a speech sequence. Table 5.3 contains a list of states (and their abbreviations) relevant for voice quality-related LVT speech phenomena. As a simplification, these states all refer to aspects of vocal tract configuration viewed at a coarse level of detail: e.g. {vfo} is any kind of vocal fold opening. The lingual states – tongue fronting {tfr}, tongue raising (back and up) {tra}, and tongue retraction (back and down) {tre} are based directly on Esling's (2005) Laryngeal Articulator Model.

The physiological relations constituting the model are of two sorts: there are synergies and anti-synergies. Synergies, denoted by {X ↔ Y}, are complementary or mutually supportive articulatory configurations between states X and Y (which may operate one or both ways, i.e. such that X supports Y,

Table 5.3 *Physiological states of the lower vocal tract*

States*	Physiological description
vfo	vocal folds open (abducted)
vfc	vocal folds closed (adducted/ prephonation)
epc	epilaryngeal constriction
epv	epilaryngeal vibration
tfr	tongue fronting
tre	tongue retraction
tra	tongue raising
tdb	tongue double bunching
↑lx	raised larynx
↓lx	lowered larynx
Hf0	increased vocal fold tension, less vibrating mass (high f0)
Lf0	decreased vocal fold tension, more vibrating mass (lower f0)

* In the text, these will appear in their abbreviated form inside { } brackets. See Figure 5.3 for the synergistic relationships of these states.

Y supports X, or that X and Y reinforce each other; detailed characterization of the directionality is reserved for future work); they do not imply a particular function but may be useful towards achieving a functional goal, such as epilaryngeal stricture. An example is the synergy between vocal fold closure (adduction) and larynx raising, symbolized as {vfc ↔ ↑lx}. Vocal fold opening (abduction), on the other hand, is synergistic with larynx lowering {vfo ↔ ↓lx}. Anti-synergies, denoted by {X ⋯ Y}, are conflicts between configurations: they do not preclude a particular combination of states, but some compensation is needed within the system (see Gick and Wilson 2006). For example, epilaryngeal vibration at higher glottal pitch {epv ⋯ Hf0} is not precluded but requires the antithetical combination of epilaryngeal constriction and longitudinal vocal fold tension (Esling 2005, Esling and Moisik 2012) needed for increasing glottal pitch. Diametrically opposed states, such as {Hf0} and {Lf0} or {↑lx} and {↓lx}, can be interpreted as being very unlikely to be combinable or outright impossible. Note that many more states could be added to cover the entire vocal tract (such as states for the lips or the velum) but these have been avoided here to place the focus on the lower (laryngeal) vocal tract, as it is most relevant to the phenomena discussed later in the chapter.

The diagram in Figure 5.3 is organized into different zones (denoted by braces), which are key facets of voice quality. These include vowel quality

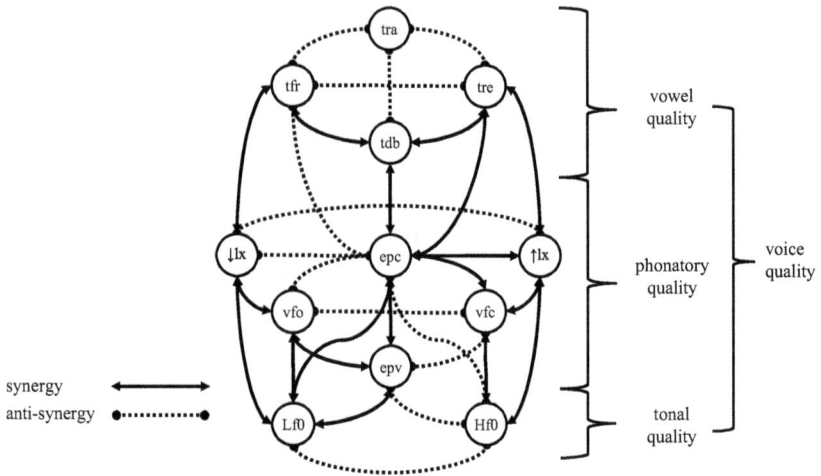

Figure 5.3 *Network of synergistic and anti-synergistic physiological relations among vocal tract states*
Physiological states defined in Table 5.3 appear inside circles. In the text, synergies are denoted with {X ↔ Y} and anti-synergies with {X ⋯ Y}, where X and Y are any given physiological states outlined in Table 5.3.

(mainly lingual states), phonatory quality (mainly laryngeal states), and tonal quality (associated with glottal f0 states). The model thus explicitly relates the interdependencies between physiological states of the vocal tract to the overlapping facets of voice quality. This is the case whether we consider a restricted-domain application of voice quality (as in a local modulation to prosodic structure, such as the syllable level) or a long-term posture (possibly pervading many syllables or even an entire utterance).

5.4   Voice Quality and Register Contrasts: A Unified Approach

Numerous languages make use of register-type contrasts that involve sets of correlated phonetic properties associated with vowel, phonatory, and tonal quality. The traditional literature contains subjective descriptors and at times contradictory or confusing terms (such as 'lax' vs. 'tense', [+ATR] vs. [−ATR], 'chest' vs. 'head', 'hollow' vs. 'choked'). In our approach, we consolidate the description of a broad set of register languages, which vary in precise detail, by appealing to the basic notion that the epilarynx serves as the articulatory nexus for relating vowel quality, controlled mainly by the tongue, to laryngeal variables such as phonatory and tonal quality. The various

languages reviewed below are thus different realizations of the same fundamental phonological potential, varying by what phonetic properties they focus
on to make the contrast (whether more oriented to vowel quality or phonatory
and/or tonal quality).

Figure 5.4 contains a simplified diagram of the phonological potential as it
relates to the physiological states of the vocal tract. There is a phonological
potential for (a) unconstricted and (b) constricted registers. The potential
unconstricted register is characterized by the absence of epilaryngeal

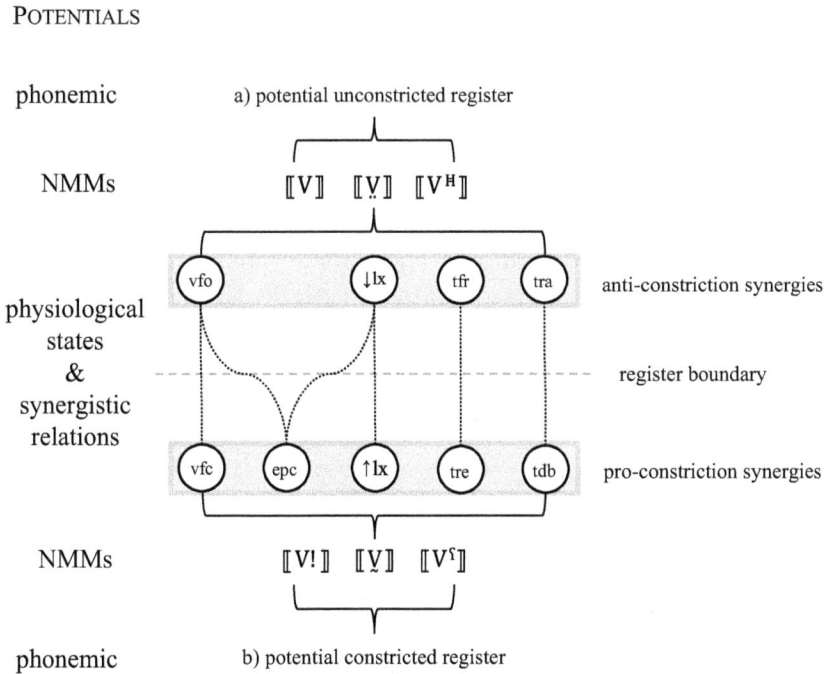

Figure 5.4 *Potential unconstricted and constricted registers*
Diagram simplifications: Brackets = broad possibilities for association (not
specific in this abstract case); Grey boxes = synergistic relations. NMMs:
[[V]] = modal; [[V̤]] = breathy; [[V^H]] = faucalized register; [[V̰]] = creaky;
[[V!]] = harsh (without epilaryngeal vibration); [[V^ˤ]] = 'raised-larynx voice'.
Abbreviations: vfo/vfc = vocal fold opening/closure (or abduction/
adduction); epc = epilaryngeal constriction; tdb = tongue double bunching;
tfr = tongue fronting (forward); tre = tongue retraction (down and back);
tra = tongue raising (up and back); ↑lx/↓lx = raised/lowered larynx. (For
simplicity, many synergistic relations have been omitted from this diagram.)

Table 5.4 *Vowel subsets in N|uu (Miller et al. 2009: 155–156), !Xóõ (Hess 1998: 176), and Ju|'hoansi (Miller 2007: 58)*

	'non-pharyngealized'			'pharyngealized'		
	i	u				uˤ
N|uu	e/ɛ	o/ɔ	eˤ			oˤ
		a/ɑ			ɑˤ	
	i i̠ iʔ	u u̠ uʔ				uˤ uˤ
!Xóõ	e e̤ eʔ	o o̤ oʔ				oˤ oˤ
	a a̤ aʔ				aˤ aˤ	
	i i̠ iʔ	u u̠ uʔ				
Ju|'hoansi	e e̤ eʔ	o o̤ oʔ			ɔˤ	
	a a̤ aʔ				ɑˤ	

constriction and association with physiological states that are anti-synergistic with epilaryngeal stricture (i.e. anti-constriction synergies in Figure 5.4). The potential constricted register is defined by the presence of epilaryngeal constriction and is associated with physiological states that synergize with epilaryngeal stricture (i.e. pro-constriction synergies in Figure 5.4). Each of these potential registers could be realized in a variety of related ways in terms of vowel, phonatory, and even tonal quality. The registers form a natural opposition (as indicated by the register boundary) suitable for phonological implementation because most of the physiological states differentiating the two registers are anti-synergistic (e.g. {↓lx ··· ↑lx}, {tfr ··· tre}, and {vfo ··· vfc}).

What follows is a survey of several languages that exhibit register-type contrast sets, each different in its own way, but each showing some realization of the synergistic relations outlined in the Phonological Potentials Model.

In Khoisan-group languages, sets of vowels are identified as either 'non-pharyngealized' or 'pharyngealized' (Table 5.4). The Khoisan vowels in the 'pharyngealized' sets, loosely grouping vowels variably described as pharyngealized, strident, and/or epiglottalized, tend towards the retracted vowels [ɑ ɒ ʌ ɔ], while [i] does not appear at all. In N|uu, non-pharyngealized mid vowels have '[–ATR]' allophones [ɛ ɔ], but the pharyngealized mid vowels are realized as '[+ATR]' [eˤ oˤ]. In !Xóõ, only correspondents of /a o u/ are found in the pharyngealized set. Ju|'hoansi has the most restricted pharyngealized set, [ɑˤ] and [ɔˤ], both of which are retracted vowels. Epilaryngeal vibration occurs in the so-called epiglottalized/sphincteric vowels of N|uu (Moisik 2013: 128–131) and !Xóõ (Traill 1986: 198). Glottalized vowels (shown in the non-pharyngealized grouping), which occur in !Xóõ and Ju|'hoansi, do not show such restrictions.

Thus, in the Khoisan-group languages, there is a divide between unconstricted (non-pharyngealized) and constricted (pharyngealized) registers, with sub-register differentiation based on phonatory quality (such as a modal or breathy set, or a set with epilaryngeal vibration). As indicated by the presence of {tre} in association with the constricted register potential, the retracted vowels [ɑ o/ɔ] appear to be the vocalic 'anchor' points of the constricted registers, but [eˤ] and [uˤ] are also attested. X-ray evidence of pharyngealized and sphincteric vowels in !Xóõ (Hess 1998: 346, 353) and auditory evaluations of epiglottalized vowels in N|uu suggest that these languages may involve Catford's double-bunching lingual configuration similar to pharyngealization in Caucasian (Catford 1983: 350, 2002: 176–177), consistent with the inclusion of {tdb} in Figure 5.4 in association with the constricted register potential.

The following language cases implicate not just vowel quality in the register contrast but tonal quality as well. Bai and Zhenhai are languages with tonal register systems in which epilaryngeal vibration occurs in a subset of tonal and vocalic environments. Bai is particularly intriguing since laryngoscopy reveals that even in [i] contexts, extreme epilaryngeal stricture and vibration can occur (Edmondson and Esling 2006: 176). Epilaryngeal vibration also tends to occur on low-tonal targets, leaving only harshness (without epilaryngeal vibration) on mid or high targets. 'Growling' (epilaryngeal vibration) is found in Zhenhai Yang tones (Rose 1989) and is restricted to relatively open oral vowels (e.g. [œˤ ɛˤ aˤ]); it can occur on close nasalized vowels and tends to be followed by a glottal stop; whisperiness, in nearly complementary distribution with growling, occurs on relatively close vowels [i̥ ẏ ɛ̥]. Whisperiness uses epilaryngeal constriction (Honda et al. 2010) but lacks epilaryngeal vibration.

The potential constricted registers are associated with retracted, open vowels via the pro-constriction synergistic relations, but nothing in the PPM precludes a vowel like /i/ from being realized in the constricted register. We would expect that this would be less typical than more compatible, synergistic vowels, such as retracted vowels (as in Khoisan 'pharyngealized' vowels). Bai is a case where epilaryngeal constriction freely combines with any vowel quality (although we cannot rule out that the tongue is not engaged in a {tdb} state, which we might predict based on the PPM, given that tongue double bunching synergizes with a fronted state of the tongue {tdb ↔ tfr}). Zhenhai Wu is very similar to Bai if we accept the analysis that the Yang tones generally use epilaryngeal constriction and hence form an instance of constricted register. However, Zhenhai shows more vowel-quality restrictions with epilaryngeal vibration (although epilaryngeal constriction still freely combines with any vowel quality, since whisper is a form of epilaryngeal constriction). The PPM can account for the tendency for growl to occur in relatively open vowel contexts: growl is synergistic with epilaryngeal stricture, epilaryngeal stricture is synergistic with retraction {epc ↔ tre}, and, critically, retraction complements open vowel production. In both Bai and Zhenhai, the tendency for epilaryngeal vibration to be limited to low-tonal targets is an expression of the synergy between epilaryngeal vibration and low f0 {epv ↔ Lf0} and the corresponding anti-synergy with high f0 {epv ⋯ Hf0}.

Many languages of Southeast Asia have register systems. Akha (Tibeto-Burman) has been described as having two registers given various names by various researchers: 'oral'/'low'/'chest' vs. 'laryngealized'/'high'/'head' (Lewis 1968, Wyss 1976, Trigo 1991: 117). Vowel and phonatory quality correlate with register. The 'chest' register gives the impression of 'hollow' or 'soft' auditory quality and 'varying degrees of breathiness', while 'head' register gives a 'tense, restrained and choked' auditory impression and is always terminated with [ʔ] when pre-pausal; (Wyss 1976: 152; see also Trigo 1991: 117). Trigo (1991: 133, n. 10) also notes that 'chest' register vowels involve 'dilated pharyngeal walls, lowered larynx and breathy voice' and are 'peripheral [i u ɑ] etc.', whereas 'head' register vowels involve 'narrowed pharyngeal walls, raised larynx and pressed voice' and are 'centralised [ɪ ʊ a] etc.'. Rengao (Mon-Khmer) has 'lax' and 'tense' registers (Gregerson 1976: 329, 333): 'lax' register exhibits pharyngeal expansion associated with tongue-root advancement, larynx lowering, and the vowels [i e ə o u], and 'tense' register has constricted pharynx associated with tongue-root retraction, larynx raising, and the vowels [eⁱ ɛ a ɔ oᵘ]. From these loose descriptions, we can infer that Akha and Rengao have a distinction between unconstricted ('chest'/'lax') and constricted ('head'/'tense') registers. Unifying these systems as register potentials allows us to move away from non-phonetic ('chest' vs. 'head'), subjective ('hollow' vs. 'choked'), and confusing or contradictory labels (e.g. using 'tense' in Rengao to describe a register containing vowels [ɛ ɔ] that are termed lax in other linguistic traditions such as Germanic).

In the PPM, Akha constricted ('head') register correlates with centralization of the vowel space, and unconstricted ('chest') register correlates with expansion or peripheralization of the vowel space. Centralization may indicate that the 'head' register vowel space is characterized by tongue double bunching {tdb}, heavily distorting lingual configuration and associated acoustics, combined with epilaryngeal constriction {epc}, since the phonatory quality is constricted (characterized as harsh or creaky). The appearance of a more front open vowel [a] in the constricted register is consistent with the {tdb} configuration. It echoes similar changes described for Caucasian languages and for pharyngeals in general being associated with a front open vowel (Moisik 2013, sec. 7.3.1). The occurrence of [ɑ] in the unconstricted register, on the other hand, illustrates the need to differentiate between pharyngeal and epilaryngeal constriction (as emphasized in the PPM). The pharynx is constricted, but the epilarynx is not, making this vowel compatible with the unconstricted register.

In northern Africa, there are several languages that employ register. Various dialects of Dinka have vocal-register contrasts involving vowel and phonatory quality, length, and tone. In Agar Dinka (Andersen 1993: 4), modal [i e ɛ a ɔ o], breathy [i̤ e̤ ɛ̤ a̤ ɔ̤ o̤ṳ], and creaky [ḭ ḛ ɛ̰ a̰ ɔ̰ o̰] registers occur, with the only vowel restriction being that /u/ is never modal or creaky. Luanyjang Dinka (Remijsen and Ladd 2008) has breathy and modal registers, both combining with its seven vowel phonemes /i e ɛ a ɔ o u/, except that /u/ is always breathy. Bor Dinka has the most elaborate system, exhibiting four registers: modal, harsh, breathy, and faucalized (Denning 1989: 68, 131, Edmondson et al. 2003, Edmondson and Esling 2006: 182–185), outlined in Table 5.5.

According to Edmondson et al. (2003), the basic vowel system of Bor Dinka is /i e a ɔ o/, but the vowels change depending on the register, as depicted in Table 5.6 (ignoring faucalized register).

Somali (Edmondson and Esling 2006: 175) also has a register-like system contrasting modal and harsh sets with correlated vowel quality (and associated

Table 5.5 *Phonetics of register in Bor Dinka based on Denning (1989: 68)*

	faucalized/ 'hollow'	breathy	normal	harsh
glottal aperture*	greatest	←	→	least
tongue root	advanced	advanced	normal	retracted
mandible	advanced, lowered	advanced, lowered	normal	retracted, lowered
larynx	lowered	normal or lowered	normal	raised
rounding	rounder if round	rounder if round	normal	normal
fauces	expanded	normal	normal	normal
vowel height	closer	←	→	opener

* Arrows indicate a continuum between the extremes.

Table 5.6 *Vowel alternations in Bor Dinka (Edmondson et al. 2003)*

Modal	Breathy	Harsh
i	i̤	i̤ɛ
e	e̤	ɛ
a	a̤	ɛ
ɔ	o̤	a̤
o	ṳ	ṳɔ

harmony processes): the modal vowel set contains /i e æ ö ʉ/ (transcription based on Saeed 1999: 11–16), while the harsh set exhibits /ɪ ɛ ɑ ɔ u/ and accompanying creakiness and raised-larynx voice quality.

Dinka dialects and Somali are cases further supporting the need for a model, such as the PPM, which associates vowel-quality changes with particular registers but which is not fixated around such changes. Agar and Luanyjang Dinka registers, although still fundamentally realizations of the unconstricted vs. constricted register potentials, are phonatory-quality rather than vowel-quality dominant. This means that they allow the combination of most vowel qualities – both [+ATR] (e.g. [e o]) and [–ATR] (e.g. [ɛ ɔ]) – with the distinctive phonatory qualities. Somali and Bor Dinka, on the other hand, present a greater degree of vowel-quality–phonatory-quality correlation. However, Bor Dinka is an extreme case where the register system has subdivided the continuum of (epilaryngeal) constriction into four registers rather than two: faucalized and harsh represent extreme opposite ends of this spectrum. A striking, PPM-affirming fact about Dinka is that /u/ is associated with the unconstricted, breathy register. This vowel is well known across languages to implement larynx lowering (Ewan 1979). It is thus not surprising that it shows a restrictive tendency towards the most unconstricted register type – breathy register. The PPM reflects this in terms of the synergistic relation between larynx lowering and vocal fold opening { ↓lx ↔ vfo}.

Many languages of Africa possess a cross-height vowel harmony system that is commonly thought to be a function of tongue-root position, typically treated with the feature [±ATR] (Welmers 1946, Halle and Stevens 1969, Stewart 1967, Painter 1973, Lindau 1975, 1978, Denning 1989, Archangeli and Pulleyblank 1994). Casali's (2008) comprehensive review of ATR-harmony languages provides a summary of these systems (Table 5.7).

The routine analysis of ATR phenomena is as a vowel-quality contrast. However, some earlier researchers framed the phenomenon in terms of phonation type (Tucker 1975, Jacobson 1980). It is frequently reported that [+ATR]

Table 5.7 *'ATR' systems based on Casali (2008)*

Type	+ATR	−ATR	Location / Families	Examples
10-V	i e ə o u	ɪ ɛ a ɔ ʊ	Saharan	Akposso, Bongo, Diola-Fogny
9-V	i e o u	ɪ ɛ a ɔ ʊ	Niger-Congo, Nilo-Saharan	Akan, Maasai; very common
7-V, 1IU	i e o u	ɛ a ɔ	West & Central Africa	Yoruba; Wolof; common
7-V, 2IU	i u	ɪ ɛ a ɔ ʊ	East Africa	Kinande; relatively rare
5-V	i u	ɛ a ɔ	West Atlantic, Bantu	Pulaar, Tsonga, Zulu

V = vowel; 1IU = one set of close vowels /i u/; 2IU = two sets of close vowels /i u/ and /ɪ ʊ/.

vowels correspond (approximately) with breathiness and [−ATR] vowels with creakiness (Stewart 1967, Painter 1973: 117, Lindau 1975, Hall and Hall 1980; see also Czaykowska-Higgins 1987: 3–5, Denning 1989, Trigo 1991: 119–120, Keyser and Stevens 1994: 213, Guion et al. 2004). Although Casali (2008) suggests that phonatory quality is 'more subtle than some of the impressionistic labels might imply' (p. 510), he also suggests that phonatory quality is probably more common than descriptions of ATR languages disclose, especially in West African languages and East African Nilo-Saharan languages. Turkana is a noteworthy case because in certain contexts, the registers coalesce on [−high, −low] vowels, yielding '[ẹ ọ]', which are produced with harsh phonatory quality (denoted in an ad hoc way by the underdot) according to Dimmendaal (1983; see also Trigo 1991: 120).

No previous phonological theory has been able to adequately 'ground' ATR around a physiological mechanism that can coherently relate these properties. The PPM can model the lingual–laryngeal relationships found in ATR because it acknowledges the role of the epilarynx as the physiological mechanism that links vocal fold state, larynx height, and lingual state together. The schematic in Figure 5.5 depicts the relationships involved in ATR for a handful of illustrative (unrounded) vowels. The typical vowels associated with [±ATR] fall on the appropriate side of the 'ATR boundary' (horizontal dashed line). This line also divides physiological states according to their synergistic relation with epilaryngeal stricture (not all associations are shown, refer to Figure 5.3). Thus, '[+ATR]' vowels (a) are associated with the physiological states that synergize with epilaryngeal anti-constriction (including {tfr}), while '[−ATR]' vowels (b) are associated with physiological states that synergize with epilaryngeal constriction (including {tre}). The key articulatory basis for

POTENTIALS

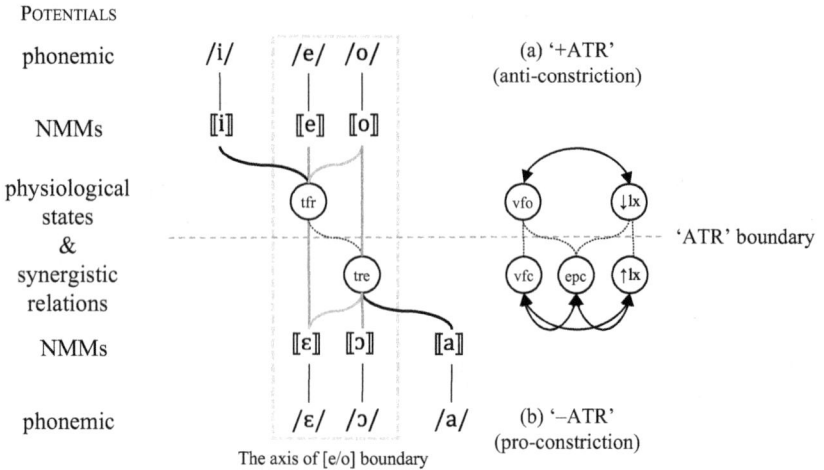

Figure 5.5 *Cross-height harmony ('ATR') in the PPM*
Greyness of the association lines represents physiological-state association
strength (e.g. [[ɛ]] involves greater tongue fronting {tfr} than retraction {tre});
Abbreviations: vfo/vfc = vocal fold opening/closure (or abduction/
adduction); epc = epilaryngeal constriction; tfr = tongue fronting (forward);
tre = tongue retraction (down and back); ↑lx/↓lx = raised/lowered larynx.

associating ATR-like systems with correlated phonatory and general voice quality effects (such as raised-larynx voice quality) is a relationship mediated by the state of the epilarynx – not the pharynx. In the PPM, physiological states relevant to phonation, such as {vfo}, are not directly associated with physiological states that are highly significant in vowel production, such as {tre}, {tfr}, and {tra} (see Figure 5.3). This signifies that ATR, unlike phonatory register, is vowel-oriented, not phonation-oriented.

As Casali's typology (Table 5.7) indicates, 'ATR' is not often realized as a simple cross-height system (as in ten-vowel systems), but rather manifests in asymmetric or 'imbalanced' ways (which is true for all of the other, non-ten-vowel, ATR-type systems listed in Table 5.7). We claim that the 'ATR' vowel system is 'imbalanced' across 'the axis of [e/o]' boundary (grey dashed box in Figure 5.5), which roughly separates vowels with {tfr} and {tra} from those with {tre} physiological states ({tra} is not included in the diagram for simplicity). The axis of [e/o] is yet another potential boundary, but it is one that exerts its main influence in the vowel domain (see Section 8.2).

To the left of the axis of [e/o] are the 'high' (close) vowels (e.g. /i/) and to the right are the 'low' (open) vowels (e.g. /a/). In Casali's typology, if any [+ATR] vowels exist in the system, they will most likely be /i u/: these vowels are found to the left of the axis of [e/o]. Likewise, the canonical [–ATR] vowel is /a/, which lies to the right of the axis of [e/o] in Figure 5.5. Thus, close vowels – especially those that are strongly {tfr} or {tra} – are attracted or biased towards to the [+ATR] set; open vowels – those that are more strongly {tre}– are attracted or biased towards the [–ATR] set.

In our approach, we follow through on Ohala's (1994: 492) contention that cross-height/ATR systems might originate as (and often persist in being) a phonation-type contrast. Related to this is Denning's (1989: 9) vocal-register implicational universal, which states that if there is a relationship between vowel height and voicing or phonation, the 'laxer' the phonation associated with the vowel, the greater the vowel's height. Denning's universal is based on a survey that includes numerous languages from Sino-Tibetan, Austroasiatic, Afro-Asiatic, Niger-Congo, Nilo-Saharan, Khoisan, Indo-European, Central Amerind and Na-Dene language groups.

Perhaps the most tantalizing aspect of Denning's proposal is that it implies a possible pathway of evolution for ATR-like systems through not just phonation type but also consonantal laryngeal contrasts and tonal quality. Denning (1989: 50–55) presents several cases, including Javanese, Lungtu, Lhasa Tibetan, Mnong, Murle, Middle Khmer, Mon, English and Buchan Aberdeenshire Scots (attributable to Stewart 1967), for which consonantal voicing correlates with relatively higher/closer vowels, lower tone level, and 'laxer'/breathier phonation, with phonetic details varying by language (cf. Huffman 1976). Much of this evidence reflects Haudricourt's (1946) theory that Mon-Khmer register originated as a voicing contrast, such that voiceless ('tense') stops are associated with [–ATR] 'head' register and voiced ('lax') ones with [+ATR] 'chest'/'breathy' register. These associations are reflected in observations by Matisoff (1968), Gregerson (1976: 328, 342, 333), and Trigo (1991: 128–129). Cohn (1993) describes the same relationship in Madurese, noting that voicing or aspiration conditions [+ATR] vowels (e.g. [birɤŋ] 'shy' and [pʰipʰiʈ] 'seed'), and unaspirated stops condition [–ATR] vowels (e.g. [pɛlɛ] 'choose') (p. 107). In the same vein, Vaux (1996), buttressing earlier arguments made by Trigo (1987, 1991: 128–131) and citing evidence from Babine, Jingpho, Kirzan Armenian, and southern dialects of Akan, argues that voiced obstruents are [+ATR] (but voiceless ones not necessarily [–ATR]).

There is thus support in the literature for drawing a connection across consonant voicing, phonatory quality, vowel quality, tonal bias, and overall voice quality. In the PPM, the connection amongst all of these properties is larynx height, as understood in relation to epilaryngeal stricture. Larynx lowering can be viewed as facilitating consonant (mainly obstruent) voicing, via the robustly substantiated aerodynamic voicing constraint (Trigo 1991: 130, Ohala 2011). It can also be viewed as favourable for vocal fold abduction. Larynx raising has the opposite effects of enhancing vocal fold adduction and inhibiting phonation.

Assuming a consonantal starting point, as in Proto Mon-Khmer (Huffman 1976), possibilities for contrast tend to fall on either side of the contrast boundary line (horizontal dashed line in Figure 5.5). The 'lax'/'tense' distinction (e.g. Denning 1989) is often a voiced/voiceless distinction, but aspirated/unaspirated voicelessness can also be split across the contrast pivot. Figure 5.6 (a) depicts a potential consonantal contrast between aspirated stops (to represent 'lax' stops and symbolized as ⟦h⟧) and unaspirated stops (to represent 'tense' stops and symbolized as ⟦₀⟧) as a starting point. These two types of stops are associated with the anti-constriction and pro-constriction physiological states, respectively.

It is typically claimed (e.g. Huffman 1976) that coarticulation with adjacent vowels begins the process of register formation. The states associated with each incipient register gradually become phonologized on the vowels when the register-inducing properties bleed off neighbouring 'lax' (voiced or aspirated) and 'tense' (voiceless or voiced unaspirated) consonants. This yields the so-called 'chest' and 'head' registers (as in Akha or Rengao). Thus, in the Figure 5.6 example, the consonantal contrast (a) develops into a register contrast (b). The result is a phonatory-quality-oriented contrast that may also have correlated vowel-quality changes. In the example, the registers resulting from 'lax' and 'tense' consonantal contrasts correspond to breathy (⟦V̤⟧) and creaky (⟦V̰⟧) vowels. The prediction of the PPM is that whatever the exact realization of the system, it will tend to settle into the familiar pattern formed by the opposition between epilaryngeal anti-constriction and pro-constriction.

Figure 5.6(c) represents the potential for register-like systems to develop into a cross-height contrast (such as 'ATR'). The [+ATR]/[−ATR] contrast is illustrated with canonical /i/ and /a/ (purely for illustration, as in Figure 5.5). To highlight the tendency for phonatory-quality association, /i/ is depicted as breathy (⟦V̤⟧), and /a/ is depicted as creaky (⟦V̰⟧). At the point of (c), the system has become vowel-oriented, but there may be concomitant phonatory, tonal, and voice quality correlates. Some languages may start to abandon the non-vocalic properties and shift towards a basic Germanic-style (non-constriction-based) tense/lax vowel contrast. Others may maintain the non-vocalic

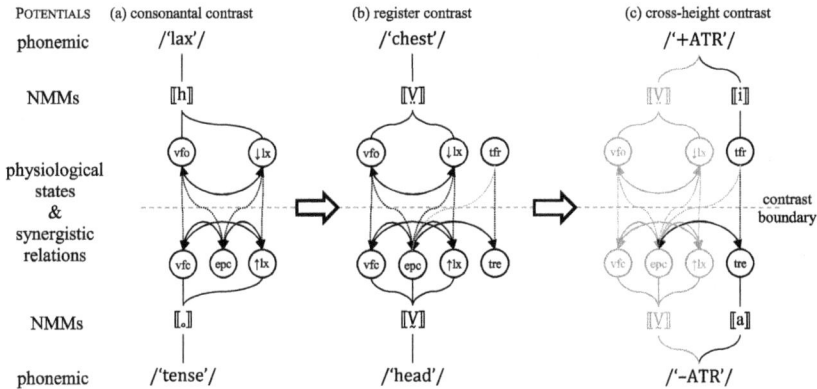

Figure 5.6 *From (a) consonantal to (b) register to (c) cross-height contrast in the PPM*
Only a few potentials are shown (e.g. 'ATR' contrast is illustrated with canonical [+ATR] /i/ and [–ATR] /a/). NMMs: ⟦h⟧ = vocal fold abduction (voiceless, as in aspirated stops); ⟦ ₒ⟧ = prephonation (voiceless, as in unaspirated stops); ⟦V̤⟧ = breathy; ⟦V̰⟧ = creaky. Abbreviations: vfo/vfc = vocal fold opening/closure (or abduction/adduction); epc = epilaryngeal constriction; tfr = tongue fronting (forward); tre = tongue retraction (down and back); ↑lx/↓lx = raised/lowered larynx. (Not all synergistic relations are represented.)

properties. The PPM satisfies the typical case of ATR-vowel correlates such that [+ATR] vowels /i e ə o u/ tend to be relatively more unconstricted in phonatory quality and voice quality, while [–ATR] vowels /ɪ ɛ a ɔ ʊ/ tend to be relatively more constricted in regard to these parameters.

Ohala's claim (1994) is that ATR languages started as a phonatory-register contrast, as in (b), and subsequently evolved into a cross-height contrast, as in (c). His claim is consistent with the PPM. We do not know whether there was an earlier consonantal stage. The only possible case of such a connection is Stewart's (1967) suggestion (see also Vaux 1996) that there is a relationship between consonant voicing and vowel quality in eastern dialects of Akan. Such a connection is not essential, since potentials might be realized at particular evolutionary stages for a time, only to be pushed out later by other forces that shape the sound system.

The PPM predicts that the systemic realignment with particular articulatory (and resulting auditory) properties will happen according to the synergistic relations associated with epilaryngeal functioning. In actual cases, languages will merge into and branch off the development path outlined in Figure 5.6; not all languages must go from (a) to (b) to (c). Factors outside of the articulatory domain, such as perceptual factors, are likely to play a significant role in the developmental pathway of individual languages. The principle of voice quality (variably emphasizing different phonetic parameters associated with vowel, phonatory, and tonal quality) provides a means to unify register and account for its historical development in a way that is consistent with phonetic facts. This is possible provided such systems are viewed as varying expressions of the basic underlying mechanism of epilaryngeal constriction (and anti-constriction), since this is the means by which the vowel, phonatory, and tonal components of voice quality become intertwined, as they are in languages with register-type contrasts.

5.5   Voice Quality in Sound Change: The Case of Southern Wakashan Pharyngeal Genesis

The PPM explicitly encodes voice quality by incorporating physiological states of the vocal tract that may not necessarily contribute independently to segmental identity but which may be superimposed over and interact with segmental content. Through time, such components can form evolutionary spandrels connecting one segment to another. In the PPM, larynx raising and tongue retraction both play an important role in voice quality characterization, reflecting laryngeal articulatory physiology. They are posited to be synergistic with epilaryngeal engagement. Accordingly, sounds which share these states are expected in the PPM to be susceptible to epilaryngeal stricture, even generating pharyngeals (or 'epilaryngeals' in general). This section examines such a case of pharyngeal genesis from the history of Southern Wakashan, where we claim that larynx raising and tongue retraction bias epilaryngeal stricture to occur (taking the form of pharyngeal consonants), and, when they combine, this bias becomes even stronger.

Pharyngeal genesis is a well-known pattern (Jacobsen 1969, Colarusso 1985: 367, Trigo 1991: 125, Davidson 2002: 75) in the diachronic phonology of Southern Wakashan languages. The key facts are as follows: Proto Southern Wakashan (PSW) uvular ejectives, *q' and *qʷ', merge into /ʕ/ in modern-day Nuuchahnulth (Nootka) and Ditidaht (Nitinaht); its uvular fricatives, *χ and *χʷ, become /ħ/ only in Nuuchahnulth; plain (non-glottalized) uvular stops do not participate in the change and are retained; and no changes occurred in the development of the southern-most Wakashan language, Makah (see Carlson et al. 2001 for an overview). Thus, both changes occurred in Nuuchahnulth, but the change only partially occurred in Ditidaht, which retains the historical

Table 5.8 *Pharyngeal genesis in the history of Southern Wakashan*

Proto-sounds		Makah	Ditidaht	Nuuchahnulth
$*q'$ $*q^{w'}$	$\rightarrow$	q' $q^{w'}$	Υ	Υ
$*\chi$ $*\chi^{w}$	$\rightarrow$	χ χ^{w}	χ χ^{w}	$\hbar$

Cognates for all three languages can be found in Trigo (1991: 125).

uvular fricatives, while Makah retains both proto-phonemes, as summarized in Table 5.8.

Moisik (2013, sec. 7.2.4) details previous traditional phonological analyses of this pattern, which tend to treat pharyngeals as modified uvular segments. No distinction can be identified to explain why plain (non-glottalized) uvular stops failed to change – plain uvular stops appearing to be as incipiently pharyngeal as uvular fricatives or uvular ejectives. Traditional models fail to predict the pharyngeal genesis pattern adequately because they do not incorporate an understanding of the epilarynx; these models treat the lower vocal tract as a single pharyngeal tube with a flat larynx at the bottom. Not only do such models get the details wrong, they also provide a misleading interpretation for why the sound change would occur in the first place. For instance, the suggestion that the change occurred because the representation was too complex, or by appealing to markedness, places the causal burden on the nature of representation, minimizing the contribution of physiological/articulatory factors.

The PPM is focused on the role of the epilarynx in phonological patterning. The pharyngeal genesis case is interpreted as evidence that some understanding of the epilarynx, its basic physiological nature, and its role in the production of pharyngeals provides insight into the Southern Wakashan sound pattern. Epilaryngeal constriction – the core operation of the lower vocal tract – is synergistic with larynx raising, i.e. $\{\uparrow lx \leftrightarrow epc\}$. However, this does not mean that larynx raising entails epilaryngeal stricture or vice versa. For example, larynx raising occurs when pitch is increased, but this does not mean that the epilarynx constricts to increase pitch. It only means that larynx raising creates conditions that are synergistic with epilaryngeal constriction. Tongue retraction also plays a role in producing uvular stricture (Namdaran 2006), synergizing with epilaryngeal stricture, i.e. $\{tre \leftrightarrow epc\}$. While velars and uvulars involve significant $\{tra\}$ activity, uvulars are drawn back towards the uvula and oropharynx by the additional strength of $\{tre\}$ engagement.

The PPM hypothesis is that the Proto Southern Wakashan uvulars form a gradient of susceptibility towards engaging epilaryngeal stricture (Table 5.9),

Table 5.9 *Gradient of uvular proneness to inducing epilaryngeal stricture*

	least prone	more prone	most prone
PSW	*q *q^w	*χ *χ^w	*q' *q'^{w}
Makah	q q^w	χ χ^w	q' q'^{w}
Ditidaht	q q^w	χ χ^w	ʕ
Nuuchahnulth	q q^w	ħ	ʕ

and this gradient is paralleled in the geographical distribution of the sound change itself, occurring most pervasively in the northern-most Nuuchahnulth languages (where uvular ejectives and fricatives underwent the change), less so in Ditidaht (where only uvular ejectives underwent the change), and not at all in Makah, the southern-most language.

The gradient nature of the change is a reflex of the degree of synergistic potential each uvular has in relation to epilaryngeal stricture (depicted in the three parts of Figure 5.7). Uvular stops (a), which require closure at the oropharyngeal isthmus, primarily have tongue raising {tra} and, of secondary importance, retraction {tre}, hence indicated with grey association lines. Retraction does synergize with epilaryngeal stricture {tre ↔ epc}, but it is relatively weak because retraction is less important than tongue raising to uvular stop production. The {epc} and {↑lx} physiological states are depicted as only indirectly associated with ⟦q⟧ via {tre}. The potential for laryngeal interaction exists; it is just relatively weak. Thus, according to the PPM, we interpret /q/ as being the least likely of the three to change into a pharyngeal. Uvular fricatives (b) are associated with less extreme tongue raising than /q/, since fricative stricture does not involve complete closure. This is depicted by stronger association of ⟦χ⟧ with {tre} than with {tra}, by means of association-line darkness. Thus, the overall more retracted position of the tongue means there is stronger synergy with epilaryngeal stricture (and correspondingly the association lines with {epc} and {↑lx} are darker than they are in /q/). Thus, in the PPM we declare that these sounds have a greater likelihood of becoming pharyngeals, as they did in Nuuchahnulth. At some point (call it 'step 1'), the uvular stricture was diminished, represented as dashed association lines in (b) and then diachronically abandoned (in 'step 2') in favour of pharyngeal stricture. Uvular ejectives (c) are the most synergistic with epilaryngeal stric-ture. Ejection ⟦'⟧ intrinsically relies on larynx raising {↑lx} and vocal fold adduction {vfc}. This reliance combined with the tongue retraction inherent to

(a) uvular stop: least prone to epilaryngeal stricture

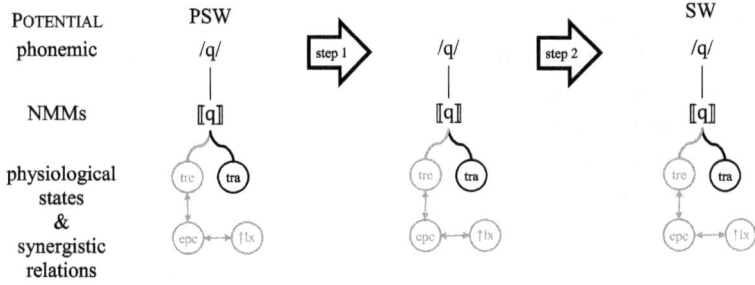

(b) uvular fricative: more prone to epilaryngeal stricture

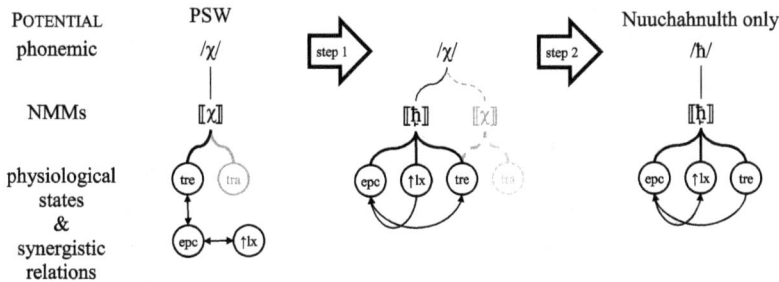

(c) uvular ejective: most prone to epilaryngeal stricture

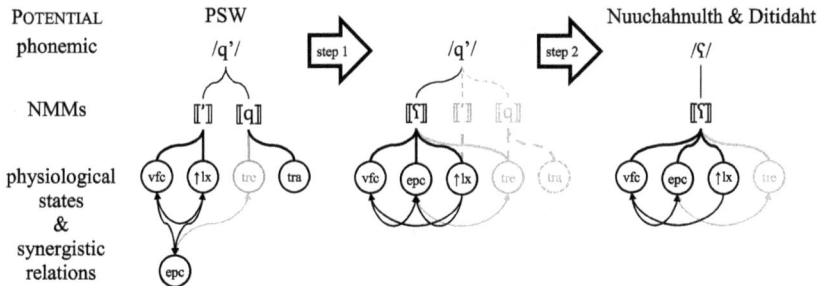

Figure 5.7 *Potential pharyngeal genesis for (a) uvular stops, (b) uvular fricatives, and (c) uvular ejectives*
PSW = Proto Southern Wakashan; SW = Southern Wakashan. Grey lines = relatively weaker physiological-state association strength; Dashed lines = 'oral depletion'/historical loss. Abbreviations: vfc = vocal fold closure/ adduction; epc = epilaryngeal constriction; ↑lx = raised larynx; tre = tongue retraction (down and back); tra = tongue raising (up and back). NMMs: [[ʕ]] = aryepiglotto-epiglottal (upper-epilaryngeal/UE) stricture; [[ħ]] = linguo-epiglotto-pharyngeal stricture; [[q]] = linguo-oropharyngeal isthmus stricture as in [q]; [[ʼ]] = ejection manoeuvre.

⟦q⟧ means that /q'/ carries the strongest potential to engage epilaryngeal stricture. Thus, /q'/ has the greatest likelihood of becoming a pharyngeal (i.e. [ʕ]). In the diagram, step 1 shows a possible transitional state in the history of Southern Wakashan at which point the oral depletion was starting to take effect (again, represented with dashed association lines) with concomitant strengthening of the vocal fold component to an epilaryngeal stricture (⟦ʕ⟧), which brings about direct association of the /q'/ with {epc}. This intermediate step may or may not have occurred; it is included in the diagram for the sake of exposition as a plausible phase, since modern-day uvular ejectives in Nlaka'pamuxcín have been shown to involve epilaryngeal stricture (Carlson and Esling 2003: 186). As in the case of /χ/ (Figure 5.7b), at some point the oral depletion becomes complete, and we are left with the pharyngeal residue. Thus, the gradient nature of the sound change is simply a matter of some uvulars showing more potential for synergizing with the substance that makes a 'pharyngeal' a pharyngeal – i.e. epilaryngeal stricture.

This example demonstrates that the PPM is a model that can help to clarify the physiological components that are implicated not only in segmental identity but also in voice quality and how these can influence patterns of change on the diachronic scale. Importantly, and in contradistinction with traditional phonological models, by expressing these physiological states as synergistically related, we have a means to capture the logic of how voice quality properties, which can operate at longer-term timescales, come to influence segmental content, which operate at shorter-term timescales.

5.6   Voice Quality in Phonology

The idea of phonological potentials and their expression as tendencies in the patterning of voice quality challenges the traditional phonological organization of the lower vocal tract. In traditional models, there is no intrinsic means to express the connectivity between lingual and glottal systems, which limits the ability of phonology to explain the intersection of phonatory, tonal, vocalic, and 'global' quality of the voice. Earlier models give us a relatively inorganic picture of lower-vocal-tract phonology. Traditional models weakly describe phonatory quality and weakly describe vowel quality but do not make the link to voice quality. Starting from the premise that the larynx is a flat one-dimensional glottis, traditional phonological approaches treat the pharynx as a single tube controlled by glottal height and 'tongue-root' position. In such models, interaction between the glottal level and the lingual level can only be treated as unexpected.

The Phonological Potentials Model (PPM) requires that phonological patterns of the lower vocal tract reflect the behaviour of the epilarynx. If phonology is not entirely substance free and can be determined by the form and functioning of the vocal tract, then the epilarynx fits as the structure that physically links the vocal folds to the rest of the vocal tract. Potentials, mediated through the epilarynx, help clarify many problems, such as how trilling through the laryngeal articulator interacts with tone and vowel subsystems, or how ejectives might bias pharyngeal genesis. The PPM lends some insight into how phenomena as seemingly diverse as consonant voicing contrasts and 'ATR harmony' are related. The connection relies on a direct characterization of those elements of vocal tract posturing which can be taken together to characterize voice quality, not just segmental identity.

Although the PPM is quite explicit about the types of phonetic behaviour predicted to occur – allowing productive work on diachronic patterns in linguistic communities, for example, or empirical work on epilaryngeal behaviour in sound systems, especially where epilaryngeal vibration is involved – perceptual and aerodynamic considerations still remain. The question is whether a unifying version of the PPM can be created that spans these domains. We suggest tentatively that there is considerable parallelism across these non-articulatory domains. A more profound formulation would aim to reconcile articulation, perception, and aerodynamics (which in some ways is the bridge between articulation and acoustics) in conjunction with other factors, such as sociophonetic influences. The mainly articulatory groundwork laid out here enables voice quality as a component of phonology, with the potential to express how speech-sound systems work and evolve over time.

6 Infant Acquisition of Speech and Voice Quality

Chapter 6 investigates the earliest steps of infants' acquisition of the phonetic capacity to speak. We present research that reveals how infants actively and systematically explore the laryngeal articulator to establish early voice quality categories throughout the first year of life. Using our model of the lower vocal tract, we demonstrate how all infants employ the same strictures and generate the same qualities in their first several months as they learn to manipulate the laryngeal vocal tract, regardless of their ambient languages. Predisposed by their laryngeal physiology, infants begin their articulatory development by making extensive use of laryngeal constriction, demonstrating that speech begins in the laryngeal articulator. To illustrate this process, we document the use of constricted and unconstricted settings in infants learning a Tibeto-Burman tonal register language compared to infants learning English. We also establish the importance of the laryngeal articulator approach to show that infants use constricted settings as a basis for later exploring unconstricted qualities and sounds produced in the oral vocal tract. Relating laryngeal articulation to voice quality acquisition, our phonetic observation of early infant speech production provides an insight into the theoretical distinctions between 'voice' (as in the voicing of a cry), 'articulatory settings' (which are originally short-term events in the infant), and 'long-term voice quality' (when long-term settings overlay shorter-term phonetic contrasts as a secondary coarticulatory background to the formation of primary oral strictures).

The Laryngeal Articulator Model (LAM) provides an indispensable phonetic framework for exploring the process of first language acquisition, speech development, and the beginnings of the awareness of articulation and quality. We examine speech development in the first year of life to demonstrate that phonetic models that lack an elaborated laryngeal mechanism inevitably overlook the growth in articulatory production that infants master during their first months. We illustrate this process with a sample of infants learning English in Canada and Bai in southwest China. These two languages differ fundamentally in their use of the laryngeal articulator. English does not employ laryngeal constriction contrastively, while, as illustrated in Chapter 4, the Bai language of Jianchuan, Yunnan, has a complex phonological inventory contrasting constricted and unconstricted tonal registers.

Regardless of the differences between the adult languages, we observe that both sets of infants take a laryngeally constricted phonetic path in their first months of life. Most sounds produced by English or Bai infants are constricted, exploiting the phonetic range of the laryngeal articulator and using laryngeal voice qualities such as harsh voice, creaky voice, raised-larynx voice, whisper, and whispery voice. As the year progresses, infants produce an increasing proportion of vocalizations with unconstricted laryngeal voice qualities, such as modal voice, breathy voice, and falsetto. Throughout the year, all infants explore degrees of constriction in 'dynamic' utterances that contain alternations between constricted and unconstricted laryngeal voice quality settings. We are able to hypothesize that the use of laryngeal voice quality in the first year of life reflects a complex interaction between the developing physiology of the infant vocal tract and the infant's innate disposition to engage in a process of vocal exploration in which laryngeal constriction plays a crucial role in speech development and in the infant's gradual attunement to the distribution of phonetic properties in the ambient language.

6.1   The Infant Vocal Tract

The disposition of the infant larynx directly impacts the nature and development of infant vocalizations in the first year of life. Most information on the disposition of the infant larynx stems from the medical literature (Crelin 1973, Sasaki et al. 1977, Fried et al. 1982, Kent and Vorperian 1995, Eckel et al. 1999, Vorperian et al. 1999), with some additional research originating from researchers with a particular interest in the relationship between infant vocal physiology and the evolution of language (Fitch and Giedd 1999, Lieberman et al. 2001). According to this body of research, the infant vocal tract differs from the adult vocal tract in five main respects. First, in contrast to the right-angled posture of the adult oral cavity relative to the pharynx, the infant oropharyngeal channel is sloped. Second, the tongue is in a retracted position, by virtue of its slope and predisposition to engage with epilaryngeal structures. Third, the vocal folds are short and the musculature that controls them is undeveloped. Fourth, compared to adults, the larynx is in a higher and more constricted position. Finally, the epiglottis rests against the soft palate, maintaining a respiratory passageway from the larynx through the posterior nares. Starting in the third month of life, the infant vocal tract undergoes significant growth and restructuring, increasing infants' vocal capacities. The larynx, epiglottis, and hyoid bone begin to descend, lengthening the vocal tract and changing the angle of the oral cavity relative to the pharyngeal cavity. This restructuring continues throughout infancy, affording infants the capacity to produce a wide range of pitch, intensity, and constriction at the laryngeal level.

Figure 6.1 illustrates the anatomy of the newborn and infant vocal tracts within the LAM, compared to the adult vocal tract (Figure 1.1). The anatomical features of the infant vocal tract make it more similar to the mature larynx of other primates than to the larynx of mature humans. Given the comparatively limited vocal abilities of other primates compared to humans – and in particular, given the absence of language among the other primates – many researchers are led to conclude that the infant vocal tract is underdeveloped compared to the adult vocal tract (Kent 1981, Thelen 1991).

While infants in the first months of life are unable to produce the range of oral sounds used in adult language, from the time they are born, infants are physiologically disposed to produce a range of stricture-based and prosodic sounds that involve laryngeal constriction, many of which function contrastively in linguistic systems (Catford 1977a, Ladefoged and Maddieson 1996, Esling and Edmondson 2002, Carlson et al. 2004, Edmondson et al. 2005, Edmondson and Esling 2006). Moreover, the right-angled, lowered larynx is not limited to humans (Fitch and Reby 2001) and is not necessarily the primary determinant in the evolution of speech and language. The disposition of the infant larynx constrains the range of sounds that infants can make, particularly in the first months of life (Benner et al. 2007). However, the way that infants use their developing vocal capacities in the lower vocal tract illustrates processes that are at least as relevant to human speech and language development as any anatomical orientation (Grenon et al. 2007). In particular, the disposition to explore emergent phonetic capacities and to build a system of contrasts at the segmental and suprasegmental levels is critical to speech development. We elaborate on these processes as they occur in the laryngeal articulator.

6.2 Vocal Exploration in Infancy

Oller (1978, 1980, 2000, 2004) has emphasized the role of 'vocal play' or 'vocal exploration' in speech development. In addition to the alternations between constricted and unconstricted utterances that we have labelled dynamic, we often observe infants between the ages of three and seven months engaging in systematic alternations between new sounds, including different

(a) Newborn (estimated based on ~3-month-old fetus)

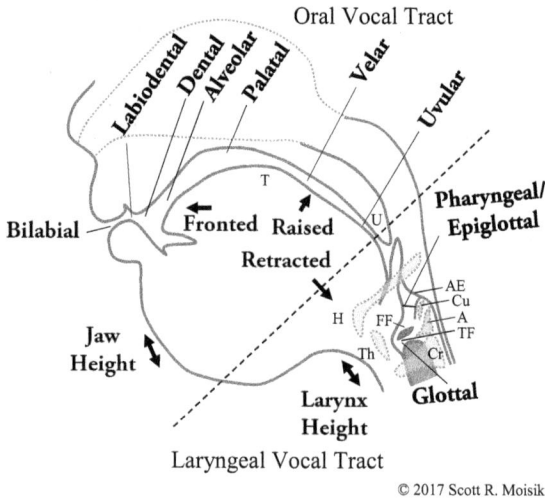

© 2017 Scott R. Moisik

(b) 7-month-old child

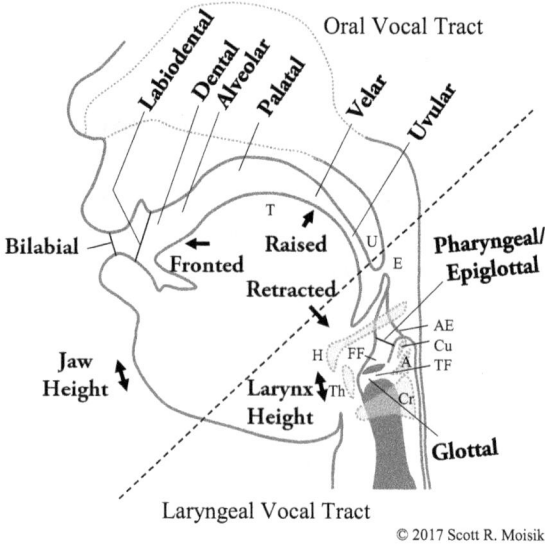

© 2017 Scott R. Moisik

Figure 6.1 *The vocal tract of (a) a newborn infant and (b) a 7-month-old infant*
T = tongue; U = uvula; E = epiglottis; H = hyoid bone; AE = aryepiglottic folds; Cu = cuneiform cartilage; A = arytenoid cartilage; FF = ventricular (false) folds; TF = vocal (true) folds; Th = thyroid cartilage; Cr = cricoid cartilage.

vowels, different pitches, and different phonation types. Oller (2000, 2004) characterizes such vocal play as the infant's first exploration in contrastive features, and thus, as the precursor to the development of linguistic categories. Buder et al. (2013) have developed an impressive taxonomy of early phonetic behaviour that includes categories for different types of 'protophones' that are posited to be precursors to speech. Other researchers have also noted increased exploratory vocalization during these months (Stark 1980, Koopmans-van Beinum and van der Stelt 1986, Roug et al. 1989, Thelen 1991). In a detailed study of the vocalizations of one English infant, Bettany (2004) highlighted the role of alternations in laryngeal voice quality in developing laryngeal control during the first six months of life, observing that the number and length of such alternations increase in the fourth month of life. Vihman et al. (1985) and Vihman (2014) have noted the production of laryngeal sounds in infant articulations and their possible role in speech and language acquisition.

Some time after, or overlapping with, the period of vocal play, infants begin to produce canonical babbling sequences, utterances that display repetitive consonant-vowel (CV) syllables. In the initial stages of babbling, sometimes referred to as 'marginal' babbling (Oller 1980), the consonants in babbling sequences do not display the timing features of adult CV(C) syllables, with stops showing longer periods of silence and longer transitions to vowels. With practice, however, CV(C) sequences begin to acquire the timing features seen in adult utterances, allowing infants to produce babbling sequences with rapidly articulated syllables. Babbling generally appears in infant vocalizations by the seventh month of life (Koopmans-van Beinum and van der Stelt 1986).

MacNeilage's 'frames, then content' theory of speech development (1998) has been profoundly influential in shaping infant speech researchers' understanding of the origins of babbling. MacNeilage and his colleagues (MacNeilage et al. 2000, MacNeilage and Davis 2001) have explored the notion that babbling originates from the jaw cyclicities involved in chewing, and thus, evolves from an adaptation of a human non-speech behaviour. The 'content' of early babbling – the specific vowels and consonants – is initially dominated by the 'frame' provided by jaw movement, making bilabial babbling sequences produced with low central vowels among the first to appear in the productions of most infants. Over time, infants begin to produce alveolar and velar babbling sequences, the latter often produced with back vowels and the former with front vowels, in keeping with the notion of 'frame dominance'. With practice, infants gain freedom in producing different combinations of consonants and vowels, allowing for the integration of language-specific 'content' in syllabic utterances, including language-specific prosody (Davis et al. 2000).

Of all the utterances infants produce in the first year of life, babbling is considered to be the most speech-like and, therefore, the most likely among infant vocalizations to reflect the influence of the ambient language. Many researchers have examined the babbling of infants from different language backgrounds, with a view to identifying language-specific features. Congruent with MacNeilage's (1998) perspective, the segments in infant babbling tend to show a remarkable consistency in early babbling, but the prosody may exhibit language-specific characteristics (Boysson-Bardies et al. 1984, Hallé et al. 1991, Nathani et al. 2003). Some aspects of laryngeal control, such as prevoicing and/or voice onset time, may begin to show in the ways that infants produce some consonants in babbling sequences (Whalen et al. 2007). Overall, however, while research suggests that infants actively explore linguistically relevant aspects of prosody in the first year (Sheppard and Lane 1968, Delack and Fowlow 1978, Hsu et al. 2000), sometimes producing utterances that resemble their ambient language (Boysson-Bardies and Vihman 1991, Hallé et al. 1991), infants do not begin to combine these elements consistently in language-specific ways until at least the second year of life (Snow and Balog 2002).

The acquisition of voice quality in infancy and childhood is seldom considered, except as reflected in a bias towards studying sounds produced with modal voice. In the past thirty-five years, infant speech researchers have paid increasing attention to the early vocalizations of infants as precursors to communication and language development. In earlier research, studies focused on identifying the most 'speech-like' early vocalizations, so many researchers focused only on earlier utterances produced with 'normal' or modal phonation (Oller 1980, 2000, Koopmans-van Beinum and van der Stelt 1986). Oller (2000) considers modal phonation as a first step in the development of control over syllable production in babbling. Buder et al. (2008) note that 'caregivers, researchers, and others primarily interested in tracking incipient language understandably attend to productions spoken with modal voice, as being indicative of emerging linguistic control, while treating "squealy" or "growly" voices as pertaining to more paralinguistic communication indicating emotion, attitude, or overall fitness' (p. 553). However, it is increasingly recognized that these squealy or growly sounds, which are non-modal sounds produced with laryngeal constriction, represent a large proportion of the sounds produced in early infancy, and that they may play an important role in the evolution of infants' communicative resources (McCune et al. 1996) and in their phonetic development (Bettany 2004, Esling et al. 2004). Moreover, some languages use laryngeal constriction contrastively (Esling and Edmondson 2002). Our analysis focuses specifically on the non-modal, constricted vocalizations in infants' speech development, with the aim of integrating them into the wider discussion of ontogenetic phonetic acquisition.

6.3　Laryngeal Voice Quality in the First Year of Life

The research in this chapter is based on 2400 infant vocalizations from our corpus, balanced over the first year (months 1–3, 4–6, 7–9, and 10–12) and between two groups of infants (four infants in English surroundings and four in Bai surroundings). Vocalizations are classified using auditory analysis, supplemented by examination of wide-band spectrograms. Utterances are classified according to laryngeal quality and utterance type. For laryngeal quality, utterances are divided into three broad categories: *constricted, unconstricted,* and *dynamic*. Constricted utterances are those produced with harsh voice, creaky voice, whispery voice, or whisper. Unconstricted utterances are those produced with modal voice, breathy voice, or falsetto. Dynamic utterances involve at least one alternation between a constricted and an unconstricted voice quality posture within a single vocalization. For utterance type, we use the categories *non-syllabic, mixed,* and *syllabic*. Non-syllabic utterances are vocalic in nature, while syllabic utterances include the production of at least one CV sequence (what is usually referred to as babbling in the literature). Mixed utterances are primarily vocalic vocalizations that include the production of a partial oral stricture (similar to what Oller refers to as 'gooing'). Figure 6.2 is an example of a dynamic non-syllabic utterance. Using auditory criteria, this utterance can be heard to start out in modal voice and end in harsh voice, visible in the increase in energy in the upper portion of the spectrum towards the end of the utterance.

Audio file 6.104 is the sound file that corresponds to the acoustic spectrum in Figure 6.2.

6.3.1　Laryngeal Quality

As laryngeal quality is endemic to infants in the first year of life, the very notion of developing phonetic distinctions parallels the development of voice quality settings at this stage. The general pattern in the development of laryngeal qualities for Bai and English infants is similar, while exhibiting some differences that may reflect the influence of the ambient target language. These common and divergent patterns are demonstrated in Figures 6.3 and 6.4 for Bai and English infants, respectively.

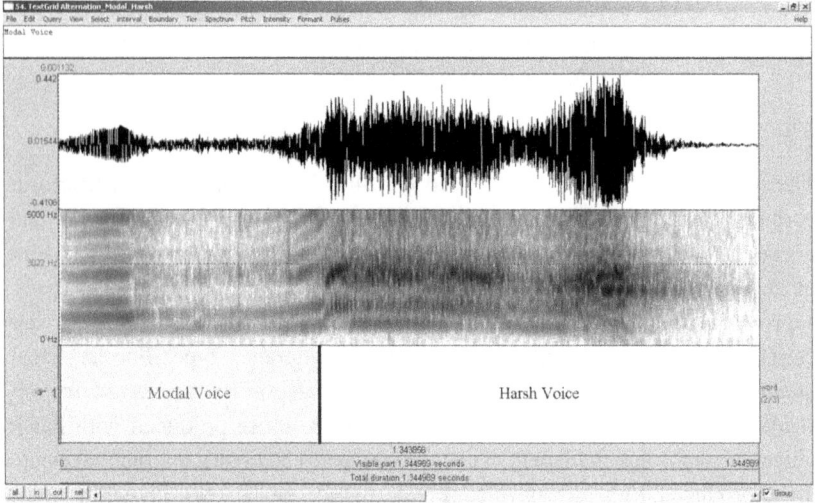

Figure 6.2 *A dynamic non-syllabic utterance, 6-month-old, English context, on an open vowel*

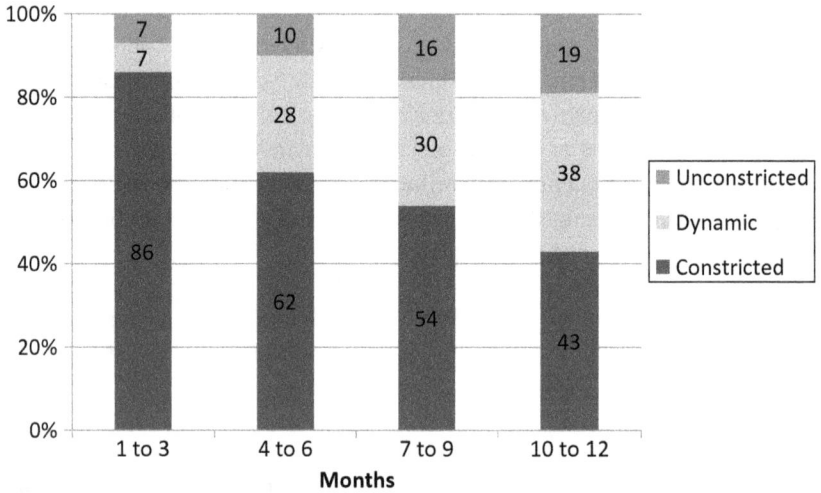

Figure 6.3 *Laryngeal voice quality in Bai infant utterances, by age and percentage of production*

Among Bai and English infants, laryngeal voice quality changes over time. For infants from both language groups, constricted vocalizations are the most frequent utterances produced throughout every period of the first year of life, though they decline linearly as the year goes on, falling slightly faster and to a

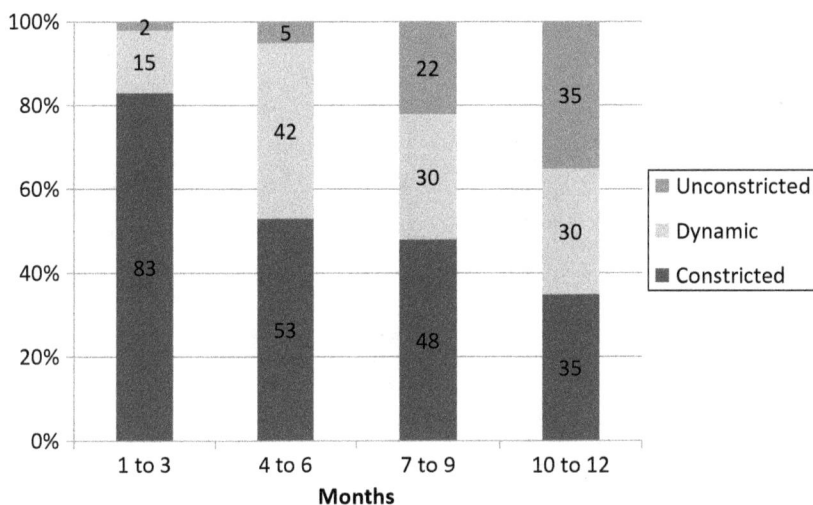

Figure 6.4 *Laryngeal voice quality in English infant utterances, by age and percentage of production*

greater extent for English infants than for Bai infants. By contrast, unconstricted utterances gradually increase for infants from both language groups, though the increase is more dramatic for English infants than for Bai infants. The number of dynamic utterances increases significantly in months 4–6 for infants of both language groups. Bai and English infants continue to produce a significant proportion of dynamic utterances throughout the first year. However, among the English infants, in the second half of the year, the proportion of dynamic utterances decreases relative to those produced in months 4–6, while for the Bai infants, dynamic utterances continue to increase during this period, with the highest incidence occurring in months 10–12.

Audio files 6.001 to 6.103 are representative files that illustrate constricted, dynamic, and unconstricted sounds produced by the English and Bai infants. For the Bai infants, files 6.001 to 6.014 are constricted sounds, 6.015 to 6.031 are dynamic utterances, and files 6.032 to 6.043 are unconstricted sounds. For the English infants, files 6.044 to 6.066 are constricted sounds, 6.067 to 6.088 are dynamic sounds, and 6.089 to 6.103 are unconstricted sounds. Earlier files in a series represent younger infants, and later files older infants. These examples are provided so that listeners can become familiar with the auditory categories used in our research.

In our organization and evaluation of the data, from constricted through dynamic to unconstricted productions, the key trend that we are tracking is how speech development progresses from dominant laryngeal constriction to

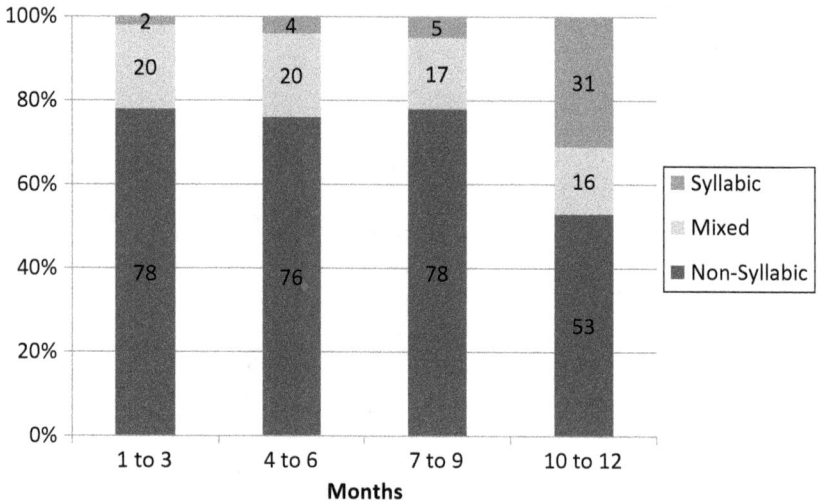

Figure 6.5 *Utterance types produced by Bai infants, by age and percentage*

sounds produced with an open, unconstricted laryngeal posture. The increasing proportion of dynamic utterances among the Bai infants, and the gradually decreasing proportion of such utterances among the English infants, in concert with the rise in unconstricted utterances in the latter group, can be hypothesized to reflect the influence of the ambient language. In terms of the use of laryngeal vocal quality, Bai is a comparatively dynamic language that makes active phonological use of laryngeal constriction and alternations between constricted and unconstricted postures. By contrast, in terms of laryngeal constriction, English is a relatively static language in which the most typical laryngeal posture is unconstricted.

6.3.2   Utterance Types

Figures 6.5 and 6.6 represent the proportion of non-syllabic, mixed, and syllabic utterances produced by Bai and English infants throughout their first year. In the first months of life and throughout the first year, Bai and English infants produce mostly non-syllabic utterances. In the second half of the year, and particularly in months 10–12, syllabic utterances increase significantly in frequency. Prior to the emergence of syllabic vocalizations in large numbers, infants from both language groups begin to produce mixed vocalizations, which involve the production of a brief oral stricture in a primarily vocalic utterance. Mixed utterances continue to comprise a substantial portion of vocalizations throughout the first year.

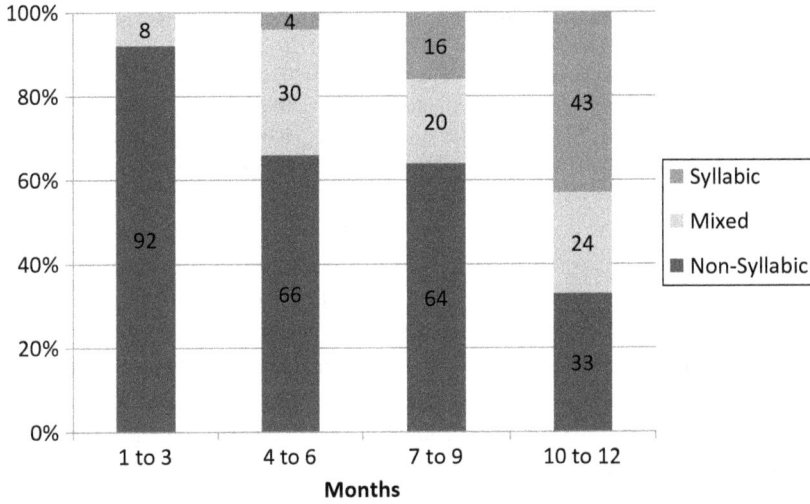

Figure 6.6 *Utterance types produced by English infants, by age and percentage*

Among Bai infants, syllabic utterances appear at least as early in speech development as they do among English infants, but they develop more slowly, showing a significant increase only by months 10–12. For English infants, once syllabic utterances begin to be produced, they proliferate. Moreover, with the exception of months 1–3, English infants produce more mixed utterances than Bai infants throughout the first year. Syllabic and mixed vocalizations involve a greater engagement of the oral vocal tract and a larger degree of integration between the laryngeal and oral vocal tracts than non-syllabic utterances.

Based on the patterns observed in our data, it appears that infants from both language backgrounds are engaged in the same processes of phonetic development, but these processes are structured differently for Bai and English infants, likely because of differences in how the laryngeal vocal tract is employed in the ambient languages of the infants. Once oral stricture and syllable structure begin to emerge, infants from both language groups are drawn to further develop these phonetic capacities. However, English infants are more attracted to the development of the oral vocal tract than are Bai infants, and they achieve some degree of integration of the oral and laryngeal vocal tracts sooner than Bai infants. We can posit that these different patterns reflect the relative importance of, and specific demands associated with, laryngeal control in the Bai sound system versus English.

Among the audio files, Bai examples by utterance type are as follows: non-syllabic (6.001–6.007, 6.015–6.020, 6.032–6.036); mixed (6.008–6.010, 6.021–6.027, 6.037–6.040); and syllabic (6.011–6.014, 6.028–6.031, 6.041–6.043). English examples by utterance type are: non-syllabic (6.044–6.058, 6.067–6.072, 6.089–6.093); mixed (6.059–6.061, 6.073–6.082, 6.094–6.098); and syllabic (6.062–6.066, 6.083–6.088, 6.099–6.103). These examples are provided to illustrate the auditory categories used in our research.

6.3.3   Distribution of Laryngeal Constriction by Utterance Type

Since both language groups produce a majority of non-syllabic utterances for most of the first year, the distribution of laryngeal voice quality categories in non-syllabic utterances essentially mirrors the data as a whole. For both language groups, constricted non-syllabic utterances decline linearly throughout the year, while unconstricted non-syllabic vocalizations steadily increase, with small differences in the degree and pace of increase between infants from the two language groups. Dynamic non-syllabic utterances gradually increase throughout the year for Bai infants, while among English infants, dynamic non-syllabic vocalizations increase dramatically in months 4–6 and then decrease slightly for the remainder of the year.

The pattern for mixed utterances – sounds that are primarily vocalic but that include a brief oral stricture – is of particular interest in that it demonstrates that emergent exploration and control of the oral vocal tract begins in the context of laryngeal constriction and of alternation between laryngeally constricted and unconstricted voice qualities. As shown in Figures 6.7 and 6.8, in months 1–3, the majority of mixed utterances are constricted for infants from both language groups. For the remainder of the year, the majority of mixed utterances tend to be associated with dynamic laryngeal voice quality for both groups. Throughout the first year of life, mixed utterances are most likely to be dynamic and least likely to be unconstricted.

Dynamic mixed utterances may play a special role in the process of speech development. In our analysis, dynamic utterances are those most likely to be associated with 'vocal play', and therefore with infants' exploration of their vocal ranges in terms of pitch and constriction. Dynamic utterances are an important medium for the development of laryngeal control of alternating postures for infants of both language backgrounds. Mixed utterances are understood as the context in which oral consonants first begin to emerge, as intermediary between non-syllabic and syllabic utterances. The fact that mixed utterances are most likely to be dynamic (alternating in laryngeal articulatory

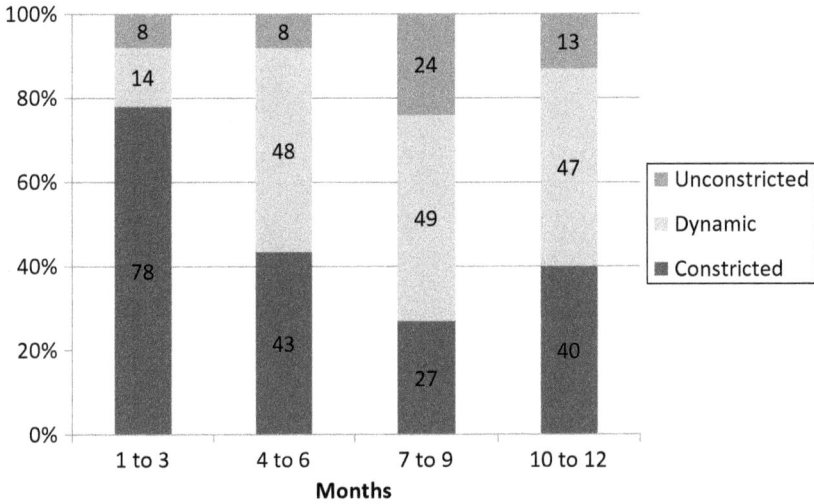

Figure 6.7 *Laryngeal voice quality in mixed utterances of Bai infants, by percentage*
Percentages in column 2 are rounded.

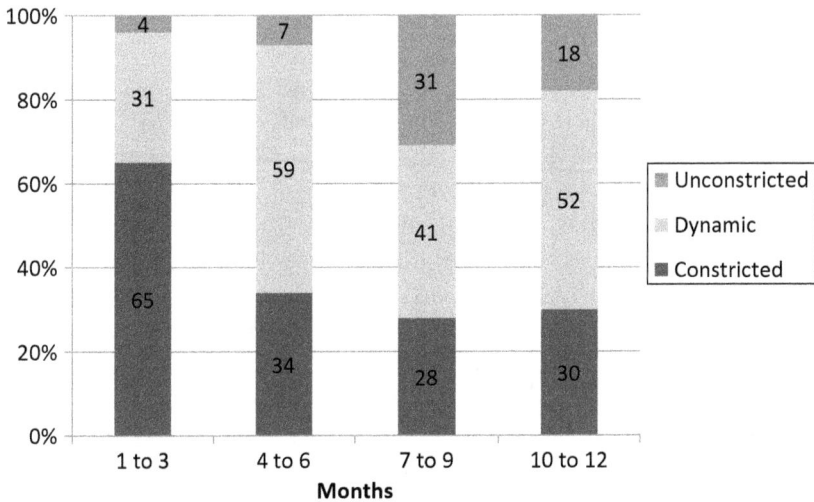

Figure 6.8 *Laryngeal voice quality in mixed utterances of English infants, by percentage*

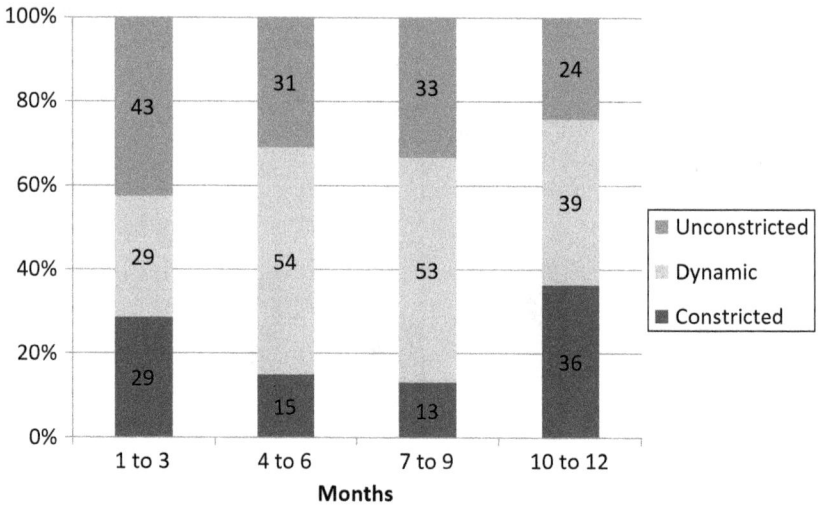

Figure 6.9 *Laryngeal voice quality in syllabic utterances of Bai infants, by percentage*
Percentages in columns 1, 3, and 4 are rounded.

posture) throughout the first year suggests that vocal play provides a medium in which infants not only develop laryngeal voice quality but are most likely to begin to integrate their emergent control of the oral vocal tract with their ongoing, developing control of the laryngeal vocal tract.

The distribution of laryngeal voice qualities in syllabic utterances – the most speech-like of the sounds in this study – suggests that, in the first year of life, infants develop a laryngeal setting that increasingly mirrors that used in their ambient language. Figures 6.9 and 6.10 show the distribution of constricted, dynamic, and unconstricted voice quality categories in syllabic utterances for Bai and English infants, respectively. Bai infants do not begin to produce syllabic utterances in significant numbers until months 10–12, making comparisons between voice qualities throughout the year difficult. However, in months 10–12, the syllabic utterances of Bai infants are distributed relatively evenly across laryngeal voice quality categories, while fully 53 per cent of syllabic utterances produced by English infants in months 10–12 are unconstricted. These patterns suggest that by the end of the first year, infants learning Bai are beginning to babble using the laryngeal voice qualities that are contrastive in their ambient language, while infants learning English are beginning to produce most of their babbling in the unconstricted laryngeal

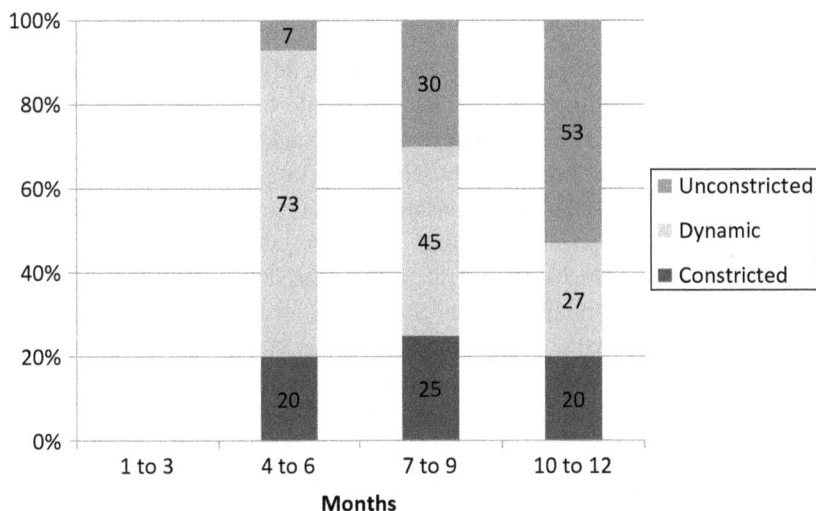

Figure 6.10 *Laryngeal voice quality in syllabic utterances of English infants, by percentage*
No syllabic utterances occurred in months 1–3.

settings that predominate in their target language, which does not use laryngeal settings contrastively. This suggests that the awareness of the need to differentiate between vocal quality as a register (within a syllabic system with the potential to carry lexical meaning) and voice quality as long-term secondary background is already beginning to be established by the end of the first year of life.

Bai examples of laryngeal voice quality by utterance type are as follows: For non-syllabic utterances, files include constricted non-syllabic (6.001–6.007), dynamic non-syllabic (6.015–6.020), and unconstricted non-syllabic 6.032–6.036. For mixed utterances, files include constricted mixed (6.008–6.010), dynamic mixed (6.021–6.027), and unconstricted mixed 6.037–6.040. For syllabic utterances, files include constricted syllabic (6.011–6.014), dynamic syllabic (6.028–6.031), and unconstricted syllabic (6.041–6.043). The corresponding examples for English: For non-syllabic, files include constricted non-syllabic (6.044–6.058), dynamic non-syllabic (6.067–6.072), and unconstricted non-syllabic (6.089–6.093). For mixed utterances, files include constricted mixed (6.059–6.061), dynamic mixed (6.073–6.082), and unconstricted mixed (6.094–6.098). For syllabic utterances, files include constricted syllabic (6.062–6.066), dynamic syllabic (6.083–6.088), and unconstricted syllabic (6.099–6.103).

6.4   Laryngeal Components of Early Babbling

The literature on infant speech production consistently chronicles the development of syllabic utterances in the first year of life for children from a wide range of language backgrounds (Grégoire 1937, Stark et al. 1975, 1993, Roug et al. 1989, Boysson-Bardies 1999, Nathani et al. 2006), normally in the context of babbling. Babbling is considered to be a universal stage in speech and language development (Jakobson 1941/1968, Oller 1978, 1980, 2000, MacNeilage 1998, MacNeilage et al. 2000, MacNeilage and Davis 2001). Koopmans-van Beinum and van der Stelt (1986) observe that syllabic utterances are produced by the seventh month of life in 90 per cent of infants. The failure to produce syllabic utterances by this time tends to be predictive of speech and language disorders (Oller et al. 1998, 1999). The Bai and English infants in our corpus, who show no signs of speech or language disorders, fit the normal pattern. All infants in the corpus had produced some syllabic utterances by the seventh month of life, as shown in Figures 6.5 and 6.6, illustrating the development of non-syllabic, mixed, and syllabic utterances for Bai and English infants, respectively, with English infants producing about 50 per cent more syllabic forms than the Bai infants.

Infants learning Bai are in the process of acquiring a tonal register language that employs both pitch and laryngeal constriction. Studies of the acquisition of tone consistently demonstrate that infants do not acquire specific lexical tones until the second year of life (Li and Thompson 1977, Ota 2003). Moreover, analyses of speech errors produced by young children, starting in the second year of life, show that infants who are learning a tone language make fewer errors in tone production than in the production of initial and final consonants (Zhu and Dodd 2000). These patterns suggest that the information conveyed in tone is highly salient for infants who are learning tone languages, and that it may be at least as salient as the information encoded in the CV(C) structures that provide the segmental foundation for syllabic utterances and that are the primary carriers of contrastive information in non-tone languages. Given that by the age of six months, infants attend preferentially to lexical words (Shi and Werker 2001), it seems likely that infants who are learning tone languages attend early on to pitch differences that create lexical contrast, including, in the case of the Bai infants, pitch-dependent changes in laryngeal vocal quality. The salience of such variations within the language, combined with the fact that infants produce similar variations as a normal part of their phonetic development, may account for the greater prevalence of non-syllabic utterances in the Bai infants' production for most of the first year of life.

Syllabic production is an essential part of speech development for infants in general, but non-syllabic utterances are not necessarily less 'developed' or less 'speech-like' than syllabic utterances for infants who are becoming attuned to pitch-dependent vocal quality contrasts that can be explored in purely vocalic utterances and later integrated into syllabic utterances. Benner (2009) reports that Bai adults consider even constricted non-syllabic utterances to sound like speech, while English adults do not. Thus, while infants from both language groups are naturally drawn to the production of syllabic utterances, the Bai infants may be just as strongly drawn to the production of non-syllabic utterances as an integral part of their phonetic and linguistic development, accounting for the greater prevalence of such utterances throughout the first year. By contrast, English infants, while engaging in considerable 'vocal play' throughout the first year, may sense fairly soon that the segmental information conveyed in syllables is more relevant to lexical contrast than pitch-dependent vocal quality variations. Thus, early in development, syllabic vocalizations may exert a stronger pull for the English infants, while discriminating laryngeal categories may exert a stronger pull for the Bai infants.

The Laryngeal Articulator Model provides an essential basis for understanding the distribution of non-syllabic, mixed, and syllabic utterances. In the LAM, we characterize the laryngeal and oral vocal tracts as distinct domains of control. In the course of speech and language development, infants develop control over the laryngeal vocal tract before they develop control over the oral vocal tract. In this sense, the laryngeal vocal tract 'primes' the oral vocal tract (Esling 2012).

Audio file 6.105 illustrates the priming of an oral stricture [m] in early babbling, where the laryngeal constrictor tightens to produce harsh voicing accompanying the nasal stop. In dynamic terms, it could be said that the utterance contains an unconstricted [m] in alternation with and in contrast to an [m] that is produced with laryngeal constriction. Audio file 6.106 illustrates the priming of an oral [t] in early babbling, where the background phonation is harsh whisperiness while the oral syllables are being produced.

The integration of the functions performed by the laryngeal and oral vocal tracts is an essential part of speech and language development. The laryngeal vocal tract carries a heavy functional load in all languages. Arguably, however, it carries a heavier functional load in pitch-dependent tone languages, and an even heavier load in a language like Bai, which employs pitch-dependent laryngeal vocal quality contrasts. This factor, in combination with the perceptual salience of laryngeal contrasts in Bai compared to English, may also serve to explain the slower development of syllabic utterances among the Bai infants. To produce syllabic utterances that begin to resemble the syllabic utterances in their ambient language, Bai infants must develop the capacity to produce rapid alternations in laryngeal vocal register from syllable to syllable. This capacity requires a higher degree of laryngeal control than is required for a language in which syllabic utterances are normally produced in a single, unconstricted voice quality. Thus, Bai infants may be motivated to invest more time than English infants in developing refined laryngeal control before they concentrate on the production of syllabic utterances, which represent a comparatively advanced integration of the oral and laryngeal vocal tracts.

Our analysis, from the perspective of laryngeal articulation, suggests a refinement of Oller's (1978, 1980, 2000) claims about the role of modal phonation in speech and language development. Among infant speech researchers, Oller is prominent for his contribution to our understanding of speech and language development as a continuous process that begins at birth. In his work on infant speech production, Oller has argued for the importance of modal voice in speech development generally and in the development of syllabic utterances in particular. Based on our findings, it is true that infants' phonetic development correlates with an increase in the frequency of production of modal voice. However, we cannot say that the production of modal voice is necessarily associated with the emergence of oral consonants or with the emergence of syllabic utterances. Rather, oral consonants and syllabic utterances first emerge in utterances produced with constricted and dynamic laryngeal voice qualities. Practising these settings produces the type of laryngeal control that allows for the eventual greater production of modal voice and the increased production of syllabic utterances. Thus, increased production of modal voice is the *effect* of developing laryngeal control, not its *cause*. A full understanding of the emergence of modal voice is only possible within a framework that includes analysis of the production of the non-modal, laryngeally constricted voice qualities that precede it.

6.5   Early Laryngeal Sounds as Foundations of Speech Development

During the first several months of life, the infant parses phonetic possibilities in a process that refines the identity of various potential individual sounds against the emerging background of laryngeal qualities, which are long term by nature. The essence of the laryngeal articulator is captured by the ontogenetic sequencing of infant speech acquisition, in which sustained pharyngealized crying precedes the development of systematic stricture to isolate an initial set of manners of articulation. Taking the laryngeal articulator as the operative model, the first stricture sound that we identify in infant speech is epiglottal stop. This conforms with the physiological requirement to close and protect the airway while breathing, eating, and speaking activities are being synchronized. Our data demonstrate that (pharyngeal) stops, fricatives, approximants, and trills are produced at the aryepiglottic constrictor by infants in the first several months. In proceeding from the original laryngeal articulator to the elaboration of strictures in the oral vocal tract, the infant recruits qualities from the laryngeal vocal tract, including sustained phonation, complex vibrations, and developing resonant qualities, to augment or prime the manners of articulation spreading through the vocal tract. We hypothesize that these various laryngeal resonances and periodicities, juxtaposed together with pitch modifications as coarticulatory accompaniments to oral strictures, are evaluated auditorily by the infant to refine the character of new consonantal sounds being produced and to coordinate their acoustic properties with articulatory-auditory productions that have already been established in the infant's repertory.

Audio files 6.107–6.120 illustrate the range of manners of articulation produced in the laryngeal articulator in early phonetic sound formation. These are samples of infants' phonetic exploration that proliferate in our database during the first months and exemplify laryngeally constricted sounds found in constricted and dynamic utterances.

Our observations and descriptions of early infant speech production reinforce the principle established by Saussure in his 'theory of the sign' (1916, 1960) that the signifier emerges and precedes the signified. In phonetic terms, this means that the sounds that the infant autogenerates become an inventory of signifiers potentially available for signified entities. In this case, the signifier is a sound image, created by the infant with phonetic predictability by obeying the physiological parameters of laryngeal anatomy. In our model, the potentiality of sound signifiers anticipates the pattern of phonological potentials, which parallel each other in that they both respond to the requirements of articulatory relationships. Infants discover these relationships during their first several months of life. Thus, one possible extension of our research in psycholinguistics would be to document how this principle unfolds with respect to early laryngeal speech sounds as potential signifiers. Our evidence, especially that relating to dynamic utterances, in which infants explore laryngeal contrasts that they later incorporate into a meaningful system in speech and language, implies that infants generate signifiers at a very early stage, even before babbling and before words.

Laryngeal qualities serve as the background to the many consonantal articulations that proliferate as speech expands. They are inherently more amenable to long-term status, as they spring from a place of articulation and a time of life that together accommodate long-term sustained production before shorter-term distinctions can be isolated and refined. As such, the distinction between voice quality and segmental identity originates in the infant vocal tract. The consonantal pieces of the matrix are defined in an ongoing relation to those qualities that preceded them and which outline them as emerging figures against the more constant background of voice quality (in the sense of Laver 1975: 2, 1980: 5) as phonation type and laryngeal posture. We propose that this developmental process lays the groundwork for the interaction between vocalic and consonantal properties and long-term voice quality settings in the mature speaking voice. Individual infants may not exploit this physiological-auditory process to the same degree or with the same cognitive outcomes, but the rudimentary exercise of articulatory-auditory parsing must take place to enable the infant to separate the short- and long-term acoustic characteristics that will become distinctive markers of their mature voices.

7 Clinical Illustrations of Voice Quality

Chapter 7 explores laryngeal and pharyngeal speech disorders, voice pathologies that depart from normal function, and the consequences of laryngeal surgery on voice quality from the perspective of the Laryngeal Articulator Model (LAM). Impairments affecting the operation of the vocal folds reveal the inherent physiological capacity to adapt epilaryngeal postures to produce new voice qualities. Many clinical disorders also affect the functioning of the laryngeal/pharyngeal articulatory mechanism directly. We explain laryngeal movements during normal vs. pathological phonation, functional abnormalities, organic lesions, and neurological movement disorders in clinical terms to demonstrate the laryngeal biomechanics of compensation behaviour. Surgical excisions of laryngeal structures are diagrammed to detail the consequences on the laryngeal articulator as a whole. We describe voice qualities resulting from various pathologies and before and after surgery and speech therapy. Compensatory behaviours identified in the aryepiglottic mechanism superior to the glottis can mimic epilaryngeal productions by speakers whose languages exploit elaborated laryngeal constrictor control. Some disorders emulate particular phonation types in our voice quality taxonomy, involving epilaryngeal structures not usually discussed in medical or anatomy texts. Vocal agility in Mongolian long song and human beatboxing performance illustrate laryngeal possibilities beyond the phonetic norm, which also exploit postures elaborated in the LAM.

With the expansion of experimental phonetics in the nineteenth century, coinciding with anatomical and physiological advances, the vaguely understood lower vocal tract became the focus of study (García 1855, Czermak 1861). Vocal fold vibration was imaged and observed to be independent of the production of vowel sounds in the upper vocal tract, but the operation of the laryngeal mechanism as a whole and its relationship to vowel production were not yet recognized. Rousselot (1904), the founder of experimental phonetics in France, can be considered the father of clinical phonetics, using acoustic, kymographic, palatographic, and photographic analysis to study the major functions underlying phonation: breathing, articulation, and dynamics. By the late nineteenth century, the term 'phonation' appeared based on physiology and included the words *voix* (voice) and *parole* (speech) in a process of *voix articulée* (articulate voice), the voice (in the sense of voicing) being considered fundamental in the production of fluent speech. It is worth pointing out that neurology (Broca 1861, Wernicke 1874) and neurolinguistics, concentrating on aphasia, clinical research, and the therapeutic management of voice and speech disorders (Gutzmann 1893, 1909) including stuttering (Chervin 1854), were fields where the study of voice per se and of speech production in general laid the critical groundwork for understanding long-term aspects of speech by examining how particular disorders deprive the speaker of long-term control. Similarly, Bell's work on speech and hearing (1908), which also concentrated on sustained production abilities in disordered circumstances, engendered interest in voice and quality in the long-term sense.

One motivation for examining pathological voice and speech is to define the limits of normal variation within linguistic phonetic systems by identifying the borders of departure from the norm. Another scientific goal is to understand how articulatory and vibratory mechanisms function in disordered or surgically altered contexts, in order to identify adaptations and compensatory strategies. Clinical goals include guiding and refining diagnosis, testing the functional efficacy of surgical treatments and rehabilitation procedures, proposing and adapting new methods of rehabilitation to overcome surgical intervention, and guiding speech therapy practices to improve vocal compensation and to facilitate social reintegration. Voice plays a significant role in social integration and in the quality of life (Laver 1980: 2–3, Preston 1992, 2006, Esling 2000, Kreiman and Sidtis 2011), and it is therefore of practical interest to restore and improve a patient's ability to present themselves verbally. The laryngeal dimension of verbal behaviour is critical, because a multitude of ailments and surgical interventions target the larynx in particular, and multiple components of voice production are affected incrementally when its function is altered.

The factors that influence the complexity of the laryngeal system include extrinsic or extralinguistic variability (the cultural and social dimensions of speech acquisition), paralinguistic variation (emotional or attitudinal implications), and intrinsic variability (individual anatomo-physiological differences in the performance of the target sound system). These levels of meaning are often conveyed through voice quality, or what has been referred to in singing-voice terminology as 'timbre' (Colton and Estill 1981, Honda et al. 1995a, Steinhauer and Estill 2008). Beyond these considerations, the boundary between the norm of a language variety and pathological departure from that norm has to be considered within Laryngeal Articulatory Model (LAM) parameters. When a pathology intervenes to cause normal targets to be altered involuntarily, the timbre inevitably changes. These changes are likely to be noticeable initially or globally as voice quality characteristics, due to their pervasive effect on vibration and sustained resonance throughout the vocal tract. Acquaintances listening to a person's voice will notice changes to what could be called the 'aesthetics' of the voice. Alterations could occur to the physiological (length and mass) or biomechanical properties of the vocal, ventricular or aryepiglottic folds and their vertical coupling, or to the physiological and dynamic characteristics of the resonance cavities, epilaryngeal and pharyngeal mucosa, mobility of the raising–lowering muscle chains, mobility of the soft palate and the tongue, and the tone of the cheeks and lips. Like fundamental frequency, timbre will vary over time depending on changes in the vibrating bodies and/or the volumes of resonance cavities as a function of the effects of disease, trauma, or surgery. Pathologies can affect vibrating sources, sequencing of chains of activity, coordination, and specific timelines. Aerodynamic forces, muscle contractions, and histo-chemical and biophysical properties of the tissues can be affected in the pathophysiology of altered voices and disordered speech. The chronicle of voice disorders necessarily starts at the glottis, with vocal fold structural pathologies (Mackenzie Beck et al. 1991).

7.1   Vocal Fold Vibration

7.1.1   Human Laryngeal Tissues

The histological structure of the vocal folds in the human larynx differs from that of other mammals. A layer of connective tissue – the 'lamina propria' between the mucosa and the vocalis muscle – is particular to humans (Hirano 1974). The lamina propria is composed of three layers. The superficial layer, beneath an external covering of stratified squamous epithelium, consists of collagen and elastin fibres and a large proportion of stroma containing hyaluronic acid. This loose tissue defines Reinke's space and allows the superficial mucosa to slide on the lining of the deeper layers so that vibration of the mucosa is independent of muscular movement. The characteristics of this space determine to a large extent the quality of voicing in glottal phonation. The intermediate and deep layers of the lamina propria constitute the vocal ligament, consisting of elastin fibres, contributing to elastic oscillation in the vibration cycle, and collagen fibres, giving a certain rigidity to the vibratory system (Kahane 1986). Contractions of the vocalis muscles determine the stiffness of the vibratory system. Another feature of the lamina propria layers is that they may regenerate thanks to the presence of structures called maculae flavae located at the end of each vocal fold at the anterior commissure and facing the vocal process (Sato et al. 2000). These structures only appear around the age of 6–7 years, explaining certain characteristics of the voice of the child.

Thus, the physiological properties of the lamina propria give the vocal folds specific vibrational qualities, responsible for the source waves that propagate through the vocal tract and fundamental to voice quality as a reflection of the spectral filter of vocal tract resonances (the timbre of the voice). This anatomo-physiological laryngeal knowledge is fundamental in formulating the relationship between structure and vocal outcomes and, above all, in preserving optimal voicing quality when performing microphonosurgery of the vocal folds, functional phonosurgery to treat a benign lesion of the glottis (Hirano 1975, Ford and Bless 1991, Giovanni et al. 2010), and more extensive laryngeal surgery. It also allows a better understanding of the pathophysiology of voice quality and of changes observed after vocal trauma or improper use (misuse or overuse) of the voice (Morrison et al. 2013).

7.1.2   The Vibratory Pattern at the Glottis
          (Oscillatory-Impedance Theories)

The oscillatory-impedance concept described by Hirano (1977) and Hirano et al. (1981) and supplemented by adjustments from Dejonckere (1981) considers the vibrator (the vocal folds) to be a low-order damped oscillator, turning the expiratory pressure from the lungs into a pulsed pressure whose repetition frequency is identical to that of the oscillator. This model derives from 'body-cover' theory (Fujimura 1981, Hirano and Kakita 1985, Titze 1991). Histologically, the body is the vocalis muscle (thyrovocalis, i.e. internal/medial thyroarytenoid) and the cover the mucosa, the two structures separated by Reinke's space for sliding and waviness over the underlying ligament-muscle structures. The passive mucosa undulates under the influence of muscle contractions and expiratory pressures during phonation (Hirano et al. 1988, Laver et al. 1992). To transform expiratory air into acoustic energy in the form of an acoustic pressure wave or voicing, either paired structures, such as the vocal folds or ventricular folds (or at least some part of their lengths), have to close against each other, or a single structure must close (again, at least partially) against another structure, in the way that the aryepiglottic folds close against either side of the tubercle of the epiglottis. Closures may be multiple, and in phase or out of phase, as we have seen for aryepiglottic trilling in Chapter 3. During each closure, subglottal air pressure momentarily increases, followed immediately by a breaching of the closure, releasing exhaled air as the structure or structures open from bottom to top, momentarily equalizing supra- and subglottal pressure, until the Bernoulli effect draws the structures together again, closing the aperture between the vibrating parts, and so the sequence repeats. As long as subglottal pressure is maintained, cyclical movements are maintained with oscillations that produce a periodic or quasi-periodic sound. Normally, this description of vibration applies to the vocal folds and defines the glottal excitation of basic modal phonation. The frequency of vibration of the vocal folds corresponds to the fundamental frequency (f0) in Hz.

Any modification of the vibratory pattern of the vocal folds themselves will have consequences for voice quality. Myoelastic and aerodynamic theories (van den Berg 1955, 1968, van den Berg et al. 1957, 1960) have explained vocal fold vibratory principles and the variation in phonatory phenomena that can result (see Titze 2006). Aerodynamic factors that regulate subglottal pressure, flow patterns, and expiratory volumes as well as glottic resistance according to degree of closure have also been elaborated (Hirose 1995, 2010). But vocal fold elasticity and the Bernoulli effect do not account completely for the precise and simultaneous regulation of the fundamental frequency of the sound and its power.

Because the buckling (folding) and vertical compression/expansion charac-teristics of the laryngeal articulator are complex (recruiting the thyromuscu-laris, i.e. external/lateral thyroarytenoid, muscles), constricted phonation, such as creakiness or harshness, introduces changes that alter periodicity, making it difficult to track f0 reliably. In adopting the LAM as an alternative to a bipartite source-filter approach, it becomes imperative to apply the principles of aerodynamics, aero-acoustics, and resonance to every possible vibrating structure within the laryngeal mechanism, to the elastic properties of its various folding surfaces, and to every resonating chamber that can be formed by its actions. Nonetheless, vocal fold vibration is the primary mechanism of voicing in speech, and the voicing–voiceless contrast is one of the most productive. Disruptions to efficient vocal fold activity are therefore among the most damaging to the ability to speak normally. Causes include the main function activities: respiratory impairments (for aerodynamic energy), neural compromise (motor control), muscular failure (contraction, movement, closure quality), tissue damage (scarring, vibratory quality, timbre). But other parts of the laryngeal articulator can also be affected by pathology or trauma, with consequences for basic vocal fold vibratory activity, supraglottic vibratory activity, or laryngeal articulator movement that can compromise normal per-formance of critical phonetic contrasts, especially in languages that make extensive use of the full extent of the mechanism. Cases of nodules or polyps of the vocal folds can result in increased mucosal stiffness, a higher threshold of phonatory pressure, and an imbalance in vibratory cycles. Damage to structures superior to the vocal folds can also impair vibratory function throughout the epilaryngeal tube, with a negative effect on pharyngeal articulation or tonal register performance. We will concentrate on impairments to the entire laryngeal articulator, not just the vocal folds.

The undulation of the vocal folds, producing primary periodic vibration, and the configuration of supraglottic structures through the epilaryngeal tube, where laryngeal constriction occurs, are examined in the clinic using either a rigid endoscope placed along the surface of the tongue or a flexible fibrescope inserted nasally. Both endoscopes are connected to a cold light source with fixed light or stroboscopic illumination (25 frames/sec) and high-speed camera imaging 500–4000 frames/sec. Normal modal phonation of the open (unconstricted) laryngeal space is taken as a baseline for comparison with clinical illustrations of disorders and surgeries.

Video 7.01 shows the adduction–abduction movements of the vocal folds (modal, open, unconstricted voicing) in a normal female larynx, followed by stroboscopic illumination emphasizing the mucosal wave. Video 7.02, of modal voicing in a normal male larynx, shows variations in the antero-posterior size and amplitude of the mucosal wave depending on pitch. The fact that the laryngeal mechanism is open and not constricted should not imply that a constricted setting of the mechanism is abnormal. The illustrations of clinical disorders in this chapter are abnormal because they are an impediment beyond the speaker's control.

7.1.3   Nonlinear Dynamic Theories

The borderline between normal and pathological voice quality is not clear. Vocal changes may occur without any obvious pathological conditions or arise in cases of asymmetrical laryngeal vibration. The development of theories of nonlinear dynamics has changed physics and modified our designs of biomechanical and physiological control processes. Chaos theory suggests that the inherent nonlinearity in each system can be the source of unpredictable, but not random, behaviour, even if the number of degrees of freedom is low. The nonlinearity of tissues and their interactions explains certain irregularities of vocal fold movement (Titze 2008), and chaos theory can provide a voice production model that would explain the pathological functioning of phonation (Herzel et al. 1994). As nonlinearity and irregularity are part of our phonatory system, it is not surprising to find aphonic episodes during normal speech.

The aero-mechanical oscillation of the two vocal folds is a nonlinear mechanism that allows the regulation and synchronization of mucosal vibration (Giovanni et al. 1999). Conventional acoustic measurements using instant instability parameters such as jitter (difference in measurements of f0 between two successive cycles) and shimmer (difference in measurements of f0 amplitude between two successive cycles) can detect instability of oscillations but are not always reliable indicators of abnormalities. Vibratory asymmetry can lead to aero-mechanical desynchronization between the vocal folds, as in pathological cases where one fold does not perform as the other. A constitutional change in the oscillator is predicted to result in a change in the mode of vocal fold vibration. Increased mass, due to the presence of a benign or malignant tumour, will lead to a lowering of f0. Increased stiffness, due to an invasive lesion or scar tissue, will increase f0 and lower amplitude. An obstacle to proper vocal fold closure, such as a lesion affecting the free edge of a vocal fold, or defective closure due to functional or organic incompetence, as in laryngeal paralysis, superimposes acoustic noise, resulting in breathy or whispery voice rather than modal voice.

7.2   Benign Pathology of the Vocal Folds with Dysphonia

7.2.1   *Functional: Muscle Tension Dysphonia, Hyper- or Hypofunction*
Muscle tension can be exacerbated by stressful communication circumstances or by the reactions of listeners. Normally, the intention to communicate verbally elicits a strategy of vocal tract optimization in coordination with adaptation to surroundings. If a speaker is nervous or pressed for time, if the message is not practised with confidence, if the audience provokes anxiety, or if the speaker is afraid of not being heard or understood, the optimization strategy can be defeated, and the speaker may adopt 'emergency behaviour', which evokes an immediate increase in muscle tension and a reduced volume of air supply. In addition, the infrahyoid muscles are recruited, and their contraction becomes visible in the neck.

Video 7.03 is an example of muscle tension dysphonia. During phonation, vocal fold adduction is accompanied by the approximation of the ventricular folds that progressively cover the upper anterior surface of the vocal folds. This extra mass disorganizes the symmetry and regularity of the glottal mucosal wave. Note that this action is a recruitment of 'valve 2' of the larynx (Edmondson and Esling 2006). It is a disorder for this particular speaker because it introduces a quality that is not his normal/previous voice. The quality is slight to moderately harsh whispery voice. In this case, the 'progressive laryngealization' across stretches of speech is pathological because it is effortful, painful, and tiring – involuntary and burdensome. The same quality used in a phonological context, for example, on syllabic- or segmental-length sounds where lexical contrast demands harsh production, or where many speakers in the same linguistic community adopt a harsh whispery voice quality, would not be considered abnormal.

Chronic muscle tension, excessive use or misuse of the voice can provoke more serious vocal dysfunction of the hyperfunctional type, resulting in vocal fold nodules. The mechanism of vocal effort is not pathological in itself, since yelling or screaming can be normal modalities of communication, but they expend more energy and should not be prolonged. If the degree of energy expenditure is not controlled, the result may be muscle tension dysphonia. Many occupational situations can be considered high risk for functional dysphonia, such as teaching, singing, and professional voice use more generally. Chronic infections or inflammatory conditions of the respiratory mucosa, chronic coughing that leads to local trauma, laryngopharyngeal reflux, certain medications, and congenital malformation of the vocal folds can also lead to functional dysphonia, including nodules.

Vocal overuse and misuse with hyper- and hypotension of the vocal folds take many anatomical shapes with corresponding acoustic characteristics (Crevier-Buchman et al. 2005). At the glottic level, the different configurations relate to a laryngeal musculature imbalance, principally between the posterior and lateral cricoarytenoid muscles, generally inducing a posterior glottic gap. In cases of imbalance with the other intrinsic laryngeal muscles (thyroarytenoid and cricothyroid), the glottis can have a medial gap or a large compression along the length of the vocal folds. Such glottal configurations can induce supraglottic compensations at the level of the ventricular folds or aryepiglottic folds, in which case the voice acquires a strained quality with intermittent non-linguistic glottal stops. Although vocal pathologies may be quite idiosyncratic and blur the lines between the core canonical categories defined in Chapters 1 and 2, there are nevertheless parallels in the way they can be described by the functioning of the laryngeal articulatory mechanism. Koufman and Blalock (1991) have described four laryngeal constrictive states according to the degree of muscle tension over the glottis and in the supraglottic region. A productive way of looking at laryngeal behaviour is to consider the postero-anterior shortening of the constrictor (narrowing the epilaryngeal-tube space), with progressive ventricular fold incursion and larynx raising, the initiation of which is shown in Figure 7.1.

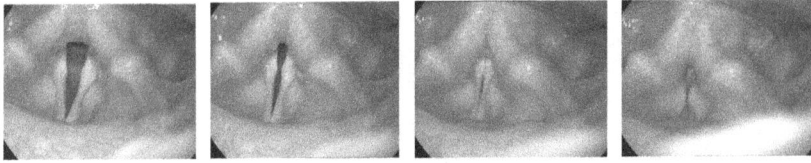

Figure 7.1 *Initiatory degrees of closure of the laryngeal mechanism Progressive moderate degrees of closure of the laryngeal mechanism that might be found in a clinical context, with gradual enhanced participation of the ventricular folds. The third image corresponds to grade 1 and the fourth image to grade 2 from Koufman and Blalock (1991). Grade 3, when the arytenoids tighten and impinge over the glottis, and grade 4, when aryepiglottic sphinctering effects strong closure against the epiglottis, are not shown.*

7.2.2   Anterior Vocal Fold Lesions: Benign Lesions: Reinke's Edema, Vocal Nodules, Polyps, Cysts, Sulci

Lesions such as vocal nodules, polyps, and Reinke's edema are related primarily to trauma to the tissues of the vocal folds and edematous swelling. The underlying causation is inadequate muscle tension and voicing hyperfunction with high subglottal pressure. The result is vibratory inefficiency with asymmetry of the mucosal wave. There are two families of benign lesions related to vocal trauma depending on the location on the vocal folds, either anterior, at the membranous or phonatory glottis, or posterior, at the cartilaginous or respiratory glottis. The former are responsible for dysphonia, and the second can cause laryngeal discomfort.

In Video 7.04a, vocal nodules are responsible for a posterior gap at low pitch and an hourglass-shaped glottic leakage at high pitch with severe dysphonia. One year after voice therapy, in Video 7.04b, the nodules are still visible, but the efficiency of glottic closure has improved, and the mucosal wave has recovered its symmetry, allowing better phonatory quality and comfort.

Nodules are bilateral lesions that occur at the longitudinal anterior third of both vocal folds, as in Figure 7.2, which is the location of significant impact during vibration, called phonotrauma. Histologically, we can find hyperplasia or parakeratosis of the superficial layer of the mucosa. During phonation, the nodules come into contact first and give an hourglass shape to the glottis. There is an air leak, with noisiness resembling whispery voice quality, lowering of f0, and laboured intensity control with softer voice. The mucosal wave is irregular, asymmetrical, and produces a quality resembling creaky voice. Voice therapy is designed to adjust the aerodynamic and musculo-mucosal balance.

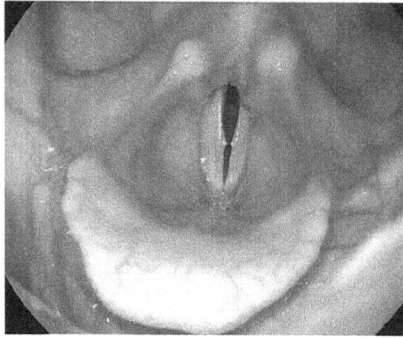

Figure 7.2 *Vocal nodules, in a state of adduction, within an unconstricted epilaryngeal space*

A polyp is a unilateral lesion located either at the anterior or posterior part of the vocal folds, when the stromal layer is modified by vascular dilation beneath the mucous membrane. Polyps can be sessile or pedunculated. Translucent polyps are called edematous, reddish polyps, angiomatous. The presence of the polyp weighs down the vocal fold, and dysphonia is variable, generally rougher than for nodules. Nodules and polyps directly affect the quality of voicing, causing irregularities to periodicity and interfering with changes in pitch, imparting the acoustic character of creaky voice. A polyp interfering with the mucosal aerodynamic function of the left vocal fold in Figure 7.3 shows effects on glottal phonation and slight tension in the aryepiglottic constrictor, resulting in increased adduction of the ventricular folds. This phonatory posture could be the individual's customary mode, a result of the polyp, or a compensatory adjustment to control or moderate voicing. Clinical observation is required to determine aetiology. A comprehensive model of epilaryngeal constriction is required to account for the postures and movements that occur.

Video 7.05a illustrates the strained behaviour of glottal voicing and the slower mucosal wave on the side with the angiomatous polyp (superior, mid portion, right vocal fold). Video 7.05b shows an anterior sessile edematous polyp resulting in visible desynchronization of the left vocal fold mucosal wave and causing irregular harsh creakiness.

Reinke's edema is characterized by significant edema with fibrosis of Reinke's space and is distinguished from edematous polyps only by the extension of this edema to the whole of the vocal folds. Generally bilateral but asymmetric, the mass of the vocal folds is increased. The voice quality is

(a)   (b)   (c)

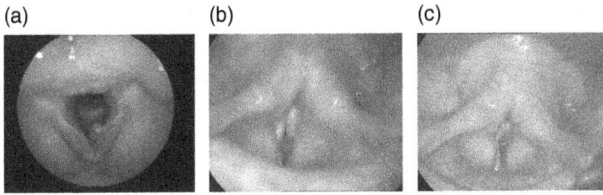

Figure 7.3 *An angiomatous polyp of the left vocal fold*
(a) during quiet breathing, (b) onset of closure for phonation, (c) tightened
phonation to overcome the glottal gap linked to the obstacle and recruiting
supraglottic structures.

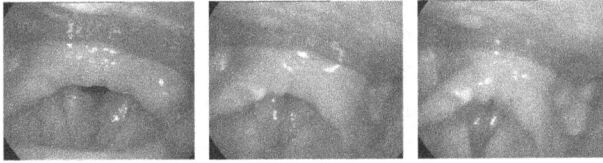

Figure 7.4 *Reinke's edema of the vocal folds, with effects on immediate*
supraglottic structures, from breathing to voicing

harsh (irregular), noisy, and low pitched. It most often results from a combination of tobacco use and voice abuse. In the case illustrated in Figure 7.4, the swelling of the vocal folds impinges upwards on the adducted ventricular folds, and the aryepiglottic structures are also swollen.

Congenital lesions such as cysts and sulci of the lamina propria can contribute to the irregularity of the mucosal wave, causing dysphonia and altering voice quality. The creaky and rough components of the voice are more severe than in benign edematous lesions. Pitch can be higher and the quality breathy or whispery, with irregularities that could be called creaky and harsh on occasions when periodicity is distorted. In all of these cases, the auditory labels resemble canonical categories that are applied to normal voices, but the articulatory/vibratory origins will not be the same – the clinical voices resulting from involuntary intrusive conditions. The presence of a benign lesion on the vocal folds can produce phonatory behaviour that resembles laryngealization or glottalization.

Video 7.06a illustrates a vocal fold cyst in a 7-year-old child. The size and mass of the cyst interfere with the mucosal wave and create a gap between the vocal folds during phonation, causing breathy offsets. Significant asymmetry results from the rigidity of the left vocal fold, where the cyst is embedded deep in the lamina propria. Video 7.06b shows a cyst in the posterior two-thirds of the right vocal fold, slightly inside the inferior edge of the free margin. The vibration of the mucosa is asymmetrical and irregular, resulting in diplophonic harsh creakiness. Two years later, without any treatment (Video 7.06c), the cyst has swollen, and the voice, though still diplophonic, has become breathy due to gaps during phonation and a wide-open epilaryngeal tube. Video 7.06d represents a bilateral sulcus glottidis – a congenital vocal fold scar – causing free margin rigidity and a gap between the vocal folds during phonation. The sulcus is a longitudinal scar, with segmental rigidity, more visible on the left VF and longer than on the right VF, responsible for the medial glottal gap.

7.2.3   Posterior Vocal Fold Lesions: Contact Ulcers, Granulomata, Laryngopharyngeal Reflux

Contact ulcers are generally bilateral lesions of the cartilaginous posterior part of the glottis at the level of the arytenoid vocal process. The dysphonia is painful. They occur when there is forceful or hyperkinetic behaviour of the larynx with arytenoid hyperadduction ('posterior hammering') contrasting with an anterior glottic gap during phonation. Voice timbre is strained, with intermittent glottal stops and adductive dysfunction causing noise. One main causal factor is laryngopharyngeal reflux, but ulcers also occur in chronic cough or throat clearing and post-intubation.

Video 7.07a is a case of a granuloma on the left interior wall of the arytenoid related to laryngopharyngeal reflux, compromising phonation. Three months after anti-reflux treatment (Video 7.07b), the granuloma has disappeared. While phonation is still produced with strong closure of the posterior glottis, it is far more efficient across the pitch range.

Similar to the contact ulcer is the granuloma, which is a rounded tumefaction located on the interior part of the arytenoid cartilage. They are of the same origin – laryngopharyngeal reflux, chronic cough and throat clearing, or after endotracheal intubation. The severity of the dysphonia is variable, depending on the degree of disturbance by the lesion to glottic approximation and to the mucosal wave. Laryngopharyngeal reflux can be responsible for inflammatory lesions of the mucosa of the larynx with diffuse erythema, swelling, and stiffness. The vibratory pattern is severely irregular with diminished amplitude of the mucosal wave. The condition can result in surfaces covered with scar tissue.

Video 7.08 is an example of synechia of the anterior commissure (scar tissue binding the vocal folds together). Phonatory quality is irregular (harsh, resembling pressed voice), with considerable high-frequency noise. There is a web joining the two vocal folds, blocking the mucosal wave, which emulates the strained phonation of harsh voice with longitudinal tension (Section 2.3.15). Video 7.09 shows the effects of chronic laryngitis with scar tissue after phonosurgery for Reinke's edema. Here again, the mucosa has lost its efficient vibratory quality, replaced by stiff and rigid scar tissue, so that phonation is uncontrollably diplophonic when altering pitch.

7.3 Malignant Laryngopharyngeal Lesions

The preceding descriptions have focused on benign modifications to the components and vibratory patterns of the mucosa and lamina propria of the vocal folds, which alter voice quality at the level of the glottis, sometimes with supraglottic effects. The following cases introduce cancerous lesions necessitating more extensive modification to the epilaryngeal tube and neighbouring structures by removing various parts of the larynx, leading to the recruitment of surviving structures for compensation.

7.3.1   Total Laryngectomy

Laryngeal cancers can affect all of the main anatomical structures of the laryngeal mechanism, with severe consequences for the production of voice and speech. Phonatory mechanisms and sound qualities after total or partial laryngectomy differ substantially from normal voices, as the shape of the lower vocal tract is altered, and vibrations occur at new sites. Total laryngectomy – the most radical treatment – results in severe alterations, adversely affecting the individual's image, physically, emotionally, and communicatively. Theodor Billroth in Vienna performed the first total laryngectomy in 1873 (Weir 1973). Total laryngectomy (TL) involves removal of the entire larynx, creating a discontinuity between the trachea and the pharynx. The airway stops at the superior level of the trachea, where it is sutured to the skin of the neck to allow breathing. This anastomosis of the trachea to the skin is called a 'tracheostomy'. As a consequence, the aero-digestive intersection changes profoundly, with the pharynx leading directly to the upper esophageal sphincter (UES) of the cricopharyngeal muscle – the cricopharyngeal sphincter. Food is supplied through the normal pathway, but breathing occurs through the stoma where the trachea is sutured to the neck. Phonation requires a replacement vibrating mechanism, since the larynx has been removed. This new vibrator is located at the UES.

A pseudo-periodic or aperiodic sound wave is produced by putting into vibration the mucosa of the UES to produce either esophageal voice (EV), when a 'sip' of air is swallowed and comes out in the form of belching (a burp), or tracheoesophageal voice (TEV), when a voice prosthesis is put in place between the trachea and esophagus (Singer and Blom 1980, Blom et al. 1982). With a prosthesis, the expiratory air comes from the lungs through the trachea and is directed to the esophagus through the device. In both EV and TEV, the UES is put into vibration, producing an irregular low-pitched source; therefore slightly harsh. The difference between these two voices is linked to air supply with different flow rates and volumes (see Hirose 1996 for a review of esophageal qualities). In the case of EV, aerodynamic energy comes from the small volume of air swallowed and belched through the mouth, with accompanying fluency disorders, as only two or three words can be produced at a time. After the removal of the aryepiglottic folds (and the entire epilaryngeal mechanism), the vibrations produced by the surviving cricopharyngeal sphincter in EV and in TEV resemble voiceless aryepiglottic trilling auditorily, due to similarities in the tissue mass and compliance of the cricopharyngeal muscle at the neoglottis.

Video 7.10 illustrates speech production after total laryngectomy, where the upper esophageal sphincter (UES) has been recruited to generate vibrations. The speaker is using TEV with a prosthesis, allowing phonation to last longer than is possible with EV. Occasionally, we hear the noise of the valve that closes the tracheostomy, enabling air from the lungs to reach the UES.

Audio 7.10a illustrates esophageal voice (EV) in a female speaker.

Audio 7.10b illustrates esophageal voice (EV) in a male speaker.

Audio 7.10c illustrates tracheoesophageal voice (TEV) in a male speaker. The quality is harsh and noisy, partly because of the vibratory characteristics of the UES and because using a finger to close the tracheostomy during phonation may create turbulence.

Audio 7.10d illustrates electrolarynx (EL) voice, using a laryngophone, in a female speaker.

In TEV, aerodynamic power comes from the lungs and provides a larger volume and adjustable flow rate, making speech more fluent and comprehensible (Brasnu et al. 1989, Crevier-Buchman et al. 1991; see Koike et al. 2002 for a comparison of rehabilitation techniques). Voicing quality, though produced by the same esophageal vibrator, is more stable, clear, and natural, and the timing of voicing for voiced consonants is easier to control. Speech fluency approaches that of normal glottal speech. A third mode of phonation is achieved by the use of an electrolarynx (EL), which generates a synthesized sound wave (Weiss et al. 1979). The electrolarynx is placed on the skin of the neck to allow the sound wave to pass through into the vocal tract, where normal articulatory shaping modulates the artificial source to generate articulate speech. EL voice is electronic-sounding with a metallic timbre, relatively disembodied, and without variations in pitch or intensity. This communication device is used in cases where the other two modes of voicing rehabilitation fail and also at the beginning of training for EV.

7.3.2 Partial Laryngectomies and Laryngopharyngeal Surgery

Surgical techniques reducing instances of total laryngectomy to partial laryngectomy have become possible through medical advances in cases where the spread of a lesion is limited. The aim is to reduce the extent of surgical resection. Functional goals are to preserve proper oral feeding, to maintain breathing through the natural airway, and to allow vocal recovery using relatively intact laryngeal mechanisms. The laryngeal categories of voice production described in Sections 2.3 and 4.1 provide guidelines to the types of vibration and resonance that can occur through the epilarynx and which can be compared with rehabilitated voices across a range of languages, including those where epilaryngeal postures contrast linguistically.

Over the course of a century, surgical techniques evolved to permit external partial laryngectomy, preserving natural respiratory tract continuity between the trachea, remaining laryngeal structures, and the pharynx. The most radical surgical technique is the supracricoid partial laryngectomy (SCPL) (Laccourreye et al. 1990, Laccourreye et al. 1995b). It replaces total laryngectomy only if arytenoid mobility is preserved and the tumour is limited to the larynx. Avoiding definitive tracheostomy represents major progress for patients, allowing social and sometimes professional reintegration and improved quality of life. To preserve swallowing, breathing, and phonation, external partial laryngeal surgeries require preservation of two fundamental anatomical structures: the cricoid cartilage, to keep the respiratory tract open for breathing, and the mobile cricoarytenoid unit, for swallowing and phonation. Different types of partial laryngectomy have been developed according to the extent of the lesion to be treated and consist of excision of the vocal folds (one or both), a variable part of the thyroid cartilage, part or all of one arytenoid cartilage, and parts of the ventricular folds and/or aryepiglottic folds of the supraglottic region, sometimes extended to neighbouring structures such as the epiglottis and the root of the tongue. Removal of each of these structures will have implications for the articulation of pharyngeals, phonatory modes that require participation of the ventricular folds or the aryepiglottic folds, the efficiency of tongue retraction, and vowel quality throughout the vocal tract. Despite technical progress in the oncological treatment of cancer, consequent changes in the length and volume of the vocal tract, particularly the lower

Supracricoid PL with CHEP (AE retained)

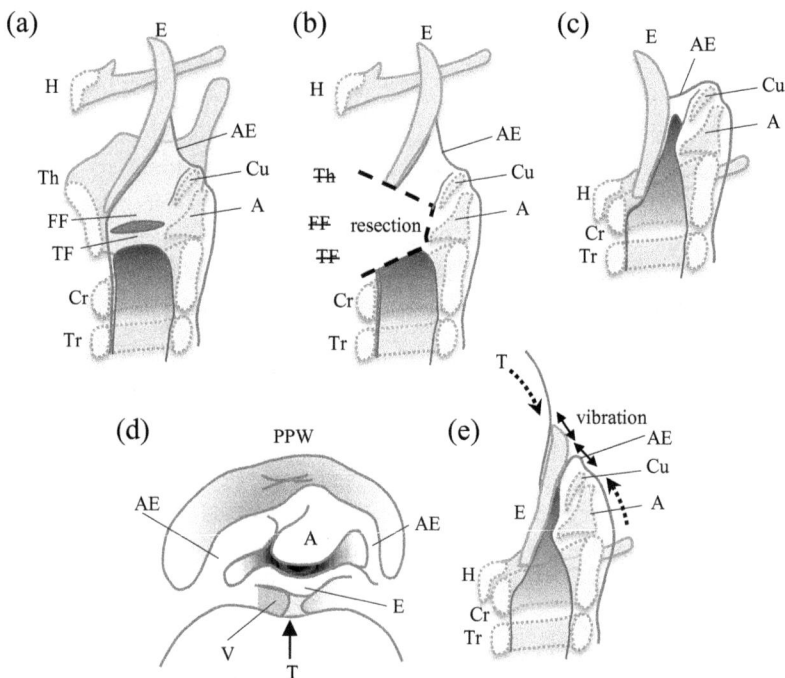

Supracricoid PL with CHP (AE removed)

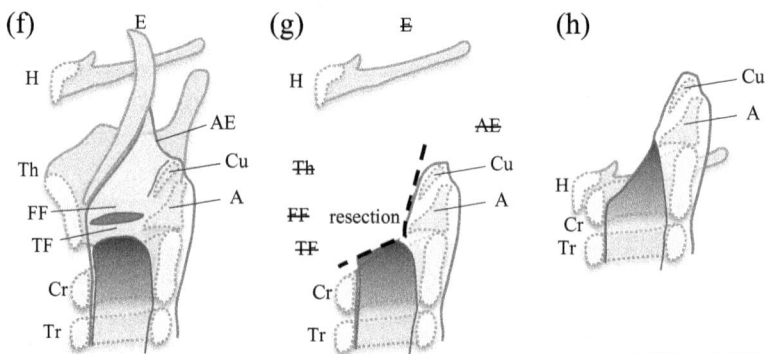

© 2018 Scott R. Moisik

Figure 7.5 *Phonatory mechanisms in voice production by the neoglottis after SCPL*
Above: Schema of laryngeal cartilages before and after SCPL with reconstruction by CHEP: (a) presurgery, (b) retained structures, (c) reconstruction result, (d) neoglottis mobilized at the front: retraction of

vocal tract, will affect voice quality and speech intelligibility. To better understand the vocal consequences of partial laryngectomy, we will frame the discussion in terms of phonatory and laryngeal mechanisms as defined in the LAM, the structures retained after surgery, and the compensatory lower-vocal-tract configurations and vibrations that emerge.

7.3.2.1 Horizontal Supracricoid Partial Laryngectomy (SCPL)

The most extensive surgical procedure is the horizontal supracricoid partial laryngectomy that removes both vocal folds, both ventricular folds, the entire thyroid cartilage and paraglottic space, and in some cases, the laryngeal portion of the epiglottis. To avoid a large gap in the neck, this surgery is followed by a reconstruction of laryngeal structures by suturing the cricoid cartilage to the hyoid bone and the remnant of the epiglottis if present. These SCPL techniques result in a modified anatomo-physiological version of the vocal tract that has been shortened by about 3 cm and is capable of producing a voice even though the glottal and immediate supraglottic structures have been removed. The critical issue for maintaining a range of laryngeal sound production is whether the aryepiglottic folds remain intact. If the aryepiglottic folds survive surgery, then a viable aerodynamic vibrator is retained in preference to an esophageal vibratory source. If the aryepiglottic folds are removed, then an important natural vibration source is lost, and other tissues that are not adapted to speech must be relied on to produce voicing, such as the base of the tongue and lateral or posterior pharyngeal walls. Any surgery altering the larynx will have variable consequences on the position of the larynx and its relation with the oropharynx. These impacts are critical to voice and speech quality as well as to compensatory behaviour. Figure 7.5 depicts how the larynx is altered by SCPL with cricohyoidoepiglottopexy (CHEP), where the cricoid cartilage is

---

Figure 7.5 (*cont.*)

the base of the tongue (T) pushing the remaining epiglottis (E), (e) neoglottis mobilized at the back: arytenoids (A) rocking forwards and inwards towards the tongue-epiglottis block. Below: Schema of laryngeal cartilages before and after SCPL with reconstruction by CHP: (f) presurgery, (g) retained structures, (h) reconstruction result. H = hyoid bone; E = epiglottis; Th = thyroid cartilage; FF = false (ventricular) folds; TF = true (vocal) folds; Cr = cricoid cartilage; Tr = trachea; AE = aryepiglottic folds; Cu = cuneiform cartilage; A = arytenoid cartilage; PPW = posterior pharyngeal wall; V = vallecula; T = tongue.
Drawings based on Traissac (1992).

sutured to the remnant suprahyoid epiglottis and hyoid bone, and with cricohyoidopexy (CHP), where the cricoid cartilage is sutured to the hyoid bone, by comparing (a) presurgery cartilaginous structures, (b) retained cartilaginous structures, and (c) the reconstruction result.

7.3.2.2   The Neoglottis and 'Substitution Voice'

Following laryngeal surgery with removal of at least one vocal fold, voicing is considered an 'alternative voice' or 'substitution voice' (Moerman et al. 2005). This terminology applies to the phonatory consequences of total laryngectomy (TL), horizontal supracricoid partial laryngectomies (SCPL), and vertical partial laryngectomies such as supracricoid hemilaryngopharyngectomy (SCHLP) and frontolateral partial laryngectomy (FLPL). After glottal voicing has been compromised in a partial laryngectomy, the voice source that is substituted will recruit available structures in the remaining epilaryngeal tube up to the aryepiglottic level.

Cricoarytenoid articulation in the neoglottis is mobilized by the posterior cricoarytenoid muscle (PCA), the lateral cricoarytenoid muscle (LCA), and interarytenoid muscle (IA). The neoglottis adopts a triangular inverted-T shape instead of the glottal-V shape of normal phonation. With surgical removal of the vocal folds, the infrastructure of the vibrator no longer consists of three distinct elements (mucosa, ligament, muscle), and no drift space (Reinke's space) remains between muscle and mucosa. The contractile possibilities and state of tension of the muscles involved in the constitution of the neoglottis determine the flexibility of the overlying arytenoid mucosa that can vibrate during phonation. Figure 7.6 illustrates arytenoid movement (where both arytenoids remain) in the closing behaviour of the neoglottis. Normally, the aryepiglottic folds are not a target of resection in SCPL, and the CHEP procedure aims to incorporate them into the reconfiguration of the neoglottis. If parts of the AE folds are removed, CHEP attempts to integrate remaining parts with other potential vibrating structures to participate in generating voicing.

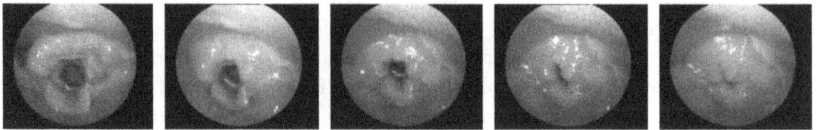

Figure 7.6 *Progression of closure of the neoglottis following CHEP*
At the front, the base of the tongue retracts, pushing the remaining epiglottis back. At the back, the arytenoids rock forwards and inwards towards the tongue-epiglottis block.

Neolarynx behaviour following SCPL with CHEP demonstrates how the upper epilarynx compensates for the loss of glottal phonatory structures. The approximation of neolarynx structures – arytenoid(s), epiglottis, and tongue root, examined videostroboscopically, remains incomplete one month post-operatively, due to: (i) transient loss of contractile properties of LCA, PCA, and IA due to surgery, (ii) modification of arytenoid position, (iii) change in epiglottis shape, and (iv) resection of the vocal folds, ventricular folds, and paraglottic spaces. Three months post-operatively, mobility of the cricoarytenoid unit from back to front and transversely gradually improves. The tongue root and remaining epiglottis ease from front to rear, and laryngeal tissues recover their intrinsic biomechanical qualities of flexibility, tension, elasticity, and mass, allowing a gradual improvement in the mobility of vibrating structures between three and six months post-operatively (Crevier-Buchman et al. 1995). Vibration of the neoglottis depends on the backward movement of the tongue root and remaining tension in the upper-epilaryngeal musculature to position the remaining epiglottis in contact with the arytenoids moving inwards and forwards. Vibration occurs at the internal and anterior edges of the arytenoid mucosa, associated with the participation of the mucosa of the aryepiglottic folds anteriorly against the epiglottis. In this new phonatory posture, the sound source resembles aryepiglottic trilling, described in Section 4.1.2.6 in singing, emphatic speech, and tonal register. Videostroboscopy suggests that independent mobility of each arytenoid, with sufficient aerodynamic flow, contributes to generating a mucosal wave, stabilized by the aryepiglottic structures. Since the mucosal surface of the arytenoid cartilage is very adherent (through the mucoperichondrium) to the underlying cartilage, vibration can be impeded, in which case an aryepiglottic vibratory mode can be cultivated with speech therapy training. The mucosal wave appears only if there is almost complete approximation either between (i) the arytenoids in the frontal plane, or (ii) the arytenoids and root of the tongue, with or without the remaining epiglottis. The mucosal wave occurs at the arytenoid level, also involving the aryepiglottic folds, with roughly vertical movement from bottom to top associated with postero-anterior displacement.

As no sliding space remains in the neoglottis to give the mucosal wave some independence from the muscle and permit individualization, every wave is asymmetrical and irregular in frequency and amplitude with occasional interruptions. This vibratory behaviour has greater inertia and mass than glottal vibration, with consequent harsh timbre (irregular vibration, often associated with mucosal edema of the arytenoid), low frequency (increase in the vibrating mass), and whisperiness (partial sphincter incompetence according to the degree of approximation of the vibrating structures), often with increased effort. The greater the amplitude of the mucosal wave, the lower and harsher the voicing. When there is some tension in the aryepiglottic folds, and arytenoid mucosal wave amplitude is reduced, the voice is higher, less rough (less irregular) but noisier (Crevier-Buchman et al. 1998). The higher voice seems to be preferred by patients, especially women, but post-operative anatomical provisions are not always predictable, and rehabilitation therapy is commonly required to nurture compensation and improve timbre. The association of the arytenoids with the aryepiglottic folds as a compensatory resource underlines the potential of the epilaryngeal structures of the laryngeal articulator in producing phonation and generating timbre in shaping the acoustic wave.

Video 7.11, two years post-CHEP surgery, illustrates the wider airway opening where structures have been removed, generating whispery quality (due to inefficient neo-glottic closure and the narrowed epilaryngeal passage). Phonation occurs via epilaryngeal compensation at the top of the epilaryngeal tube, where aryepiglottic vibration is more active on the right. The quality resembles harsh whispery voice with aryepiglottic trilling in a normal larynx, although the structures involved in post-operative neovibration have been reconfigured.

In the first two years after surgery, the higher position of the larynx and shortened vocal tract generate higher formant frequencies and compensatory lingual articulatory strategies to produce target vowels while at the same time maintaining voicing contrasts for consonants. For vowel production, the voicing gesture (aryepiglottic phonation) is a priority over articulatory tongue position. For consonant articulation, patients tend to favour the articulatory position of the tongue instead of the laryngeal mechanism responsible for devoicing consonants (Crevier-Buchman et al. 1999, 2000, 2001, 2002, 2003).

7.3.2.3 Supraglottic Partial Laryngectomy (SGPL)

In the horizontal plane, the supraglottic partial laryngectomy (SGPL) is a much less aggressive surgery in terms of vocal-ventricular fold modification. It corresponds to the resection of the epiglottis, sometimes extended to the root of the tongue and thyroid horns, but remains above the glottic level, as shown in Figure 7.7. The resulting phonation is not considered substitution voice, as both vocal folds are preserved. Although phonatory quality may not be modified, the epilaryngeal vocal tract acquires new and variable resonating properties depending on the modifications to anatomical structures, substantially altering holistic voice quality.

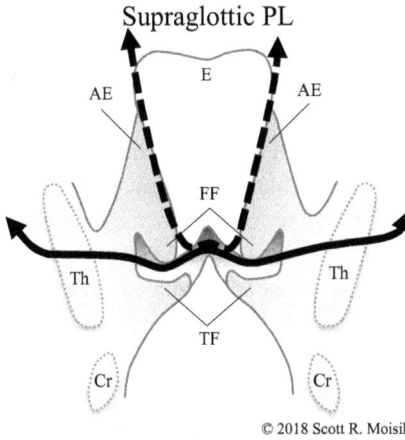

Figure 7.7 *Schema of the resection line for a supraglottic partial laryngectomy*
Showing removal of the two ventricular folds and various supraglottic anatomical structures (the wide part of the epiglottis, base of the tongue, lateral pharyngeal region). The dashed line represents minimal resection (of the epiglottis), and the solid line represents the most extensive SGPL. E = epiglottis; AE = aryepiglottic folds; Th = thyroid cartilage; FF = ventricular (false) folds; TF = vocal (true) folds; Cr = cricoid cartilage.

Video 7.12 is an example of a wide supraglottic partial laryngectomy where the epiglottis is removed as well as the anterior part of the ventricular folds and the anterior part of the left vocal fold. A gap is therefore created at the anterior commissure. The effect on phonatory quality is persistent breathiness, due to inefficient glottal closure and the lack of supraglottic compensation by the loss of the anterior part of the ventricular folds. The breathy quality intensifies to whisperiness when sphincteric narrowing increases. Lack of supraglottic structures impairs the resonance characteristics that the laryngeal articulator would normally impart. Like SCPL, the tendency to compensate using what remains of the laryngeal articulator is strong, but unlike SCPL, the function of the anterior portion of the aryepiglottic constrictor has been lost, reducing natural vibratory options.

7.3.2.4 Vertical Partial Laryngectomies

Whereas the surgical resection line in horizontal laryngectomies parallels the glottal plane, the surgical resection line in vertical laryngectomies is in the sagittal plane, perpendicular to the glottal plane. An external cordectomy, as in Figure 7.8(a), is an open surgical procedure, more extensive than endoscopic laser surgery, accessing the vocal fold through the thyroid cartilage. In frontolateral partial laryngectomy (FLPL), as in Figure 7.8(b), the access procedure through the thyroid cartilage is the same, removing one whole vocal fold and the anterior commissure as well as a small anterior part of the contra- lateral vocal fold (Biacabe et al. 1998). Unlike horizontal partial laryngec- tomies, the glottis keeps its V shape in respiration. During phonation, there is a partial joining of the ventricular folds and sometimes an approximation of the remaining vocal fold and the fibrous scar located in the resection bed. The voice has similar characteristics to dysphonia, with generally whispery voice, due to the tendency to narrow the epilaryngeal channel to compensate for the larger airway opening, but not low pitched or harsh as with SCPL, mainly because vibration remains at the level of the glottis and not at the level of the aryepiglottic folds (Biacabe et al. 1999, 2001, Wallet et al. 2009). In FLPL, both arytenoids and both ventricular folds remain, as well as the median and posterior part of one healthy vocal fold. To overcome the gap at the glottis and achieve voicing, the remaining vocal fold is assisted by ventricular fold and epilaryngeal-tube approximation. Expanded laryngectomies such as anterior frontal partial laryn- gectomy (AFPL), where both vocal folds are removed, as in Figure 7.8(c), achieve the voiceless–voiced contrast through relative degrees of opening– closure through the neoglottis. Voicing is compensated for by ventricular fold and aryepiglottic fold action, with the assistance of the remaining arytenoid(s).

Cases of partial laryngeal surgery incurring vertical alterations more aggres- sive than FLPL include supracricoid hemilaryngopharyngectomy (SCHLP). In the case of SCHLP, as in Figure 7.8(d), an entire hemilarynx is removed, resulting in a 'surgical model' of a unilateral vibrator with one vocal fold, one

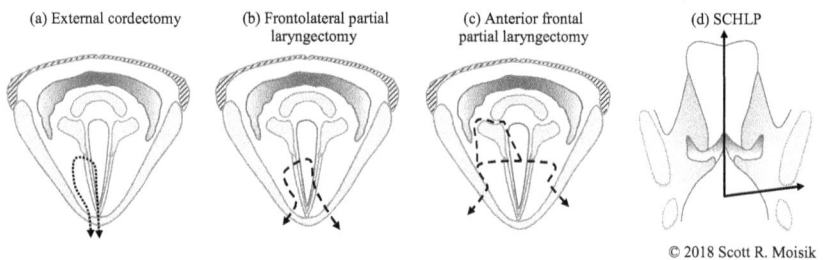

(a) External cordectomy   (b) Frontolateral partial laryngectomy   (c) Anterior frontal partial laryngectomy   (d) SCHLP

© 2018 Scott R. Moisik

Figure 7.8 *Transverse schematic of progressive vertical surgical resectioning*
(a) external cordectomy, (b) frontolateral partial laryngectomy, and
(c) bilateral anterior frontolateral partial laryngectomy; anterior at bottom
of diagrams. Diagram (d) represents a coronal schematic of a supracricoid
hemilaryngopharyngectomy; posterior-to-anterior view.

ventricular fold, one arytenoid, one aryepiglottic fold, and half of the epiglottis (Laccourreye et al. 1987, Laccourreye et al. 1995a). Videostroboscopic obser- vations demonstrate that voicing is produced not by the remaining vocal fold but by an approximation of the preserved hemilarynx against the rebuilt opposite pharyngeal wall and that the acoustic wave is generated by the undulation of the mucosa of the remaining arytenoid and aryepiglottic fold. To accomplish this, the hemilarynx must swivel inwards and forwards. This mobility appears in the third post-operative month, and the mucosal wave is regularized by the sixth post-operative month. This configuration inevitably invokes the participation of supraglottic structures that produce vibrations that are harsh rather than modal and with narrowed and raised-larynx spectral characteristics, as in varieties of harsh voice, aryepiglottic trilling, pharyngea- lized voice, or raised-larynx voice. If the mucosa are lax, a large-amplitude wave is generated, and the voice is low with harsh irregularity. A tight hemi- larynx, with the contralateral pharyngeal wall sutured so that the vocal tract is relatively narrow, produces a more high-pitched voice with the same charac- teristics found in laryngeally constricted modes. The higher-pitched configur- ation is found more commonly in women, where the larynx has a smaller diameter. In general, the quality of voicing produced after SCHLP is less harsh and less low pitched than after SCPL, probably because the hemilarynx is vibrating against the relatively firm structure of the rebuilt pharyngeal wall. Here again, the neoglottis has a V shape, with closure on a transverse axis and movement going from external to internal, contrary to SCPL, where closure is back to front at the level of the arytenoids towards the remnant of the epiglottis and/or base of the tongue. We conclude that the high functionality of the laryngeal articulator is robust enough against extremely invasive surgery that it still provides an optimal mechanism to generate voicing. Even when parts of the vocal folds remain, compensation by epilaryngeal constrictor structures is commonly observed to occur.

In Video 7.13 of SCHLP, corresponding to Figure 7.8(d), remaining left hemilarynx (glotto-supraglottic) structures compensate for the loss of right hemilarynx (vocal- ventricular) structures, as the hemilarynx swivels inwards and forwards to achieve vibration.

7.3.3 Endoscopic Laser Surgery (Cordectomy)

In the 1970s, transoral endoscopic laser cordectomy was introduced for tumours limited to a vocal fold (Weinstein et al. 2000: 165–170, 171–174). This surgery has grown, in preference to external (open) surgeries, because of its many advantages, such as positive oncologic and vocal results, lack of visible scarring on the neck, and rapid functional recovery. The resulting voice quality depends on the extent of the resection. There are five types of cordectomies (Remacle et al. 2000): subepithelial cordectomies (type I), subligamental cordectomies (type II), transmuscular cordectomies (type III), total cordectomies (type IV), and extended cordectomies (type Va, when the lesion extends towards the anterior commissure, and Vb, when the lesion extends more posteriorly). When a tumour is located at the anterior commissure and the anterior part of both vocal folds, a modified cordectomy (type VI) has been proposed (Remacle et al. 2007). The six types are illustrated in Figure 7.9. Cordectomy type I involves the epithelium of the vocal folds and resembles the surgical removal of benign lesions. Voice timbre is temporarily altered, with some roughness and noise during the first month of healing and is dependent on mucosal wave regeneration and symmetrization with the contralateral vocal fold. Cordectomy type II (subligamental) is indicated for in situ or microinvasive carcinomas of the lamina propria. The resection includes the epithelium and vocal ligament with the three layers of the lamina propria. Cordectomy type III (transmuscular) is a surgery indicated for a tumour limited to one vocal fold and lesions of the middle third of the vocal fold, involving resection of the epithelium, the lamina propria, and a variable part of the vocal muscle. The

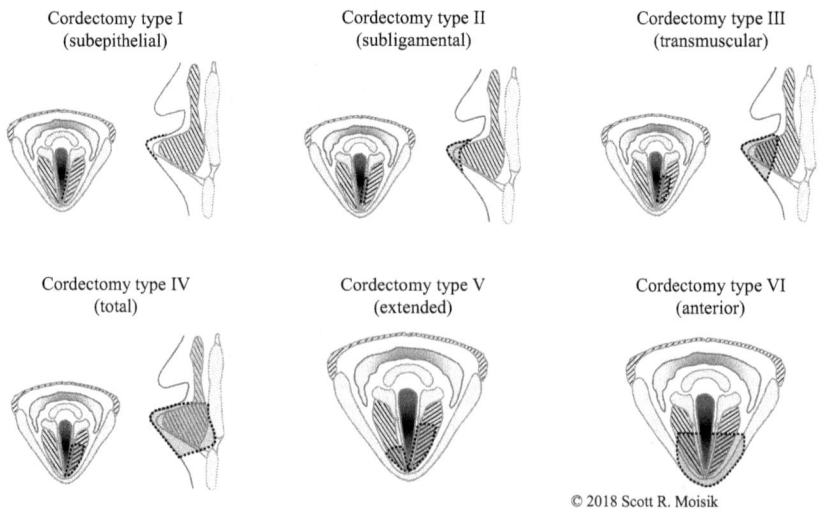

Cordectomy type I
(subepithelial)

Cordectomy type II
(subligamental)

Cordectomy type III
(transmuscular)

Cordectomy type IV
(total)

Cordectomy type V
(extended)

Cordectomy type VI
(anterior)

© 2018 Scott R. Moisik

Figure 7.9 *Types of cordectomies, transverse and coronal views*
Based on Remacle et al. (2000, 2007).

modification of the internal structure of the affected vocal fold is responsible for an asymmetry, desynchronized vibration, and a decrease of the vibrating mass, which together cause a perturbation of the frequency and amplitude of the vibratory cycle and turbulence during phonation from a glottal gap. Cordectomy type IV is a total cordectomy removing the entire muscular vocal fold up to the thyroid cartilage perichondrium. Cordectomy type V corresponds to an anterior or posterior extension of the resection with removal of part of the anterior commissure or the vocal process of the arytenoid. Cordectomy type VI removes the anterior commissure and the anterior part of both vocal folds. The wider the removal at the glottis, the more compromised the voice quality, mainly due to glottal insufficiency and increased friction. The effects of surgery could induce tubular friction that generates whisperiness more than breathiness. A principal acoustic modification is a higher fundamental frequency, which increases with the type of cordectomy (Crevier-Buchman et al. 2007). For cordectomies I–III, voice quality improves during the first three months. Alterations to the vibratory pattern from stiffness related to scar tissue replacing the vocal fold(s) increase in severity with cordectomies III–VI.

Video 7.14a. Cordectomy II. Presurgery: the lesion within the left vocal fold is rigid and does not vibrate, suggestive of a cancerous tumour within the layers of the fold. There is also a growth at the lower level of the anterior commissure, suggesting that a type VI cordectomy might also be required. Phonatory quality is whispery because of the glottal gap and irregular/harsh because of the inability of the left vocal fold to participate in medial vibration. Video 7.14b. Cordectomy II, six months post-surgery. The left vocal fold has been resectioned and much of the left and part of the right ventricular folds removed to have a clear view of the anterior commissure and the extent of the lesion beneath. Healing and speech therapy have restored some vibratory facility in the left vocal fold. Phonatory quality is less harsh and more breathy.

7.4 Movement Disorders

7.4.1 Vocal Fold Paralysis

Vocal fold paralysis is a voice disorder that causes one or both vocal folds to fail to open or close properly, resulting in voicing impairment and potentially breathing and swallowing problems. Vocal fold movement relies on two branches of the cranial vagus nerve (CN X). The recurrent laryngeal nerve (RLN) innervates various laryngeal muscles responsible for glottal opening and closing and tight closure during swallowing. On the left side, the RLN descends into the chest cavity and curves back into the neck to reach the larynx.

On the right side, the RLN stays in the neck. The superior laryngeal nerve (SLN) carries motor signals to the cricothyroid muscle, responsible for adjusting vocal fold tension to increase pitch. SLN paralysis results in abnormalities in pitch control and generally low and harsh voice quality. Some patients with SLN paralysis may have a normal speaking voice but an abnormal singing voice.

Paralysis of the laryngeal muscles can result from vagus nerve, RLN, or SLN damage during skull base, neck, or upper thoracic surgery, or from viral infections and certain cancers (Yamada et al. 1983). Sometimes no aetiology is found, and the vocal fold paralysis is called 'idiopathic'. Most often, paralysis is unilateral (Crumley 1994), and the resulting phonatory quality is breathy due to paramedian or lateral blocking of the affected vocal fold so that complete glottal adduction for phonation is not achieved. Voicing quality can also be irregular and weak in intensity with pitch instability (Laccourreye et al. 1998b, Borel et al. 2004, Hartl et al. 2005). There may be compensatory recruitment of the epilaryngeal mechanism, initially of the ventricular folds, when the vocal folds are paralysed. The respiratory protective mechanism depends on efficient closure of some combination of the vocal folds, ventricular folds, aryepiglottic folds, arytenoids, and tongue/epiglottis. When the usual glottal abductors and adductors are paralysed, neural control of the laryngeal mechanism can still function as compensation if only the RLN is paralysed rather than all of CN X.

Treatment for vocal fold paralysis involves surgery or injections to media-lize the paralysed side (Laccourreye et al. 1998a, Laccourreye et al. 1999, 2001, 2003, Nishiyama et al. 2002, Hartl, et al. 2003, 2009, Michel et al. 2003, Nouwen et al. 2004). Voice therapy can be productive in reducing excessive compensatory behaviour through the epilaryngeal tube, to try to induce the healthy vocal fold to overshoot the midline using supraglottic muscular struc-tures, and to reduce the glottal gap to restore a regular mucosal wave (Walton et al. 2017). Paresis is the partial interruption of neural impulses, resulting in weak or intermittent contractions of the laryngeal muscles.

Video 7.15a is an examination of idiopathic paralysis of the right vocal fold, probably from virus infection, performed two weeks after the onset of severe dysphonia due to the paralytic episode, showing low-intensity whispery voice and shortness of breath. Ventricular fold incursion is recruited as a compensatory behaviour for loss of vocal fold control. Two months later, during voice therapy training (Video 7.15b), closure has improved and the voice is less breathy. Three months after the onset of paralysis (Video 7.15c), vocal fold contact has improved, and the mucosal wave has recovered in amplitude and regularity.

Video 7.16 illustrates paresis. The left vocal fold at first appears paralysed, but eventually, as phonation continues, muscle tension instability causes irregular movements of the left arytenoid and vocal fold, resulting in interruptions to phonation, involuntary pitch changes, and harshness due to irregularities in the mucosal wave.

More rarely, both vocal folds can be paralysed (diplegia) either in open position (abduction) with very breathy voice quality, or in closed position (adduction) with primary symptoms presenting as breathing difficulty (Hans et al. 2000). Diplegia is a particular pathological problem where it becomes difficult or impossible to unfold (open up) the laryngeal constrictor mechanism. Specifically, diplegia is bilateral laryngeal paralysis or unilateral paralysis in a near-median position with very little contralateral mobility. It is as if, in a normal larynx, the laryngeal constrictor gets 'stuck' once it folds into a tight position, and the ability to reopen the mechanism has 'seized' and failed to work. The disordered condition can occur after thyroid surgery with recurrent nerve injury. It can be dramatic, with an urgent need for a tracheotomy and intensive care. In abduction position, phonation elicits strong compensatory contraction of the epilaryngeal region, with one ventricular fold covering the vocal fold to augment glottal closure from above. As a result, phonatory quality is strained: harsh and whispery. In an adducted posture, breathing may be compromised, while excessive abduction risks losing voicing. Remedial procedures are designed to balance improved breathing without worsening the voice (Gorphe et al. 2013).

In Video 7.17, the left vocal fold is paralysed in paramedian position, and the right vocal fold has very limited opening movements at the arytenoid. The right ventricular fold adducts over the vocal fold as a compensatory gesture. It is the left arytenoid muscles (LCA, PCA) that are paralysed; therefore, the left arytenoid is functionally immobile, and structures from the right overcompensate.

7.4.2 Parkinson's Disease

Parkinson's disease (PD) is a chronic and progressive movement disorder associated with degenerative lesions of the extrapyramidal areas of the brain. Parkinson's disease primarily affects the nigrostriatal neuronal system that produces dopamine, a chemical that sends messages to the part of the brain that controls movement and coordination. Primary motor signs of Parkinson's disease may include: tremor of the hands, arms, legs, jaw, face and larynx; bradykinesia or slowness of movement; muscle rigidity or stiffness; postural instability or impaired balance and coordination; and speech changes with soft phonation, fast speed, slur or hesitation before talking, and monotone speech. Voice issues per se are secondary to several complex pathophysiological mechanisms involving the intrinsic and extrinsic muscles of the larynx and the subglottic respiratory muscles controlling the aerodynamic component of phonation, which may result in abnormal vocal function (Blumin et al. 2004). Phonatory dysfunctions are related to an alteration of muscle tone equilibrium with hypokinesia (slow movement), hypertonia (rigidity), and vocal tremor – modifications associated with asymmetric muscle contractions. The main effects that can be seen in videostroboscopic examination are diminished vocal fold movement and lack of complete closure, with a glottic gap and a bowed aspect to the glottal area, abnormal phase closure in the anterior and middle portion of the vocal folds, mucosal waveform phase asymmetry and reduced amplitude, and posterior laryngeal tremor located at the level of the arytenoid cartilages (Perez et al. 1996).

Acoustically, in PD, as in many benign vocal fold lesions, harshness (often referred to as hoarseness or roughness) co-occurs with whisperiness due to vibratory irregularities at the same time that closure is incomplete. Voicing is weak and short in duration. During phonation, the vocal processes are hyperadducted, and the larynx is slightly rolled forward, with an asymmetry of the arytenoid and corniculate cartilages. The ventricular folds appear compressed during phonation, having the effect of limiting posterior vibration of the vocal folds and narrowing or reducing the glottic gap during phonation. This supraglottic contraction can be considered a compensatory behaviour, since the glottis is not the only site affected or where phonatory quality is generated. Many autonomically driven laryngeal actions are compromised as a result of PD, but the dominant posture of the laryngeal constrictor largely responsible for the sound of the voice is moderately tight with severely adducted ventricular folds (and potentially increased vocal-ventricular coupling). Autonomic control of all of the constricting structures throughout the epilaryngeal tube can also be affected by PD.

In the Parkinson's case in Video 7.18, repeated over-closure of the vocal processes has caused epithelial damage, evidenced by a persistent mucosal string to actual nodules. Whether or not this individual had a constricted laryngeal setting (and therefore harsh voice) before the onset of Parkinson's symptoms, the rigidity that goes with the disease can provoke epilaryngeal-tube tightening to compensate for the glottal gap, increasing constricted quality.

7.4.3   Tremor, Dystonia, Spasmodic Dysphonia, Myoclonus

Essential vocal tremor causes a regular wavering of the voice. Vocal tremor may occur alone or in combination with other neurologic conditions, particularly laryngeal dystonia. Typically, speaking with essential vocal tremor is not effortful, in contrast to laryngeal dystonia, where speaking often entails effort. Laryngeal dystonia is a benign neurological condition affecting the larynx, associated with voice disturbance or, less commonly, with breathing disturbance. Dystonic tremor is almost always accompanied by other manifestations of dystonia, such as phonatory dropouts or whisper. The entire epilaryngeal tube can be involved in uncoordinated contractions. Dystonic tremor may worsen under specific circumstances – with stress, fatigue, or on the telephone, for example. Dystonic tremor is often (though not always) more pronounced in modal voice register than in falsetto register. Spasmodic dysphonia belongs to a family of disorders called focal dystonia (Crevier-Buchman et al. 1997). When a single muscle or small group of muscles contracts spontaneously and irregularly without good voluntary control, those muscles are dystonic. The most common type of laryngeal dystonia is spasmodic dysphonia, when the glottal adductor muscles spasm intermittently during speech – also called strain strangled voice. Irregular contractions occur throughout the entire epilaryngeal tube, though the spasms disappear during whispery phonation. In this set of disorders, when glottal function is impaired, commonly observed compensation involves tighter laryngeal constriction upwards through the epilaryngeal tube, often with ventricular fold adduction. This also demonstrates that the structures of the epilaryngeal tube within the laryngeal articulator are a cornerstone of our ability to adapt to pathological or surgical laryngeal trauma.

In the case of essential vocal tremor in Video 7.19, after a short phase of laryngeal muscle stability at voice onset, the amplitude of tremor augments, causing loss of control in adductory stability with epilaryngeal narrowing as a compensatory mechanism.

The case of dystonia-dyskinesia in Video 7.20 illustrates glottal tremor as well as involuntary contraction throughout the epilaryngeal tube, which could be related to abduction spasmodic dysphonia with involuntary opening of the vocal folds during voicing and compensatory epilaryngeal tube contraction.

In spasmodic dysphonia in Video 7.21a, spasms pervade the entire epilaryngeal tube but disappear during whisper phonation. As the speaking task is prolonged, these voices take on noticeably tight laryngeal constriction with extremely adducted ventricular folds (and potentially increased vocal-ventricular coupling), as in other movement disorders, which is a common compensatory strategy. Video 7.21b illustrates a combination of vocal tremor and spasmodic dysphonia.

Myoclonus (myoclony) refers to rapid involuntary muscle twitching, which may occur because of a neurological disorder, such as epilepsy, a metabolic condition, a reaction to a medication, or following a stroke. The symptoms are often described as jerks, shakes, or spasms that are sudden, brief, involuntary, variable in intensity and frequency, and localized to one part of the body or over the entire body. Effects on all laryngeal structures can interfere with speaking, mainly disrupting the temporal domain. In virtually all of these cases of disorders, it is impossible to describe the condition's localization, effects, or treatment without reference to the structures and actions of the laryngeal articulator as a whole.

In our example in Video 7.22, diffuse oropharyngeal and laryngeal myoclonus occurred after a stroke.

7.5   The Professional Voice: Adaptive Laryngeal Articulator Possibilities

7.5.1   *Mongolian Long Song*

Professional voice artists have refined the ability to manipulate the articulators, particularly the laryngeal mechanism, as it is a part of the vocal tract that offers widely extended capabilities to vocal performance styles. Many singers cited in Chapter 4 exploit laryngeal articulations to define their own style or to perform sounds in auditory contradistinction to predominantly oral articulator sounds, such as the many varieties of throat singing around the world. One singing style that illustrates particularly well the effect of the epilaryngeal tube on auditory quality is Mongolian long song. The virtuosity of the singer also highlights the rapid movements that can be achieved in the laryngeal articulator and the capacity of epilaryngeal configurations to complement glottal production, just as many cases of speech disorders presented earlier in this chapter recruit the ready availability of the epilarynx to compensate for impaired glottal production.

Mongolian long song is a traditional ancient singing style composed of a basic melody, embellished by improvisations using vibratos, 'trills', glissandos, and yodelling effects. Long song is a difficult style to master involving a wide vocal range and requiring long training. The extreme laryngeal agility necessary to produce ornamentations such as rapid alternating vibratos in a wide tessitura requires perfect control of different levels of laryngeal movements, each level acting as an independent articulator. Two main laryngeal behaviours characterize the ornamentations: 'lyrical' vibratos mobilizing the entire larynx, and 'Mongolian trills' with supraglottic vibrator movements, the arytenoids being mobilized independently from the rest of the larynx with asymmetrical and transverse movement (Crevier-Buchman et al. 2012). These are also a kind of vibrato rather than pure aryepiglottic trilling as defined in Section 2.3.14 or 4.1.2.6, since the frequency of oscillation is much slower than in aryepiglottic fold trilling. In vibrato, distance does not vary between left and right arytenoids on the transverse axis, the movement being symmetrical and postero-anterior towards the epiglottis with periodic regular oscillations of about 7 Hz. Thus, the artistic technical feat selects epilaryngeal valve action to decorate the high-pitched sound source produced at the glottic level.

The Mongolian singer in Video 7.23a has stabilized her glottic vibrator to produce high pitch, using the supraglottic aryepiglottic structures for ornamentations.

Video 7.23b isolates the production of vibrato: the rapid postero-anterior periodic constriction of the aryepiglottic constrictor to influence vocal pitch. The arytenoids are moving in a rocking motion somewhat akin to modifications of the laryngeal constrictor for changing (lowering) pitch, but with much finer and more rapid control. It is the aryepiglottic constrictor moving as the primary agent of the manoeuvre, not the vocal folds. The arytenoid cartilages are in the centre of the image, and the prominent round tubercles are the cuneiform cartilages within the aryepiglottic folds (the pivot of the aryepiglottic constrictor).

Video 7.23c isolates ornamental 'trilling': the regular transverse pumping of the arytenoids and aryepiglottic border of the top of the epilaryngeal tube – akin to regular subtle applications of the laryngeal constrictor for pharyngealization. The large round cuneiform tubercles of the aryepiglottic folds adduct and abduct somewhat asymmetrically, without closing against the tubercle of the epiglottis.

Interestingly, the Mongolian trills of long song parallel the kinds of supraglottic compensatory manoeuvres used by supracricoid partial laryngectomy patients. Both generate vocal qualities that rely on complex laryngeal valving configurations above the glottic level, and both generate resonances similar to pharyngealized voice as a result of sphincteric constriction of the laryngeal tube at the aryepiglottic level (Esling and Harris 2005). Linguists and clinicians are often more familiar with symmetrical glottal adduction–abduction and arytenoid stability in producing phonatory quality, but many of the languages and styles reviewed in Chapter 4 demonstrate asymmetries, non-glottal vibrations, and epilaryngeal tube adjustments that contribute quite normally to the phonologies of those languages or the registers of those styles. The independent right and left arytenoid mobilization and aryepiglottic contractions during the Mongolian trills can be seen in patients after SCPL (Crevier-Buchman et al. 1995). SCPL patients need to compensate for the loss of the glottis by creating a vibrating neoglottis at the level of the mobile arytenoid cartilages, the aryepiglottic folds, and the remaining epiglottis. The rehabilitation process enabling SCPL patients to recover some voicing by acquiring posterior laryngeal and aryepiglottic agility resembles the art of the trill in long song. The common raised-larynx anatomical situation after SCPL (Laccourreye et al. 1990) also parallels the raised-larynx voice quality of Mongolian long song. In theory, the compensatory recovery of SCPL patients speaking Bai, Zhenhai, Yi, 'ATR' or Khoisan languages and having to relearn laryngeal function would require not just voicing to be re-established but phonological contrasts to be reformulated.

7.5.2   Human Beatboxing

Human beatboxing (HBB) is a traditional and also a hip-hop singing style – a form of vocal percussion where the vocalist imitates drumbeats and the sounds and rhythms of various musical instruments. It may also involve singing and the simulation of horns, strings, and machine sounds. The beatboxer manipulates the oral cavity as well as the laryngeal cavity, including the epilaryngeal tube. In theory, the articulatory structures are used very similarly to the way vowel quality or consonant stricture is articulated in speech. In practice, beatboxing artists are performers, as are professional singers or chanters, whose mastery of the intricacies of articulatory combinations and timing surpasses normal speaking ability. Drum sounds typically rely on short-term plosive and fricative combinations, and instrument sounds exploit the long-term vibratory and resonance capabilities of the oral and laryngeal vocal tracts. The virtuosity of HBB extends to simultaneity – the superposition of multiple tiers of sounds from different vocal tract origins. For certain sounds, the principle is to manipulate the speed of transition between registers.

HBB tends to alternate egressive with ingressive airflow to allow for continuity of production and a certain degree of independence between breathing and rhythm patterns. To illustrate the complex laryngeal behaviour of HBB and its relationship to voice quality in general, the videos illustrate isolated sounds (percussion, 'bass sounds', the kick, snare, and hi-hat drum sounds), instrumental sounds (wind and string musical instruments), and style effects (the muted trumpet, electric guitar, and saturated electric guitar), and electronic sounds from the DJ 'scratch' technique.

The behaviour of the epilaryngeal tube figures prominently in all of these productions, which are described by Torcy et al. (2014). Narrowing is essential to produce the degree of constriction required for pulsed impressions such as the 'beatboxed kick', where an oral [p] suddenly released in coordination with the piston-like laryngeal pumping transforms the sound into a non-pulmonic ejective, or the 'beatboxed snare'. From an open and low laryngeal starting position, the epilaryngeal tube constricts in volume, the ventricular folds compress as the glottis closes, and the larynx pumps upwards. It is significant that the narrowed tube and valve positions are maintained to generate the percussive effect. In the largely voiceless 'beatboxed hi-hat', the epilaryngeal tube constricts to achieve the sustained whisper turbulence as short-term 'segmental' events fluctuate. Similar but less constricted postures (therefore less whispery) produce 'beatboxed whistle scratch'.

Video 7.24a: 'beatboxed kick' (ejective mode, ventricular adduction)
Video 7.24b: 'beatboxed snare' (ejective mode, slight ventricular adduction)
Video 7.24c: 'beatboxed hi-hat' (pulmonic egressive, ingressive)
Video 7.24d: 'beatboxed whistle scratch' (oral sibilants, voiceless glottal abduction)
Video 7.24e: 'beatboxed muted trumpet' (falsetto, pharyngeal constriction, arytenoid trills)
Video 7.24f: 'beatboxed electric guitar' (voiced ventricular phonation, pharyngeal constriction)
Video 7.24g: 'beatboxed saturated electric guitar' (harsh voice, high pitch, ventricular incursion, larynx raising)
Video 7.24h: 'beatboxed vocal scratch' (harsh voice, varying pitch, larynx raising)

Configurations that emulate musical instruments such as trumpet or guitar demonstrate an exaggerated 'tubularized' channelling of the entire laryngeal vocal tract, through the epilaryngeal tube and continuing to the tip of the posteriorly curled tubular epiglottis. The wrap-around muscles of the pharyngeal walls assist in the circular rounding of the internal tube. The performance of 'beatboxed muted trumpet' illustrates particularly well the parallel with raised-larynx-voice speech registers, as in Yi, Akan, or Kabiye (Section 4.3.3), and what the mute does to the sound of a trumpet and how that effect is realized imitatively by narrowing the epilaryngeal tube over the glottis. Similar hypertubularization with unusual lateral pinching characterizes 'beatboxed electric guitar', where coupled vibrations of the mucosa on the folds at the bottom of the epilaryngeal tube add to the effect.

Tight lower-epilaryngeal-tube vibratory sources also occur with enhanced longitudinal tension, as in 'pressed' laryngeal constriction at high pitch (Section 2.3.15), in what can be called the 'quasi-sphincter' posture of 'beatboxed saturated electric guitar'. The same vibratory and postural conditions apply to the production of 'beatboxed vocal scratch', where the narrowing of the constrictor is even more exaggerated and the larynx more raised as the background quality for a series of complex stops. The overall posturing of the laryngeal articulator carries the long-term 'drone' quality, in an analogy to bagpipes, while the rapid closing and opening alternations at the glottal and/or ventricular level interact with articulations in the oral vocal tract to 'play the tune' as the chanter does in bagpiping. The laryngeal postures adopted by beatboxers are the same articulatory options available to speakers using the laryngeal mechanism for linguistic contrast, although beatboxers excel at practised control and extend the boundaries of what the laryngeal mechanism can achieve. HBB is an example of the agility and adaptability of the larynx to perform innovative vocal techniques and to produce wide-ranging sounds – some rare, but many found in understudied languages.

8 Laryngeal Articulation and Voice Quality in Sound Change, Language Ontogeny and Phylogeny

Chapter 8 summarizes the ramifications of the Laryngeal Articular Model for the phonetic description of voice quality and investigates its place in phonetic theory. Revising the description of speech-sound production in the lower vocal tract is relevant in explaining the intrinsic relationship between vowel quality, tonal quality, and voice quality. The phonetic concepts of voicing, vocal register, and long-term quality are integrated through the interpretation of how infants acquire the speech-production capacity, beginning in the laryngeal articulator, alternating and combining forms through dynamic utterances, and expanding in vocal tract geography to the oral articulators while still maintaining a laryngeal foundation. The layering of secondary (even multiple) articulations is shown to be endemic – an inherent and necessary property of how human speech is acquired ontogenetically. We argue that there is a parallel between the coarticulatory path that infants follow in their earliest speech development and the elements necessary for the process of phonetic sound change. In this interpretation, the laryngeal articulator is essential in enabling sound change, and we propose that infants are the engine of that change. The categories and combinations of articulation produced in the larynx exceed those of earlier models. We postulate that phonetic change is enabled as infants develop their perceptual and productive phonetic capacities, in interaction with speakers around them, and that laryngeal articulation evolves naturally into all three strands of accent – segmental articulations, intonational overlay, and long-term voice quality. We review and evaluate implications for the phylogenetic origin of human speech from the perspective of our description of laryngeal phonetic behaviour. These hypotheses, derived from our findings on laryngeal behaviour, are put forward for critical examination.

The following sections explore areas of phonetic theory where the construct of laryngeal articulation has a potential impact. One responsibility of voice quality theory is to explain the role of long-term postural settings and their auditory/acoustic consequences for how vowel-quality distinctions are realized. One question would be to determine whether vowel shifts carry with them postural traits that become generalized beyond one or two particular vowels and begin to characterize longer stretches of speech in the accent. One example of this would be the vowel quality in Canadian Raising of the /au/ diphthong in voiceless-coda contexts such as 'out, about, south, doubt' (Chambers 1973, 1979, 1989). Is there a voice quality parameter that accounts for the more [o]-like onset in Nova Scotia accents, the [ε] onset tendency in the Ottawa Valley, and the more central [ʌʊ] in Prairie accents? A corollary question is whether the collective lingual, labial, and mandibular postures over the long term reflect the centre of the vowel space. Another is whether long-term voice quality follows the direction of preponderant vowel shifting as vowels mutate over time. We have not answered these questions, and we have not demonstrated conclusively how or where the three strands of accent interact. But we have laid a foundation of articulatory interaction that can be examined based on a more reliable account of the laryngeal mechanism. Although the role of long-term settings in sociolinguistic, phonological, historical, and evolutionary processes requires continued research, building convincing theories will depend on an elaboration of the role of voice quality, particularly the contribution of the larynx with its flexibility to modulate, often simultaneously, phonatory, tonal, vowel, and overall voice quality (such as resonance changes brought about by raised- and lowered-larynx positions).

8.1   Salience and Context

We speak of voice quality as a 'quasi-permanent', more or less persistent characteristic of accent, but much of what we perceive may be more intermittent than permanent. The qualities that we identify most 'saliently' (as Abercrombie 1967 put it) may occur at certain predictable points in the stream of speech. Stress positions or the codas of intonational phrases may carry a larger load of where certain types of resonance, noise, or vibrations are at their maximum. For example, types of phonation may become most salient in the codas of sequences of intonational phrases, especially if duration plays a role, where the length of time a particular phonation type lasts is extended. Despite inevitable temporal variation in the intermittence of qualities in the stream of speech, the laryngeal articulator exerts a geographically 'upstream' influence on quality as the airstream flows through the vocal tract, so that traces of laryngeal effects persist in varying degrees even as 'downstream' modifications fluctuate under changing oral and prosodic conditions. These interconnected relationships are the same propensities that underlie the PPM outlined in Chapter 5. The LAM differs from previous source-filter conceptualizations in elaborating the articulatory possibilities of the larynx beyond merely the manner of vocal fold vibration at the glottis, identifying a wider range of qualities that originate 'upstream'.

The laryngeal constrictor is an intermediate dual phonator/articulator with multiple outcomes, depending on how it is used in the context of the language. An example can be drawn from an early sociophonetic study of voice quality in Edinburgh (Esling 1978). The findings showed that creaky voice predominated at the upper end of the social scale in Edinburgh English (with nasal voice and apical lingual articulation and close jaw orally), while harsh voice, with suggestions of pharyngeal or faucal constriction and raised-larynx voice, predominated at the lower end (with laminal lingual articulation and protruded jaw orally). At the time, auditory judgements of pharyngealization, faucalization, and raised and lowered larynx were relatively new and tentative, while judgements of phonation type were better supported instrumentally – acoustically and with EGG. In terms of the LAM, we can say that the presence of creakiness in the higher-status Standard Edinburgh English population represents slight aryepiglottic tightening for the purpose of shortening the vocal folds, but with enough vertical coupling through the epilaryngeal tube to enable creaky phonation. Phrase codas that lower in pitch intensify creakiness through lower aerodynamic pressure. On the other hand, the presence of harshness in the broad Edinburgh Scottish English population represents greater compression and tension throughout the laryngeal constrictor mechanism, predisposing vertical coupling, likely with higher pressure. When phrase codas lower in pitch, the harsh state of the constrictor is maintained even if phonation becomes creaky. The LAM allows us to characterize more elegantly the phonetic differences in the social differentiation of English in Edinburgh. The Standard Edinburgh English speakers employ the laryngeal mechanism as a phonatory device, and the broad Edinburgh Scots dialect speakers employ the laryngeal mechanism as an articulatory device. These two varieties have developed along distinctly different historical paths and are perhaps better viewed as historically distinct rather than just synchronically socially differentiated varieties. Their phonetic traits, especially their laryngeal propensities, may be compared with other varieties to which they are closely related to gain insight into their phonetic origins as well as into the ways that laryngeal function influences sound change.

8.2   The Axis of [e/o]

One particularly important consequence of the description of laryngeal articulator action is what happens to vowels that are *not* constricted. Germanic varieties are a particularly salient example of what we call the 'axis of [e/o]'.

The English mid vowels /e/ and /o/, as in FACE and GOAT, function as auto-identifying determinants of voice quality – as an auditory/acoustic cue for normalizing the rest of the vowel space. That is, hearing a close [eː] or [oː] quality in English cues the listener that the accent is Scottish; open [ɛː] or [ɔː] quality could indicate a Northern English accent; while diphthongized [ʌɪ ʌʊ] or [æɪ əʉ] could be the markers of a London or an Australian accent (cf. Cox and Palethorpe 2007). The way that the /e/ and /o/ vowels interact with lower-vocal-tract resonance and vibratory characteristics gives a good indication of how other vowels in the system integrate vowel quality with vocal quality or with tonal quality. Since the vowels run across the middle of the vowel space, they are neither close nor open, and are therefore neutrally affected by laryngeal constriction, or indeed by larynx height adjustments. More open vowels – those right of the axis in Figure 5.5 – are more compatible with laryngeal constriction, including larynx raising, and the potential for accumulating the effects of a more compacted lower vocal tract increases. Closer vowels – those left of the axis in Figure 5.5 – are less compatible with the effects of laryngeal constriction, and the potential for accumulating traits opposite to a constricted laryngeal posture increases. This includes a more open airway setting, larynx lowering, and various innovative labial and lingual adjustments to augment vowel quality. The special distinctive status of [i] and [u] vowels as vocal-tract-normalizing points is familiar from the work of Nearey (1978). Similarly, open (retracted) vowels, in the opposite corner of the vowel space from [i], are easily confused (Peterson and Barney 1952). The LAM prompts us to consider two issues: what happens to [i] under conditions of vowel shift; and whether laryngeal constriction parameters interfere with the perception of retracted vowels. We consider these issues below.

Close vowels in Germanic languages, particularly /i/, are subject to different affinities for laryngeal adjustment from open vowels. For instance, a broad Edinburgh Scots pronunciation of 'carrots and peas', where [a] has a non-lowered-larynx quality but /i/ is rendered as lowered-larynx (pharynx-expanded) [i̞], illustrates how the axis differentiates quality (from open to close on the IPA vowel chart), where open vowels predispose a narrowed laryngeal posture, while close vowels predispose an open, expanded laryngeal posture. An example of the contrast in Danish English is the pronunciation of open /æ/ and /ɑ/, where constriction dominates, vs. close /i/ and /u/, where lowered larynx is dominant (Willerslev 2011, 2013). The LAM provides the explanation that open vowels are maximally susceptible to the effects of constriction, such as raised-larynx quality and aryepiglottic trilling, while close vowels are minimally susceptible to constriction and favour airway opening and pharynx expansion as secondary complements. This split in vowel behaviour is also observed in German English (Gresky 2016), e.g. 'sharp' vs. 'see, group'. The same larynx lowering can occur on close vowels in North American English for paralinguistic emphasis. Levon Helm's Arkansas accent in the songs of The Band (1968) also distinguishes the /iː/ vowel from other vowels, especially open vowels, by applying a lowered-larynx quality. In *The Weight*, the line 'Well Luke, my friend' begins with aryepiglottic trilling, and the line 'What about young Anna. . .' is also constrictively trilled, especially open /æu/ and /æ/, the /iː/ of 'Lee' is distinctively expanded with larynx lowering. The same pharynx-expanded quality applies to 'free' and 'me'. These laryngeal synergies are affinities, and the potential for them to emerge is also governed by position and force in the prosodic phrase.

Audio files 8.01–8.02 illustrate the effect of constriction on open vowels that can occur in Danish English (Willerslev 2013): 'part, past'. Audio files 8.03–8.06 illustrate the effect of opening and larynx lowering on close vowels: 'unique, meeting, between, distribution, peoples, group, east, speak'. In audio files 8.07–8.10, the constricted-larynx quality on open vowels in 'partly, haplo, sampled, arm, far' contrasts with the lowered-larynx quality on close vowels in 'east, group, piece, Europeans, east'. Audio file 8.11 illustrates the larynx-lowered (expansion) effect on /ʊ/ 'look' and /iː/ 'see' in North American English in stressed position.

The LAM clarifies why open vowels should be eminently susceptible to laryngeal constriction and the various qualities it enables, since tongue retraction and jaw opening are synergistic with aryepiglottic tightening. Since tongue fronting or raising and jaw closing accompany close vowels, they are less likely to be laryngeally constricted. We might ask why close front vowels (or close vowels as a whole) should undergo larynx lowering at all. Labov has identified a number of acoustic adaptations that alter the quality of peripheral vowels in chain shifts as well as some of the articulatory strategies that are responsible for them (Labov 1994, Labov and Kim 2015). These pressures would explain the auditory/acoustic stimulus, if not the precise sociolinguistic motivation, for vowels at the close front corner of the conceptual vowel envelope to acquire novel elements to distinguish them. One option is to diphthongize, but other effects related to secondary articulation and to voice quality may play a role. Diphthongization is captured in Labov's Upper Exit Principle (1994: 283), where one of two high peripheral morae becomes non-peripheral in a chain shift. Labov describes the effect on the FLEECE vowel in the Southern (US) Chain Shift, where the gliding quality reduces and lowers. Labov and Kim (2015) describe shifts of /iː/ to [ej] in Prague Czech, to [aj] in

Romansch, to [ei] in Slovenian and Kajkavian dialects, and to [ej] in Old Prussian and East Latvian. They characterize the vowel shifts in these varieties as strongly influenced by Germanic. The Australian treatment of the /iː/ vowel not only diphthongizes but also sometimes reinforces lingual movement with unilateral labial raising (viz. Section 4.2.5.4). This adaptation might serve to 'expose' the oral vocal tract, raising F1 and F2. From the voice quality perspective, such a gesture may be limited to certain vowels or prosodic positions, or it may extend beyond the duration of any single vowel. The Australian example makes a case for the generalization of unilateral labial raising over longer stretches of speech, especially taking into account that intonational phrasing or emphasis might enhance and sustain the posture.

In Swedish, another type of articulatory adjustment has affected the pronunciation of /iː/ in some regions and social groups, creating a new variant that de-peripheralizes the vowel. The 'Viby-i' Swedish vowel variant, summarized from the Swedish literature by Björsten and Engstrand (1999), is lower and more reduced than /e/, as the front of the tongue is lowered and the lower part of the tongue backed (Westerberg 2016). The speech of the character Anja in the Swedish TV series *Wallander* illustrates this realization of /iː/ (Nilsson 2006). Fricativization is also reported in the end-phase of the vowel, presumably as the shape of the front of the tongue directs the airstream against the teeth. Its higher F1 and lower F2 are more suggestive of constriction than of larynx lowering. The reported tongue articulation (Westerberg 2016: 91–95) resembles the double-bunched posture reported for constricted productions of close vowels (Esling et al. 2016), where the tongue is cinched in the middle with one mass forward in the oral cavity and one mass lowered and backed towards the larynx.

8.3   Sound Change

We argue that the laryngeal articulator as a secondary or coarticulatory option provides a viable mechanism for sound change. A primary gesture is inevitably accompanied by numerous accompanying articulations, beginning, as we have shown, with infants using the laryngeal articulator to prime the production of oral sounds. Presumably, listeners who hear sounds with overlapping components need to distinguish consonants, vowel quality, and pitch elements from voice quality. This is particularly important if we follow Laver's (1980) principle that voice quality is the background against which the moving figures of segments are discriminated and identified. This argument is reminiscent of Ohala's (1993) proposal that listeners may attend to varying elements in particular sound categories; the selection of a novel hearing of a pronunciation may result in sound change. Vowel-quality perception is also influenced by speaking rate (Lindblom 1963), and Harrington (2012: 119) concludes that 'listeners do not parse coarticulation from the signal in the same way'. Interpreting our MRI results from Chapter 3, we observe that laryngeal qualities play a complex and overlapping role with different sets of vowels. We argue that vowel quality is not a stable percept uninfluenced by voice quality and that laryngeal configuration can be a significant influence on a listener's perception of a sequence of sounds. What we take to be a 'vowel', produced by the tongue in the upper vocal tract, could in fact also be a laryngeal articulation.

We propose that the laryngeal articulator has a key role to play in the variable perception of sounds, because of its positioning in the vocal tract as a source, its articulatory propensity to generate numerous differentiating qualities, and its ability to sustain long-term effects as a background to more rapid articulations. One example is the uvular genesis of pharyngeals in Wakashan languages (Jacobsen 1969), discussed in Section 5.5. It has been proposed that when a primary sound is accompanied by a subtle but potentially powerful secondary gesture, the first lingual and the other laryngeal, the second gesture has the potential to be perceived as primary (Carlson and Esling 2003). This is what we suspect occurred in Wakashan; that certain uvulars acquired secondary pharyngealization, and that the pharyngeal component eventually became the primary articulation, replacing the former uvular with a pharyngeal segment. Ohala alludes to this possibility in the dissimilation of sounds that are not immediately adjacent to each other (2012: 29). Another example is the emergence of Athabaskan tone, where opposite tones in different languages replaced the same Proto-Athabaskan contrast between stem-final glottalic vs. non-glottalic consonants (Kingston 2005). We contend that the variety of articulatory accompaniments available in the laryngeal articulator beyond just [voice] provides ample opportunity for overlapping qualities, generating the possibility for listeners to hear multiple combinations. Whereas nasality has often been shown to create an environment for reinterpreting the quality of a vowel or even a consonant (Ohala 2012: 31), the laryngeal articulator produces many qualities that can 'colour' the way a given oral sound is perceived.

With regard to the social process of sound change, we emphasize that the interaction between single-articulatory strictures and secondary articulatory background is best viewed with reference to ontogeny. Despite the fact that different speakers from differing backgrounds contribute varying mosaics of pronunciation to social discourse and that different listeners may hear those elements in varying combinations, sound change needs to be explained in the context of how infants initially acquire the capacity to form speech. This is because infants initiate the process of formulating the components of quality and the durational divisions between the strands of speech. They also use the laryngeal mechanism to ground the operation of the vocal tract. In this sense, they are the potential drivers of sound change. Labov has remarked on the intergenerational nature of language change (2001: 463), and Trudgill reminds us that 'the historical-linguistic consequences of the social phenomena of colonisation and contact are impacted on by ... the innate language-learning abilities of human children, which are not totally shared by adolescent and adult members of the same species; and the innate biological basis of human interactional synchrony' (2010: 192). Our caveats are to approach the social forces that drive language change with the knowledge of how infants acquire the phonetic capacity in their very first months, and to approach the structural aspects of change with the knowledge of the complex array of phonetic structures that are available within the laryngeal articulator. The importance of the infant as a phonetic determiner reappears in our discussion of the phylogeny of speech.

8.4   Phylogeny

The laryngeal mechanism is an active articulator, that is, the aryepiglottic structures approximate and form stricture against the tubercle of the epiglottis. From a phonetic perspective, the epiglottis is a passive articulator. It is equally compelling to view the laryngeal mechanism as an articulatory foundation for the initial generation of speech sounds largely related to its airway-closure function. This has been shown to be the case ontogenetically in Chapter 6. Negus (1949) postulated an evolutionary imperative for this airway-closure role, summarized in Section 1.6.3, surmising that the aryepiglottic valve evolved to control airflow to enable independent use of the forelimbs. Fink's (1975) rejoinder, however, that the evolution of the hominin larynx advantaged spring-like recoil of the folding structures to *open* the airway, quickly and widely, suggests opening not closing of the airway as the evolutionary imperative. The contact mechanisms involved in his spring-loading theory may have been exapted as stabilization mechanisms in the motor control of the larynx (Moisik and Gick 2017), just as lingual-molar bracing provides degree-of-freedom-reducing stabilization in the motor control (Gick et al. 2017). Laitman and Reidenberg (2009: 33) concur that the larynx may have evolved to provide increased air intake and oxygen, to service burst and endurance running or increased brain function (the upright running scenario being more likely, since the increase in human brain size postdates the key stages of laryngeal development). In the relatively flat angle of the vocal tract of a canine, the large epiglottis is in firm contact with the undersurface of a long and massive soft palate; the arytenoidal and aryepiglottic structures almost touch the back of the palate; the epiglottis is prevented from actively retracting by the pressure of the palate, but the aryepiglottic structures immediately behind the palate are free to approximate the epiglottis. Aryepiglottic folds are increasingly prominent in the evolution of bears, dogs, apes, and humans; and in the canine family, the cuneiform cartilages hold the aryepiglottic folds parallel to the epiglottis and perpendicular to the glottis, giving the larynx a characteristically T-shaped appearance (Negus 1949: 84–86). One paralinguistic function of aryepiglottic trilling is growling, or imitating growling, and this ability appears to be due to the anatomical evolution of the aryepiglottic folds, manipulated around the raised cuneiform cartilages. To whatever degree climbing, upright walking, forelimb use, or providing ready oxygen to serve running requirements might have triggered the way a multiple-valve pseudo-sphincter evolved in humans, it is clear from the ontogenetic evidence that this adapted arrangement of structures created the possibility for a greater range of sounds to be produced within the laryngeal articulator – for an elaborated array of manners of articulation to be generated. In other words, this adaptation created the laryngeal articulator (the larynx as an articulator).

According to Negus, in carnivore species (e.g. the large cats), the function of the epiglottis is associated with olfaction and not with swallowing, to allow continuous nasal respiration while eating and drinking (1949: 29, 77). In these species, the folds of the thyroarytenoid muscles themselves are capable of acting in a valvular manner at the glottis, as the primary sphincter mechanism (p. 99). Surrounding the glottis in those species where breathing is not interrupted by swallowing, prominent lateral epiglottic folds are present to channel food and fluids around the glottis (pp. 78–80). These lateral folds are lost in species that have evolved aryepiglottic folds with interpositioned cuneiform cartilages. As a consequence, humans have 'a fairly big but degenerate epiglottis; degenerate because of immobility and lack of function' (Negus 1949: 182). Reviewing the anatomical process of deglutition, 'during swallowing, contraction of the sphincteric muscle fibres contained between the layers of the aryepiglottic folds closes the aperture of the larynx and prevents inundation. The inner surface of the aryepiglottic fold is smooth, as it passes down towards the thyro-arytenoid fold, which bounds the glottis or respiratory aperture' (p. 163). 'In deglutition, the abductor muscles play a passive role, and by their relaxation allow the arytenoids to be drawn forwards towards the base of the tongue' (p. 169); 'it is not only the vocal cord but also the aryepiglottic fold which is affected in cases of recurrent nerve paralysis, whether the disordered action concerns the dilator muscles alone or the sphincteric group as well; the vocal cord is moved by certain fibres of the sphincteric muscles, which are not, however, specialized for vocal purposes. Protective closure during deglutition is effected, in man, by the aryepiglottic folds and not at the level of the glottis' (pp. 203–204). This anatomical account clarifies that the epiglottis is not the active articulator, but that the aryepiglottic folds are (through complex folding by multiple musculature); and it underlines that sound generation is achieved by the same mechanism that is responsible for swallowing. Regarding musculature, we should point out that postero-anterior closure of the epilarynx and adduction and vertical compaction of the ventricular folds into the vocal folds is still possible even though the aryepiglottic muscles are found to be sparse or even non-existent (Reidenbach 1997, 1998a, 1998b). This conclusion is also supported by computational biomechanical modelling (Moisik and Gick 2017). Leaving open the question of how the larynx evolved as it did, the anatomical accounts make it clear that the direction of evolution led to a sophisticated development of the epilaryngeal/supraglottic mechanism from a breathing-assisting, food-channelling, nasally-oriented pathway to a breath-regulating, airway-controlling, articulatorily-independent lower vocal tract. Fink (1975) also points out the advantages for speech resonance of vertical larynx mobility. The matter of how speech sounds could be produced in the lower vocal tract, and linguistically implemented, provokes a re-examination of the origins of speech.

The LAM provides a new perspective by which to measure theories of the origin of speech (e.g. MacNeilage 2008). Without a description of the laryngeal articulator, theories are limited to discussing the actions of the oral articulator; but given the evolutionary prominence of the aryepiglottic sphincter mechanism outlined above, discussing the laryngeal articulator has to figure as one of the first considerations in exploring the development of speech sounds. The question that has not yet been answered is: why in the context of hominin evolution do modern human infants use the laryngeal articulator for their first speech? It is tempting to speculate that this behaviour pattern has not changed since hominin speech has existed. And, if we have always developed ontogenetically by using the laryngeal articulator, then could the laryngeal mechanism have been the trigger that combined with cognitive capacity to enable our first awareness of speech sound in general? The exploration of the ontogeny of speech in Chapter 6 also gives us good reason to suppose that this awareness, when it did arise, would have occurred in the same infant–caregiver environment in which it occurs today.

Burling's (2005) account of the evolution of language, and of speech, makes many points that are strengthened by our research. The assertion that human speech sounds have conventional meaning rather than just being iconic from an early stage is supported by our account of phonetic ontogeny. What our research adds is that infants acquire motor control over contrastively useful parcels of speech at a surprisingly early age and in a reflexively rich but visually hidden part of the vocal tract. Basically, because speech sounds are observed to begin ontogenetically in the lower vocal tract, we must ask whether the laryngeal generation of speech sounds was a phenomenon that was also present at a phylogenetically critical time. Reflecting on Burling's account, it is important to point out that we are talking about infants in both cases rather than adults. It seems likely that speech representations did not start with early hominins who had already reached adulthood. At any point in time, the likely path of developing the speech forms that would be used for spoken language was always a question of an infant interacting with adults, while generating (laryngeal) speech spontaneously. In our methodology, it has become clear that adults become intensely aware of the human sound-producing capability when they have infants who are generating the basic elements of phonetic motor production during the first several months of life. The elements become familiar to the adults, but the infant is the driving force; that is, the sounds are created by each infant in a logical progression of how sounds can be produced in the lower vocal tract rather than being taught to the infant. Another way of putting this is that we all learn phonetics 'experimentally' (cf. Catford 2001). Early hominin infants, once they began to possess the required cognitive criteria for language development that Burling enumerates, could be expected to have generated sounds similar to those pharyngeal sounds that every infant generates today, refined into durations short enough to serve for linguistic meaning; the vehicle for drawing the phonetic and the semantic processes together being the dynamic of the infant–caregiver interaction. Burling's observation that 'it is the parent, not the child, who is the imitator' (2005: 110) gains support from our observations of each infant's remarkable control and early mastery of our innate sound-producing instrument.

Any theory based on the oscillatory patterns of articulators – a concept put forward by MacNeilage (1998) – needs to take into account how initial articulatory closing and opening gestures develop in the lower vocal tract, since the laryngeal articulator defines the earliest exploration of manners of articulation. A second crucial issue to resolve is to what extent those earliest laryngeal gestures become cyclical movements; but there is no reason to suppose that the concept of 'syllable' cannot be generated by the larynx. Infant production often pairs laryngeal stricture with a following resonant, and many languages contain pharyngeal-vowel CV sequences. We have noted that infants in the reflexive laryngeal stage produce closing-opening patterns, such as [ʔəʔəʔə] or [ħɑħɑħɑ], or systematically add and drop pharyngeal quality on a vowel [ɑ ɑˤ ɑ ɑˤ ɑ] or [ʕə ʕə]. Another physiological question to address is whether laryngeal articulatory patterns progress developmentally to the jaw and the oral cavity, or whether these areas are under separate and independent control. Whatever the neurological pathways, the existence of autogenerated articulatory patterns in the larynx provokes speculation about early hominins. The cornerstone of MacNeilage's frame/content theory is that 'the motor frame first appears at the onset of canonical babbling' (2008: 188). Given our evidence that speech production progresses from birth to become a salient and self-observed behaviour, cognitive motor frames may be enabled earlier in development than in babbling; and it is reasonable to search for them in the earliest laryngeal productions. MacNeilage's assertion that 'the first and most momentous move an infant makes towards acquiring speech-like forms is to begin babbling at about seven months of age' (2008: 107) needs to be qualified to incorporate what infants control within the laryngeal articulator before oral babbling begins. The processes observed in babbling (Davis and MacNeilage 1995, MacNeilage and Davis 2005) have a foundation within the larynx. Close–open alternations appear in the laryngeal articulator throughout the first several months of life when infants produce dynamic sequences, turning laryngeal constriction on and off. To address MacNeilage's criteria (2008: 244) and reframe them within the context of the LAM: *reduplication* appears before babbling, in cycles of laryngeal constriction and as vibratory oscillations of the aryepiglottic valve; and *variegation* occurs when infants alternate dynamically between laryngeally tight and open forms, binarily in vocal play. We contend that not only labial consonants and central vowels should form the basis of the frame/content concept, but also laryngeal consonants at the deep and primary end of the vocal tract.

Video 8.1 illustrates jaw opening accompanying laryngeal constrictor stricture in a 4-month-old. We posit that the jaw opening is secondary to the primary action of the laryngeal articulator, but related through the hypoglossal nucleus in the medulla shared by the hyoglossus (tongue retracting), thyrohyoid (larynx raising), and geniohyoid (jaw opening).

We concur with MacNeilage that 'the modern human infant reflects the most fundamental properties of the speech-production system' and that 'these bodily properties must therefore have been at the base of emerging mental representations of sound structures in hominids' (2008: 261). We would point out that if the first hominin speakers had infant-like speech patterns, it is because they were infants when they acquired the phonetic capacity, presuming that modern-day infants have very likely continued the same ontogenetic process since then. We take the ontogenetic origin of speech in the epilarynx as an indication that early speech patterns began in the laryngeal vocal tract. The development of the phonetic production capacity in the infant is a quintessential instance of the body (and its sound-generating movements) exerting a formative influence on the mind – which is a fundamental requirement of MacNeilage's theory (2008: 264). Infants auto-produce sounds with the laryngeal mechanism and then attend to and exercise them. We anticipate that further research into ontogenetic phonetic production will explore how these physical components are interfaced with the mental components of the system, shedding light on the process throughout evolution. Since MacNeilage maintains that 'a *totally* closed mouth is the modal early form' (2008: 289), we are bound to ask whether a totally closed laryngeal articulator ([ʔ]) at the other end of the vocal tract is part of that form, or perhaps even more primal. Relating sound production to the biological imperatives in the laryngeally motivated order suck, swallow, and then (some time later in development) chew, would seem to have more evolutionary potency than 'chew, suck, and lick' (MacNeilage 2008: 294).

Our explanation of the LAM and its importance in early infant speech production changes our opinion of early hominin speech. Although velum-epiglottis overlap and a short oropharynx in Australopithecus may have limited the production of a wide range of oral sounds (Laitman and Reidenberg 2009), the ability of modern human infants to acquire a range of manners of laryngeal articulation within a limited and nasally dominant vocal tract suggests that the similar vocal tract of early hominins could have produced comparable sounds. Evidence is building that speech among human progenitors may have been more common than formerly thought. 'The Neanderthal vocal tract, however, has more "speech" ability than the nonhuman primates ... It can produce vowels like /ɪ/, /e/, /ʊ/, and /æ/ ... in addition to the reduced schwa vowel ... Dental and labial consonants like /d/, /b/, /s/, /z/, /v/, and /f/ are also possible' (Lieberman and Crelin 1971: 217). They conclude: 'If Neanderthal man were able to execute the rapid, controlled articulatory maneuvers that are necessary to produce these consonants and had the neural mechanisms that are necessary to perceive rapid formant transitions . . . he would have been able to communicate by means of sound' (p. 217). Ours is a very different view from the emphasis on oral vowel production found in Lieberman and Crelin, as we inject a number of laryngeal phonetic quantities into the discussion. From a purely phonetic point of view, early hominins could presumably produce at least a close vowel and an open vowel, by means of jaw opening, and surely used labialization (cf. chimpanzee vocalizations). Laryngeal strictures co-occur naturally with open vocalization, and the available range of manners of laryngeal articulation co-occurring with a single open vowel sound would have been enough to establish several contrasts. A close jaw vowel, physiologically less likely to occur with constriction, would have added more contrasts. As the cognitive incentive evolved for early hominin infants to recognize (a) that a sound has been produced and (b) that one sequence can be made to contrast with another, they could have begun the process of auto-discovery and phonetic experimentation that every human infant experiences today.

Our focus is on the laryngeal vocal tract rather than on the oral vocal tract, and our emphasis on articulations in the larynx does not hinge on the question of the descent of the larynx per se. Laitman and Reidenberg (2009: 24) observe that the elongated larynx in certain nonhuman species retains its relative position from the basiocciput to C2-C3, that the cervical vertebrae are also elongated, and that the velum or epiglottis is similarly elongated (to maintain palatal contact and the two-tube system for uninterrupted breathing). They stress that these species have modified a basic plan, not changed it, whereas human larynx descent differs due to the anatomical and functional disengagement of the soft palate from the epiglottis and the consequently enlarged oropharynx. Given that both oral and laryngeal Neanderthal vocal tracts resemble those of newborn modern human infants, our contention is that if their supralaryngeal vocal tracts have been thought inadequate to produce a range of speech articulations, then their similar laryngeal vocal tracts should nevertheless be assumed capable of producing the range of laryngeal articulations that infants are capable of today. Importantly for this argument: the larynx is not just a source of vocal fold vibration; the supralaryngeal vocal tract is not the only formant-/noise-generating space in the vocal tract; modern infants also have nasal predominance, but they still produce stricture contrasts plus vowel quality; and if the small vocal tract area of an infant can generate these sound shapes, then the Neanderthal lower vocal tract (and similar physiology) must have been capable of them. Even more importantly, scaling down Lieberman and Crelin's reconstruction of the volume of a Neanderthal vocal tract to infant size (p. 210) would closely match the volume of a modern newborn vocal tract. Comparing the infants of both lineages lends merit to the hypothesis that the exploitation of the sound-producing capabilities of the infant laryngeal articulator was an ontogenetic process experienced by early hominin infants as it is today. Based on the articulatory comparison, it is reasonable to suspect that such a process occurred in the last common ancestor of modern humans and Neanderthals.

Taking the argument one step further, if early hominins had even the sound-producing capacity of modern infants, then they also had voice quality. That is, the process of autogeneration of speech would have also involved steps towards the discrimination and differentiation of the strands of the medium – separating out isolated articulations, as speech develops, against the background qualities already established in the primary, laryngeal, articulator.

Despite suggestions that mutations in the shape of the pharyngeal vocal tract might have been selected and retained for their advantage in proliferating more distinctive acoustic signals (Lieberman and Crelin 1971: 218), it is doubtful that natural selection was based on sound-producing abilities (Nishimura et al. 2006). As Laitman and Reidenberg (2009) put it, 'the human larynx did not evolve *for* speech . . . we have garnered a number of rather special laryngeal modifications that have allowed us to develop this decidedly human ability' (p. 19). Lending support to our position on the parallel between infant laryngeal development throughout evolution and the comparison of adult vocal tracts, Laitman and Reidenberg explain that 'the unique characteristics of the adult human larynx reflect both a distinctive developmental path as well as an evolutionary one. Whereas Ernst Haeckel's "Biogenetic Law" – that "ontogeny recapitulates phylogeny" – has long been proven untrue (we decidedly do not demonstrate exact stages in our development that reflect specific evolutionary periods), features of development may offer insight into evolutionary scenarios that can only be hypothesized' (p. 25). In this same vein, we contend that infant phonetic development, specifically in the way our first speech sounds are constructed within the laryngeal articulator, offers insight into an evolutionary scenario about which we can form new hypotheses.

Since Lieberman and Crelin's (1971) estimations, new research has revealed 'evidence from linguistics, genetics, paleontology, and archaeology clearly suggesting that Neandertals shared with us something like modern speech and language' (Dediu and Levinson 2013: 1). The similar pattern of birth and slow infant development between Neanderthals and modern humans is evidence of the nurturing during the prolonged childhood necessary for the transmission of speech and language. This pattern could have already been developing in a common ancestor as long as 800,000 years ago. Four consider-ations make it likely that our recent ancestors had already evolved spoken language: early hominin vocal tract shape, estimates of sound-production capacity in early hominins, the time depth of the lengthy infant-nurturing period, and the articulatory sound-production capability of the larynx by modern humans in their earliest infancy. First, the vocal tract reconstructions of Neanderthal by Lieberman and Crelin (1971) propose a similar structure to human newborns and to our model of the modern laryngeal vocal tract. The pharyngeal reconstruction and casts of the air passages of a child, Neanderthal and modern humans by Lieberman and Crelin indicate that the laryngeal air space was substantial in Neanderthals. The reconstructions of Australopith-ecus, particularly of the laryngeal space, by Laitman and Heimbuch (1982) – also illustrated in Lieberman (1984: 308–311) – and Laitman and Reidenberg (2009) match quite closely the Laryngeal Articulator Model of the larynx, suggesting the same speech-production capacity as the modern laryngeal mechanism. Second, Lieberman and Crelin's estimation of the range of Nean-derthal vowel and consonant production, however limited, is in itself far greater than the production capability of the laryngeal articulator alone. This range of oral sounds, added to laryngeal sounds, and given jaw-opening capabilities, yields an estimated articulatory production, which over 400,000 years ago could have sufficed to construct a very plausible sound system to carry meaning. This view is strengthened by the estimates of monkey vocal tract area functions and the conclusion that they are capable of producing speech-like sounds (Fitch et al. 2016). Boë (2013) contends that anatomy is not the limiting factor that Lieberman and Crelin suppose, and Boë et al. (2017) believe that a range of vowel sounds could have been produced by very early common ancestors, despite their high larynx position, adding to the argument that speech sounds have been available for linguistic exploitation even millions of years earlier than previously imagined. We have argued that there is no justifiable reason to assume that a low-larynx position in and of itself should be required to produce the kinds of speech sounds that humans produce, based on our evidence that infants produce sounds initially using only the laryngeal articulator and inherently high larynx position, producing consonant strictures while expanding vowel sounds. Demolin and Delvaux (2006) point out that all primate larynxes are more diverse and variable (necessarily in laryngeal articu-lation, we might add) than previously thought by primate researchers. Third, the developmental similarities documented between early hominins and modern humans by Dediu and Levinson (2013) imply that infant development has been similar over the last 500,000 years, supporting the evolution of a complex representational system. Finally, our elaboration of the articulatory and speech-production capabilities of the laryngeal vocal tract demonstrates that the specialized machinery for speech production has been present within the laryngeal mechanism, even if not yet to a large scale in the oral vocal tract, for the time period reviewed by Dediu and Levinson (2013, 2018), where they argue that Neanderthals were fully articulate and that language evolution was gradual. Our findings that human newborns embark on a systematic pattern of phonetic discovery through their own self-generated production, within a vocal tract structure that parallels a long line of hominid ancestors, does not contradict, on phonetic grounds, the hypothesis that language mediated by speech had its origins at least half a million years ago.

To address MacNeilage's (2008: 301) criteria for 'speechlikeness' (and Lieberman and Crelin's criteria for 'articulate speech'), we can confirm that, like songbirds in MacNeilage's example, 'hearing one's own vocalizations makes a contribution to learning' also applies to the attention infants pay to their own production. The productions that occur during the first two months are, articulatorily, more elaborate than just phonation as in Oller's 'phonation stage' (2000: 63–64). In the 'primitive articulation stage' (1–4 months), infants explore the vocal tract phonetically, to exploit the range of articulatory manners that are available within the laryngeal articulator. Within the 'expansion stage' (3–8 months), we emphasize that infants generate laryngeal articulations *because* they are available to them, and there need not be specific inciting stimuli. Our observation of phonetic vocal play suggests that laryngeal articulations and their contrasting pairings in dynamic utterances are voluntary. We must demonstrate more comprehensively, however, that rhythmic frames – 'biphasic rhythm generation' as a product of a central pattern generator (MacNeilage 2008: 309) – appear during this laryngeal articulation stage, varying manner of articulation, airflow and phonatory quality, and pitch contrasts within the laryngeal articulator. Notwithstanding these requirements, we have shown that the laryngeal mechanism is capable of articulation, that the range of manners of articulation it can produce is broad, and that the voice qualities it generates can function as secondary background to later-emerging pieces of sound (in addition to the facility of timing that it enjoys). These observations provide a phonetic argument that the articulatory tools to engage with an emerging language capacity have existed within the laryngeal articulator, even with limited oral vocal tract elaboration, since *H. heidelbergensis* 500,000 years ago, as Dediu and Levinson contend (2013: 2–3). Since we now know that infants use the laryngeal mechanism to build a set of phonetic units (as well as a set of 'baseline' qualities) that can appear with different timing in speech sequences, we hypothesize that this same heuristic process has been a part of hominin vocal development for the same length of time. The fact that elaborated oral articulations preserve a combined articulated laryngeal base, as in laryngeal priming (Chapter 6), makes it impossible to ignore the essential role of the larynx in ontogeny or in phylogeny. The larynx is the infant's phonetic toolbox. It provides an anatomically and physiologically stable basis on which the phonetic component of the complex adaptive system that is language could have evolved. We contend, on phonetic grounds, that the vocal tract, in particular the lower vocal tract, was ready to adapt the essential components of speech sounds whenever the cognitive circumstances arose (over 100,000s of years of successive infants).

References

Abercrombie, David (1967) *Elements of General Phonetics*. Edinburgh: Edinburgh University Press.

Adamson, Benetta (1981) A spectrographic analysis of pharyngeal consonants in Sudanese Arabic. *Work in Progress* 3. University of Reading Phonetics Lab, 81–96.

Al-Ani, Salman H. (1970) *Arabic Phonology: An Acoustical and Physiological Investigation (Janua Linguarum 61)*. The Hague: Mouton.

(1978) An acoustical and physiological investigation of the Arabic /ʕ/. In Salman H. Al-Ani (ed.), *Readings in Arabic Linguistics*. Bloomington: Indiana University Linguistics Club, 89–101.

Ali, Latif H. and Raymond G. Daniloff (1972) A contrastive cinefluorographic investigation of the articulation of emphatic-non-emphatic cognate consonants. *Studia Linguistica* 26, 81–105.

Allen, Elizabeth L. and Harry Hollien (1973) A laminagraphic study of pulse (vocal fry) register phonation. *Folia Phoniatrica* 25, 241–250.

Andersen, Torben (1993) Vowel quality alternation in Dinka verb inflection. *Phonology* 10, 1–42.

Anderson, Peter, Sidney Fels, Negar M. Harandi, Andrew Ho, Scott Moisik, C. Antonio Sánchez, et al. (2017) FRANK: A hybrid 3D biomechanical model of the head and neck. In Yohan Payan and Jacques Ohayon (eds.), *Biomechanics of Living Organs: Hyperelastic Constitutive Laws for Finite Element Modeling*. Oxford: Academic Press, 413–447.

Annan, Brian (1972) The 'articulation base' and Chomsky's 'neutral position'. In Rigault and Charbonneau (eds.), 1080–1082.

Aralova, Natalia, Sven Grawunder, and Bodo Winter (2011) The acoustic correlates of tongue root vowel harmony in Even (Tungusic). In Lee and Zee (eds.), 240–243.

Archangeli, Diana, and Douglas Pulleyblank (1994) *Grounded Phonology*. Cambridge, MA: MIT Press.

Ball, Martin J., John H. Esling, and B. Craig Dickson (2000) The transcription of voice quality. In Kent and Ball (eds.), 49–58.

(2018) Revisions to the VoQS system for the transcription of voice quality. *Journal of the International Phonetic Association* 48, 165–171.

Basbøll, Hans (2014) Danish stød as evidence for grammaticalisation of suffixal positions in word structure. *Acta Linguistica Hafniensia* 46, 137–158.

Bel, Bernard and Isabelle Marlien (eds.) (2004) *Actes des XXVes Journées d'Étude sur la Parole*. Fès, Morocco: AFCP.

Bell, Alexander Graham (1908) *The Mechanism of Speech*. New York: Funk & Wagnalls.

Bell, Alexander Melville (1867) *Visible Speech: The Science of Universal Alphabetics*. London: Simpkin, Marshall & Co.

Bell-Berti, Fredericka and Lawrence J. Raphael (eds.) (1995) *Producing Speech: Contemporary Issues: For Katherine Safford Harris*. Woodbury, NY: AIP Press.

Benítez, Andrés, Vikram Ramanarayanan, Louis Goldstein, and Shrikanth Narayanan (2014) A real-time MRI study of articulatory setting in second language speech. In *Proceedings of Interspeech*, Singapore.

Benner, Allison (2009) *Production and Perception of Laryngeal Constriction in the Early Vocalizations of Bai and English Infants*. Doctoral dissertation, University of Victoria.

Benner, Allison, Izabelle Grenon, and John H. Esling (2007) Infants' phonetic acquisition of voice quality parameters in the first year of life. In Trouvain and Barry (eds.), vol. 3, 2073–2076.

Bergan, Christine C., Ingo R. Titze, and Brad Story (2004) The perception of two vocal qualities in a synthesized vocal utterance: Ring and pressed voice. *Journal of Voice* 18, 305–317.

Bertinetto, Pier Marco, and Michele Loporcaro (2005) The sound pattern of Standard Italian, as compared with the varieties spoken in Florence, Milan and Rome. *Journal of the International Phonetic Association* 35, 131–151.

Bessell, Nicola J. (1992) *Towards a Phonetic and Phonological Typology of Post-Velar Articulation*. Doctoral dissertation, University of British Columbia.

Bettany, Lisa (2004) *Range Exploration of Pitch and Phonation in the First Six Months of Life*. Master's thesis, University of Victoria.

Bgažba, Xuxut Solomonovich (1964) *Bzybskij Dialekt Abxazskogo Jazyka (the Bzyb Dialect of the Abkhaz Language)*. Tbilisi, USSR.

Biacabe, Bernard, Lise Crevier-Buchman, Ollivier Laccourreye, and Daniel Brasnu (1998) Laryngectomie partielle verticale avec reconstruction glottique: résultats carcinologiques et fonctionnels. *Ann. Otolaryngol. Chir. Cervicofac.* 115, 189–195.

Biacabe, Bernard, Lise Crevier-Buchman, Stéphane Hans, Ollivier Laccourreye, and Daniel Brasnu (1999) Vocal function after vertical partial laryngectomy with glottic reconstruction by false vocal fold flap: Durational and frequency measures. *Laryngoscope* 109, 698–704.

Biacabe, Bernard, Lise Crevier-Buchman, Ollivier Laccourreye, Stéphane Hans, and Daniel Brasnu (2001) Phonatory mechanisms after vertical partial laryngectomy with glottic reconstruction by false vocal fold flap. *Annals of Otology, Rhinology & Laryngology* 110, 935–940.

Billington, Rosey (2017) *The Phonetics and Phonology of the Lopit Language*. Doctoral dissertation, University of Melbourne.

Birkholz, Peter (2005) *3D-Artikulatorische Sprachsynthese*. Doctoral dissertation, Universität Rostock.

(2011) A survey of self-oscillating lumped-element models of the vocal folds. In Bernd J. Kröger and Peter Birkholz (eds.), *Studientexte zur Sprachkommunikation: Elektronische Sprachsignalverarbeitung 2011*. Dresden: TUDPress, 47–58.

Björsten, Sven and Olle Engstrand (1999) Swedish 'damped' /i/ and /y/: Experimental and typological observations. In Ohala et al. (eds.), 1957–1960.

Blom, Eric D., Mark I. Singer, and Ronald C. Hamaker (1982) Tracheostoma valve for postlaryngectomy voice rehabilitation. *Annals of Otology, Rhinology & Laryngology* 91, 576–578.

Blumin, Joel H., Dana E. Pcolinsky, and Joseph P. Atkins (2004) Laryngeal findings in advanced Parkinson's Disease. *Annals of Otology, Rhinology & Laryngology* 113, 253–258.

Boë, Louis-Jean (2013) Anatomy and control of the developing human vocal tract: A response to Lieberman. *Journal of Phonetics* 41, 379–392.

Boë, Louis-Jean, Frédéric Berthommier, Thierry Legou, Guillaume Captier, Caralyn Kemp, Thomas R. Sawallis, et al. (2017) Evidence of a vocalic proto-system in the Baboon (Papio papio) suggests pre-hominin speech precursors. *PLoS ONE* 12(1): e0169321. doi:10.1371/journal.pone.0169321.

Boff-Dkhissi, Marie-Christine (1983) Contribution à l'étude expérimentale des consonnes d'arrière de l'arabe classique (locuteurs marocains). *Travaux de l'Institut Phonétique de Strasbourg* 15.

Borel, Stéphanie, Lise Crevier-Buchman, Christophe Tessier, Stéphane Hans, Ollivier Laccourreye, and Daniel Brasnu (2004) Quality of life before and after thyroplasty for vocal fold paralysis. *Revue de Laryngologie Otologie Rhinologie* 125, 287–390.

Borroff, Marianne L. (2007) *A Landmark Underspecification Account of the Patterning of Glottal Stop*. Doctoral dissertation, SUNY, Stony Brook.

Boysson-Bardies, Bénédicte de (1999) *Comment la parole vient aux enfants: de la naissance jusqu'à deux ans* (éd. revue et corrigée). Paris: Editions Odile Jacob.

Boysson-Bardies, Bénédicte de, Laurent Sagart, and Catherine Durand (1984) Discernible differences in the babbling of infants according to target language. *Journal of Child Language* 11, 1–15.

Boysson-Bardies, Bénédicte de and Marilyn M. Vihman (1991) Adaptation to language: Evidence from babbling and first words in four languages. *Language* 67, 297–319.

Brasnu, Daniel, Marshall Strome, Lise Crevier-Buchman, Marie-Claude Pfauwadel, and Henri Laccourreye (1989) Voice evaluation in myomucosal shunt after total laryngectomy: Comparison with esophageal speech. *American Journal of Otolaryngology* 10, 267–272.

Bravi, Paolo (2017) Diverse notes: The origin of variation of the quality of voice in singing voices. Paper presented at *AISV 2017*, Pisa.

Broca, Pierre Paul (1861) Perte de la parole, ramollissement chronique et destruction partielle du lobe antérieur gauche du cerveau. *Bulletin de la Société Anthropologique* 2, 235–238.

Brown, Penelope and Stephen Levinson (1987) *Politeness: Some Universals in Language Usage*. Cambridge: Cambridge University Press.

Brücke, Ernst (1860) Beiträge zur Lautlehre der Arabischen Sprachen. *Wiener Sitzungs-berichte Philologisch Historische Classe* XXXIV, 307–356.

Brunelle, Marc, Duy Duong Nguyễn, and Khac Hùng Nguyễn (2010) A laryngographic and laryngoscopic study of Northern Vietnamese tones. *Phonetica* 67, 147–169.

Brunner, Jana and Marzena Żygis (2011) Why do glottal stops and low vowels like each other? In Lee and Zee (eds.), 376–379.

Bruyninckx, Marielle, Bernard Harmegnies, Joachim Llisterri, and Dolors Poch (1994) Language-induced voice quality variability in bilinguals. *Journal of Phonetics* 22, 19–31.

Buder, Eugene H., Lesya B. Chorna, D. Kimbrough Oller, and Rebecca B. Robinson (2008) Vibratory regime classification of infant phonation. *Journal of Voice* 22, 553–564.

Buder, Eugene H., Anne S. Warlaumont, and D. Kimbrough Oller (2013) An acoustic phonetic catalog of prespeech vocalizations from a developmental perspective. In Beate Peter and Andrea A. N. MacLeod (eds.), *Comprehensive Perspectives on Speech Sound Development and Disorders: Pathways from Linguistic Theory to Clinical Practice.* Hauppauge, NY: Nova Science, 103–134.

Bukshaisha, Fouzia (1985) *An Experimental Phonetic Study of Some Aspects of Qatari Arabic.* Doctoral dissertation, University of Edinburgh.

Burling, Robbins (2005) *The Talking Ape: How Language Evolved.* Oxford: Oxford University Press.

Butcher, Andrew and Kusay Ahmad (1987) Some acoustic and aerodynamic character-istics of pharyngeal consonants in Iraqi Arabic. *Phonetica* 44, 156–172.

Camper, Peter (1779) Account of the organs of speech of the orangoutan. *Philosophical Transactions of the Royal Society London* 69, 139–159.

Carlson, Barry F. and John H. Esling (2000) Spokane. *Journal of the International Phonetic Association* 30, 101–106. (Erratum: vol. 31, 298.)

  (2003) Phonetics and physiology of the historical shift of uvulars to pharyngeals in Nuuchahnulth (Nootka). *Journal of the International Phonetic Association* 33, 183–193.

Carlson, Barry F. and Pauline Flett (1989) *Spokane Dictionary.* Missoula: University of Montana Press.

Carlson, Barry F., John H. Esling, and Katie Fraser (2001) Nuuchahnulth. *Journal of the International Phonetic Association* 31, 275–279.

Carlson, Barry F., John H. Esling, and Jimmy G. Harris (2004) A laryngoscopic phonetic study of Nlaka'pamux (Thompson) Salish glottal stop, glottalized reso-nants, and pharyngeals. In Donna B. Gerdts and Lisa Matthewson (eds.), *Studies in Salish Linguistics in Honor of M. Dale Kinkade. Occasional Papers in Linguistics* No. 17. Missoula: University of Montana Press, 58–71.

Casali, Roderic F. (2008) ATR harmony in African languages. *Language and Linguis-tics Compass* 2, 496–549.

Catford, J. C. (1964) Phonation types: The classification of some laryngeal components of speech production. In D. Abercrombie, D. B. Fry, P. A. D. MacCarthy, N. C. Scott, and J. L. M. Trim (eds.), *In Honour of Daniel Jones.* London: Longmans, Green & Co., 26–37.

(1968) The articulatory possibilities of man. In Bertil Malmberg (ed.), *Manual of Phonetics*. Amsterdam: North-Holland, 309–333.

(1977a) *Fundamental Problems in Phonetics*. Edinburgh: Edinburgh University Press.

(1977b) Mountain of tongues: The languages of the Caucasus. *Annual Review of Anthropology* 6, 283–314.

(1983) Pharyngeal and laryngeal sounds in Caucasian languages. In Diane M. Bless and James H. Abbs (eds.), *Vocal Fold Physiology: Contemporary Research and Clinical Issues*. San Diego: College Hill Press, 344–350.

(1990) Glottal consonants . . . another view. *Journal of the International Phonetic Association* 20(2), 25–26.

(2001) *A Practical Introduction to Phonetics* (2nd edn). Oxford: Oxford University Press.

(2002) On Rs, rhotacism and paleophony. *Journal of the International Phonetic Association* 31, 171–185.

Chambers, Jack K. (1973) Canadian Raising. *Canadian Journal of Linguistics* 18, 113–135.

(1979) Canadian English. In Jack K. Chambers (ed.), *The Languages of Canada*. Montreal: Didier, 168–204.

(1989) Canadian Raising: Blocking, fronting, etc. *American Speech* 64, 75–88.

Chao, Yuen-Ren (1930) A system of 'tone-letters'. *Le Maître Phonétique* 45, 24–27.

(1968) *A Grammar of Spoken Chinese*. Berkeley: University of California Press.

Chervin, Claudius (1854) *Guérison des bègues, prompte et radicale, sans remède ni opération, mais par l'imitation*. Lyon: A. Brun.

Chomsky, Noam and Morris Halle (1968) *The Sound Pattern of English*. New York: Harper & Row.

Clements, G. Nick (1985) The geometry of phonological features. *Phonology Yearbook* 2, 225–252.

(1989) *A Unified Set of Features for Consonants and Vowels*. Manuscript, Cornell University.

Clements, G. Nick and Elizabeth V. Hume (1995) The internal organization of speech sounds. In John A. Goldsmith (ed.), *The Handbook of Phonological Theory*. Oxford: Blackwell, 245–306.

Coey, Christopher, John H. Esling, and Scott R. Moisik (2014) *iPA Phonetics*, Version 1.0 [2014]. Department of Linguistics, University of Victoria, Canada.

Cohn, Abigail C. (1993) Voicing and vowel height in Madurese: A preliminary report. *Oceanic Linguistics Special Publications* 24, 107–121.

Colarusso, John (1985) Pharyngeals and pharyngealization in Salishan and Wakashan. *International Journal of American Linguistics* 51, 366–368.

Collins, Beverley and Inger M. Mees (1998) *The Real Professor Higgins: The Life and Career of Daniel Jones*. Berlin: Mouton de Gruyter.

Colton, Raymond H. and Jo A. Estill (1981) Elements of voice quality: Perceptual, acoustic, and physiologic aspects. In Norman J. Lass, *Speech and Language: Advances in Basic Research and Practice*, vol. 5. New York: Academic Press, 311–403.

262   *References*

Coupe, A. R. (2003) *A Phonetic and Phonological Description of Ao: a Tibeto-Burman Language of Nagaland, North-East India.* Canberra: The Australian National University, Research School of Pacific and Asian Studies.

Cox, Felicity and Sallyanne Palethorpe (2007) Australian English. *Journal of the International Phonetic Association* 37, 341–350.

Crelin, Edmund S. (1973) *Functional Anatomy of the Newborn.* New Haven: Yale University Press.

Crevier-Buchman, Lise, Marie-Claude Pfauwadel, Eric Chabardes, Ollivier Laccourreye, Daniel Brasnu, and Henri Laccourreye (1991) Etude comparative des paramètres temporels des voix sans larynx (oesophagienne et trachéo-oesophagienne). *Ann. Otolaryngol. Chir. Cervicofac.* 108, 261–265.

Crevier-Buchman, Lise, Ollivier Laccourreye, Gregory Weinstein, Dominique Garcia, Véronique Jouffre, and Daniel Brasnu (1995) Evolution of speech and voice following supracricoid partial laryngectomy. *Journal of Laryngology & Otology* 109, 410–413.

Crevier-Buchman, Lise, Ollivier Laccourreye, Jean-François Papon, Dominique Nurit, and Daniel Brasnu (1997) Adductor spasmodic dysphonia: Case reports with acoustic analysis following botulinum toxin injection and acupuncture. *Journal of Voice* 11, 232–237.

Crevier-Buchman, Lise, Ollivier Laccourreye, Floris L. Wuyts, Marie-Claude Monfrais-Pfauwadel, Claire Pillot, and Daniel Brasnu (1998) Comparison and evolution of perceptual and acoustic characteristics of voice after supracricoid partial laryngectomy with cricohyoidoepiglottopexy. *Acta Oto-Laryngologica* 118, 594–599.

Crevier-Buchman, Lise, Daniel Brasnu, and Jacqueline Vaissière (1999) Voice intelligibility after supracricoid partial laryngectomy. In Ohala et al. (eds.), 1815–1818.

Crevier-Buchman, Lise, Shinji Maeda, Daniel Brasnu, Philippe Halimi, and Jacqueline Vaissière (2000) Phonetic consequences of supracricoid partial laryngectomy: Phonation-articulation tradeoff: articulatory compensation. *5th Seminar on Speech Motor Control*, Kloster Seeon.

Crevier-Buchman, Lise, Shinji Maeda, Natacha Bély, Ollivier Laccourreye, Jacqueline Vaissière, and Daniel Brasnu (2001) Compensations articulatoires après laryngectomie partielle supracricoïdienne avec cricohyoïdoépiglottopexie. *Ann. Otolaryngol. Chir. Cervicofac.* 118, 81–88.

Crevier-Buchman, Lise, Jacqueline Vaissière, Shinji Maeda, and Daniel Brasnu (2002) Etude de l'intelligibilité des consonnes du français après laryngectomie partielle supracricoïdienne. *Revue de Laryngologie Otologie Rhinologie* 123, 307–310.

Crevier-Buchman, Lise, Shinji Maeda, Daniel Brasnu, and Jacqueline Vaissière (2003) Perceptual and acoustic correlation in consonant identification after partial laryngectomy. In Solé et al. (eds.), 2361–2364.

Crevier-Buchman, Lise, Christophe Tessier, Alexandra Sauvignet, Sylvie Brihaye-Arpin, and Marie-Claude Monfrais-Pfauwadel (2005) Diagnostic d'une dysphonie non organique de l'adulte. *Revue de Laryngologie Otologie Rhinologie* 126, 353–360.

Crevier-Buchman, Lise, Isabelle Colomb, Stéphane Hans, Jacqueline Vaissière, and Daniel Brasnu (2007) Evolution de la voix et de la qualité de vie après cordectomie au laser CO_2 par voie endoscopique. *Revue de Laryngologie Otologie Rhinologie* 128, 315–320.

Crevier-Buchman, Lise, Claire Pillot-Loiseau, Annie Rialland, Coralie Vincent Narantuya and Alain Desjacques (2012) Analogy between laryngeal gesture in Mongolian Long Song and supracricoid partial laryngectomy. *Clinical Linguistics and Phonetics* 26, 86–99.

Crumley, Roger L. (1994) Unilateral recurrent laryngeal nerve paralysis. *Journal of Voice* 8, 79–83.

Czaykowska-Higgins, Ewa (1987) *Characterizing Tongue Root Behavior*. Manuscript, MIT, Cambridge, MA.

(1998) The morphological and phonological constituent structure of words in Moses-Columbia Salish. In Ewa Czaykowska-Higgins and M. Dale Kinkade (eds.), *Salish Languages and Linguistics*. Berlin: Mouton de Gruyter, 153–195.

Czermak, Johann N. (1861) *On the Laryngoscope and Its Employment in Physiology and Medicine*. London: New Sydenham Society.

Davidson, Matthew (2002) *Studies in Southern Wakashan (Nootkan) Grammar*. Doctoral dissertation, SUNY, Buffalo.

Davis, Barbara L. and Peter F. MacNeilage (1995) The articulatory basis of babbling. *Journal of Speech and Hearing Research* 38, 1199–1211.

Davis, Barbara L., Peter F. MacNeilage, Christine L. Matyear, and Julia K. Powell (2000) Prosodic correlates of stress in babbling: An acoustical study. *Child Development* 71, 1258–1270.

Davis, Stuart (1995) Emphasis spread in Arabic and grounded phonology. *Linguistic Inquiry* 26, 465–498.

Dediu, Dan and Stephen C. Levinson (2013) On the antiquity of language: The reinterpretation of Neandertal linguistic capacities and its consequences. *Frontiers in Psychology* 4, 397.

(2018) Neanderthal language revisited: Not only us. *Current Opinion in Behavioral Sciences* 21, 49–55.

Dediu, Dan and Scott R. Moisik (2019) Pushes and pulls from below: Anatomical variation, articulation and sound change. *Glossa: A Journal of General Linguistics* 4(1), 7.

Deguchi, Shinji, Yuki Kawahara, and Satoshi Takahashi (2011) Cooperative regulation of vocal fold morphology and stress by the cricothyroid and thyroarytenoid muscles. *Journal of Voice* 25(6), e255–e263.

Dejonckere, Philippe H. (1981) *Theorie oscillo-impédantielle de la vibration des cordes vocales*. Thèse d'agrégation de l'enseignement supérieur, Université Catholique de Louvain.

Delack, J. B. and P. J. Fowlow (1978) The ontogenesis of differential vocalization: Development of prosodic contrastivity during the first year of life. In Natalie Waterson and Catherine E. Snow (eds.), *The Development of Communication*. Chichester: Wiley, 93–110.

Delattre, Pierre (1971) Pharyngeal features in the consonants of Arabic, German, Spanish, French, and American English. *Phonetica* 23, 129–155.

Delattre, Pierre and Donald C. Freeman (1968) A dialect study of American r's by x-ray motion picture. *Linguistics* 6, 29–68.

Demolin, Didier and Véronique Delvaux (2006) A comparison of the articulatory parameters involved in the production of sound of bonobos and modern humans. In Angelo Cangelosi, Andrew D. M. Smith, and Kenny Smith (eds.), *The Evolution of Language*. Singapore: World Scientific, 67–74.

Denning, Keith (1989) *The Diachronic Development of Phonological Voice Quality, with Special Reference to Dinka and the Other Nilotic Languages*. Doctoral dissertation, Stanford University.

DiCanio, Christian T. (2009) The phonetics of register in Takhian Thong Chong. *Journal of the International Phonetic Association* 39, 162–188.

    (2012) Coarticulation between tone and glottal consonants in Itunyoso Trique. *Journal of Phonetics* 40, 162–176.

Dickson, B. Craig (1980) *An Investigation of Theories and Parameters Pertaining to Speaker Recognition*. Master's thesis, University of Victoria.

Dimmendaal, Gerrit Jan (1983) *The Turkana Language*. Dordrecht: Foris.

Dzhejranishvili, E. F. (1959) Faringalizovanye Glasnye v Tsakursko-Rutul'skom i Udinskom Jazykakh. *Iberijsko-Kavkazkoe Jazykozananie* 11, 339–359.

Eckel, Hans E., Jürgen Koebke, Christian Sittel, Georg M. Sprinzl, Claus Pototschnig, and Eberhard Stennert (1999) Morphology of the human larynx during the first five years of life studied on whole organ serial sections. *Annals of Otology, Rhinology and Laryngology* 108, 232–238.

Edmondson, Jerold A. and John H. Esling (2006) The valves of the throat and their functioning in tone, vocal register, and stress: Laryngoscopic case studies. *Phonology* 23, 157–191.

Edmondson, Jerold A., Ziwo Lama, John H. Esling, Jimmy G. Harris, and Li Shaoni (2001) The aryepiglottic folds and voice quality in the Yi and Bai languages: Laryngoscopic case studies. *Mon-Khmer Studies* 31, 83–100.

Edmondson, Jerold A., John H. Esling, Jimmy G. Harris, Deborah Martin, Edward C. Weisberger, and Lesa Blackhurst (2003) The role of the glottic and epiglottic planes in the phonetic qualities of voice in the Bor Dinka language (Sudan) and other phonetic features: A laryngoscopic study. Retrieved from http:// ling.uta.edu/_jerry/dktry.pdf

Edmondson, Jerold A., John H. Esling, Jimmy G. Harris, and James Wei (2004) A phonetic study of Sui consonants and vowels. *Mon-Khmer Studies* 34, 47–66.

Edmondson, Jerold A., John H. Esling, Jimmy G. Harris, and Huang Tung-chiou [Akiyo Pahalaan] (2005) A laryngoscopic study of glottal and epiglottal/pharyngeal stop and continuant articulations in Amis – an Austronesian language of Taiwan. *Language and Linguistics* 6, 381–396.

Edmondson, Jerold A., Cécile M. Padayodi, Zeki Majeed Hassan, and John H. Esling (2007) The laryngeal articulator: Source and resonator. In Trouvain and Barry (eds.), vol. 3, 2065–2068.

Edmondson, Jerold A., Yueh-chin Chang, Feng-fan Hsieh, and Hui-chuan J. Huang (2011) Reinforcing voiceless finals in Taiwanese and Hakka: Laryngoscopic case studies. In Lee and Zee (eds.), 627–630.

Edmondson, Jerold A., John H. Esling, and Ziwo Lama (拉玛兹偓) (2017) Nuosu Yi. *Journal of the International Phonetic Association* 47, 87–97.

Eklund, Robert (2008) Pulmonic ingressive phonation: Diachronic and synchronic characteristics, distribution and function in animal and human sound production and in human speech. *Journal of the International Phonetic Association* 38, 235–324.

El-Halees, Yousef (1985) The role of F1 in the place-of-articulation distinction in Arabic. *Journal of Phonetics* 13, 287–298.

Ellis, A. J. (1869–89) *On Early English Pronunciation* (5 parts). London: Asher & Co. and Trüber & Co.

Esling, John H. (1978) *Voice Quality in Edinburgh: A Sociolinguistic and Phonetic Study*. Doctoral dissertation, University of Edinburgh.

    (1984) Laryngographic study of phonation type and laryngeal configuration. *Journal of the International Phonetic Association* 14, 56–73.

    (1991) Sociophonetic variation in Vancouver. In Jenny Cheshire (ed.), *English Around the World: Sociolinguistic Perspectives*. Cambridge: Cambridge University Press, 123–133.

    (1996) Pharyngeal consonants and the aryepiglottic sphincter. *Journal of the International Phonetic Association* 26, 65–88.

    (1999) The IPA categories 'pharyngeal' and 'epiglottal': Laryngoscopic observations of pharyngeal articulations and larynx height. *Language and Speech* 42, 349–372.

    (2000) Crosslinguistic aspects of voice quality. In Kent and Ball (eds.), 25–35.

    (2005) There are no back vowels: The Laryngeal Articulator Model. *Canadian Journal of Linguistics* 50, 13–44.

    (2010) Phonetic notation. In Hardcastle, Laver, and Gibbon (eds.), 678–702.

    (2012) The articulatory function of the larynx and the origins of speech. *Annual Meeting of the Berkeley Linguistics Society* 38, University of California, Berkeley, 121–149 (via LSA eLanguage).

Esling, John H. and Jerold A. Edmondson (2002) The laryngeal sphincter as an articulator: Tenseness, tongue root and phonation in Yi and Bai. In Angelika Braun and Herbert R. Masthoff (eds.), *Phonetics and Its Applications: Festschrift for Jens-Peter Köster on the Occasion of his 60th Birthday*. Stuttgart: Franz Steiner Verlag, 38–51.

    (2011) Acoustical analysis of voice quality for sociophonetic purposes. In Marianna Di Paolo and Malcah Yaeger-Dror (eds.), *Sociophonetics: A Student's Guide*. London: Routledge, 131–148.

Esling, John H. and Jimmy G. Harris (2003) An expanded taxonomy of states of the glottis. In Solé et al. (eds.), 1049–1052.

    (2005) States of the glottis: An articulatory phonetic model based on laryngoscopic observations. In Hardcastle and Mackenzie Beck (eds.), 347–383.

Esling, John H. and Scott R. Moisik (2012) Laryngeal aperture in relation to larynx height change: An analysis using simultaneous laryngoscopy and laryngeal ultrasound. In Dafydd Gibbon, Daniel Hirst, and Nick Campbell (eds.), *Rhythm, Melody and Harmony in Speech: Studies in Honour of Wiktor Jassem* (vol. 14/15). Poznań: Polskie Towarzystwo Fonetyczne, 117–127.

Esling, John H. and Rita F. Wong (1983) Voice quality settings and the teaching of pronunciation. *TESOL Quarterly* 17, 89–95. Reprinted in Adam Brown (ed.) *Teaching English Pronunciation*. London: Routledge, Chapman and Hall, 288–295.

Esling, John H., Bernard Harmegnies, and Véronique Delplancq (1991) Social distribution of long-term average spectral characteristics in Vancouver English. *Actes du XIIème Congrès International des Sciences Phonétiques*, vol. 2. Aix-en-Provence: Université de Provence, 182–185.

Esling, John H., Lynn M. Heap, Roy C. Snell, and B. Craig Dickson (1994) Analysis of pitch-dependence of pharyngeal, faucal, and larynx-height voice quality settings. In *ICSLP 94*. Yokohama: Acoustical Society of Japan, 1475–1478.

Esling, John H., Allison Benner, Lisa Bettany, and Chakir Zeroual (2004) Le contrôle articulatoire phonétique dans le prébabillage. In Bel and Marlien (eds.), 205–208.

Esling, John H., Katherine E. Fraser, and Jimmy G. Harris (2005) Glottal stop, glottalized resonants, and pharyngeals: A reinterpretation with evidence from a laryngoscopic study of Nuuchahnulth (Nootka). *Journal of Phonetics* 33, 383–410.

Esling, John H., Chakir Zeroual, and Lise Crevier-Buchman (2007) A study of muscular synergies at the glottal, ventricular and aryepiglottic levels. In Trouvain and Barry (eds.), vol. 1, 585–588.

Esling, John H., Scott R. Moisik, and Christopher Coey (2015) *iPA Phonetics*: Multimodal iOS application for phonetics instruction and practice. In Scottish Consortium (ed.), paper 263.

Esling, John H., Scott R. Moisik, and Lise Crevier-Buchman (2016) Putting the larynx in the vowel space: Studying larynx state across vowel quality using MRI. Paper presented at BAAP 2016, Lancaster.

Ewan, William G. (1979) Laryngeal behavior in speech. *Report of the Phonology Laboratory* 3, Berkeley: University of California.

Ewan, William G. and Robert Krones (1974) Measuring larynx movement using the thyroumbrometer. *Journal of Phonetics* 2, 327–335.

Fairbanks, Grant (1960) *Voice and Articulation Drill-book* (2nd edn). New York: Harper & Row.

Fels, S. Sidney, Florian Vogt, Bryan Gick, Carol Jaeger, and Ian Wilson (2003) User-centered design for an open source 3D articulatory synthesizer. In Solé et al. (eds.), 179–183.

Fink, B. Raymond (1974a) Folding mechanism of the human larynx. *Acta Oto-Laryngologica* 78(1–6), 124–128.

(1974b) Spring mechanisms in the human larynx. *Acta Oto-Laryngologica* 77(1–6), 295–304.

(1975) *The Human Larynx: A Functional Study*. New York: Raven Press.

Fischer-Jørgensen, Eli (1989) Phonetic analysis of the stød in standard Danish. *Phonetica* 46, 1–59.

Fitch, W. Tecumseh and Jay Giedd (1999) Morphology and development of the human vocal tract: A study using magnetic resonance imaging. *Journal of the Acoustical Society of America* 106(3), 1511–1522.

Fitch, W. Tecumseh and David Reby (2001) The descended larynx is not uniquely human. *Proceedings of the Royal Society of London* 268, 1669–1675.

Fitch, W. Tecumseh, Bart de Boer, Neil Mathur, Asif A. Ghazanfar (2016) Monkey vocal tracts are speech-ready. *Science Advances* 2: e1600723.

Ford, Charles N. and Diane M. Bless (eds.) (1991) *Phonosurgery: Assessment and Surgical Management of Voice Disorders*. New York: Raven Press.

Foulkes, Paul and Peter French (2012) Forensic speaker comparison: A linguistic–acoustic perspective. In Lawrence M. Solan and Peter M. Tiersma (eds.), *The Oxford Handbook of Language and Law*. Oxford: Oxford University Press, 557–572.

Fourcin, Adrian J. (1974) Laryngographic examination of vocal fold vibration. In Barry Wyke (ed.), *Ventilatory and Phonatory Control Systems*. London: Oxford University Press, 315–333.

(2003) Phonetics and measurements of voice quality. Abstract, In *VOQUAL'03*, 11, ISCA.

Fried, M. P., J. H. Kelly, and M. Strome (1982) Comparison of the adult and infant larynx. *The Journal of Family Practice* 15, 557–561.

Fujimura, Osamu (1981) Body-cover theory of the vocal fold and its phonetic implications. In Stevens and Hirano (eds.), 271–281.

Fujimura, Osamu and Minoru Hirano (eds.) (1995) *Vocal Fold Physiology: Voice Quality Control*. San Diego: Singular Publishing.

Fujimura, Osamu and Masayuki Sawashima (1971) Consonant sequences and laryngeal control. *Annual Bulletin, Research Institute of Logopedics and Phoniatrics, University of Tokyo* 5, 1–6.

Fuks, Leonardo (1999) *From Air to Music: Acoustical, Physiological and Perceptual Aspects of Reed Wind Instrumental Playing and Vocal-ventricular Fold Phonation*. Doctoral dissertation, KTH, Stockholm.

Fuks, Leonardo, Britta Hammarberg, and Johan Sundberg (1998) A self-sustained vocal-ventricular phonation mode: Acoustical, aerodynamic and glottographic evidences. *KTH TMH-QPSR* 3/1998, Stockholm, 49–59.

Gao Man (2002) *Tones in Whispered Chinese: Articulatory Features and Perceptual Cues*. Master's thesis, University of Victoria.

Gaprindashvili, Sh. G. (1966) *Fonetika Darginskogo jazyka*. Tbilisi: Metsniereba.

García, Manuel (1855) Observations on the human voice. *Proceedings of the Royal Society (London)* 7: 399–420.

Garellek, Marc (2012) The timing and sequencing of coarticulated non-modal phonation in English and White Hmong. *Journal of Phonetics* 40, 152–161.

(2013) *Production and Perception of Glottal Stops*. Doctoral dissertation, UCLA.

(2015) Perception of glottalization and phrase-final creak. *Journal of the Acoustical Society of America* 137, 822–831.

Gauffin, Jan (1977) Mechanisms of larynx tube constriction. *Phonetica* 34, 307–309.

Gauffin, Jan and Johan Sundberg (1978) Pharyngeal constrictions. *Phonetica* 35, 157–168.

Gerratt, Bruce R. and Jody Kreiman (2001) Toward a taxonomy of nonmodal phonation. *Journal of Phonetics* 29, 365–381.

Ghazeli, Salem (1977) *Back Consonants and Backing Coarticulation in Arabic*. Doctoral dissertation, University of Texas at Austin.

Gick, Bryan (2016) Ecologizing dimensionality: Prospects for a modular theory of speech production. *Ecological Psychology* 28, 176–181.

Gick, Bryan and Ian Stavness (2013) Modularizing speech. *Frontiers in Psychology*, doi.org/10.3389/fpsyg.2013.00977.

Gick, Bryan and Ian Wilson (2006) Excrescent schwa and vowel laxing: Cross-linguistic responses to conflicting articulatory targets. In Louis Goldstein, Doug H. Whalen, and Catherine T. Best (eds.), *Papers in Laboratory Phonology VIII: Varieties of Phonological Competence*, vol. 8. Berlin: Mouton de Gruyter, 635–659.

Gick, Bryan, Ian Wilson, Karsten Koch, and Clare Cook (2004) Language-specific articulatory settings: Evidence from inter-utterance rest position. *Phonetica* 61, 220–233.

Gick, Bryan, Ian Wilson, and Donald Derrick (2013) *Articulatory Phonetics*. Oxford: Wiley-Blackwell.

Gick, Bryan, Blake Allen, François Roewer-Després, and Ian Stavness (2017) Speaking tongues are actively braced. *Journal of Speech, Language, and Hearing Research* 60, 494–506.

Giovanni, Antoine, Maurice Ouaknine, Bruno Guelfucci, Ping Yu, Michel Zanaret, and Jean-Michel Triglia (1999) Nonlinear behavior of vocal fold vibration: The role of coupling between the vocal folds. *Journal of Voice* 13, 465–476.

Giovanni, Antoine, A. Lagier, and M. Remacle (2010) Fonochirurgia dei tumori benigni delle corde vocali. *EMC – Tecniche Chirurgiche – Chirurgia ORL e Cervico-Facciale* 14, 1–14.

Gobl, Christer and Ailbhe Ní Chasaide (2000) Testing affective correlates of voice quality through analysis and resynthesis. In *ISCA Tutorial and Research Workshop (ITRW) on Speech and Emotion, 2000*.

(2003) The role of voice quality in communicating emotion, mood and attitude. *Speech Communication* 40, 189–212.

Gordon, Matthew and Peter Ladefoged (2001) Phonation types: A cross-linguistic overview. *Journal of Phonetics* 29, 383–406.

Gorphe, Philippe, Dana M. Hartl, Adi Primov-Fever, Stéphane Hans, Lise Crevier-Buchman, and Daniel Brasnu (2013) Endoscopic laser medial arytenoidectomy for treatment of bilateral vocal fold paralysis. *European Archives of Oto-Rhino-Laryngology* 270, 1701–1705.

Gregerson, Kenneth J. (1976) Tongue root and register in Mon-Khmer. *Oceanic Linguistics Special Publications* 13, 323–369.

Grégoire, Antoine (1937) *L'apprentissage du langage: les deux premières années*. Paris: Félix Alcan.

Grenon, Izabelle, Allison Benner, and John H. Esling (2007) Language-specific phonetic production patterns in the first year of life. In Trouvain and Barry (eds.), vol. 3, 1561–1564.

Grønnum, Nina (1998) Danish. *Journal of the International Phonetic Association* 28, 99–105.

Grønnum, Nina, Miguel Vazquez-Larruscaín, and Hans Basbøll (2013) Danish stød: Laryngealization or tone. *Phonetica* 70, 66–92.

Guion, Susan G., Mark W. Post, and Doris L. Payne (2004) Phonetic correlates of tongue root vowel contrasts in Maa. *Journal of Phonetics* 32, 517–542.

Gutzmann, Hermann (1893) *Vorlesungen über die Störungen der Sprache und ihre Heilung: gehalten in den Lehrcursen über Sprachstörungen für Aerzte und Lehrer*. Berlin: Kornfeld.

(1909) Stimme und Sprache ohne Kehlkopf. *Zeitschrift für Laryngologie, Rhinologie und ihre Grenzgebiete* 1, 221–242.

Hall, Beatrice L. and R. M. R. Hall (1980) Nez Perce vowel harmony: An Africanist explanation and some theoretical questions. In Robert M. Vago (ed.), *Issues in Vowel Harmony*. Amsterdam: John Benjamins, 201–236.

Halle, Morris (1995) Feature geometry and feature spreading. *Linguistic Inquiry* 26, 1–46.

Halle, Morris and Kenneth N. Stevens (1969) On the feature 'Advanced Tongue Root'. *MIT Research Laboratory of Electronics Quarterly Progress Report* 94, 209–215. (1971) A note on laryngeal features. *MIT Research Laboratory of Electronics Quarterly Progress Report* 101, 198–212.

Halle, Morris, Bert Vaux, and Andrew Wolfe (2000) On feature spreading and the representation of place of articulation. *Linguistic Inquiry* 31, 387–444.

Hallé, Pierre A., Bénédicte de Boysson-Bardies, and Marilyn M. Vihman (1991) Beginnings of prosodic organization: Intonation and duration patterns of disyllables produced by Japanese and French infants. *Language and Speech* 34, 299–318.

Hans, Stéphane, Jacqueline Vaissière, Lise Crevier-Buchman, Ollivier Laccourreye, and Daniel Brasnu (2000) Aerodynamic and acoustic parameters in CO_2 laser posterior transverse cordotomy for bilateral vocal fold paralysis. *Acta Oto-Laryngology* 120, 330–335.

Hansen, Gert Foget (2015) *Stød og stemmekvalitet: En akustisk-fonetisk undersøgelse af ændringer i stemmekvaliteten i forbindelse med stød*. Doctoral dissertation, Københavns Universitet, Det Humanistiske Fakultet.

Hardcastle, William J. (1976) *Physiology of Speech Production: An Introduction for Speech Scientists*. London: Academic Press.

Hardcastle, William J. and Janet Mackenzie Beck (eds.) (2005) *A Figure of Speech: A Festschrift for John Laver*. Mahwah, NJ: Lawrence Erlbaum Associates.

Hardcastle, William J., John Laver, and Fiona E. Gibbon (eds.) (2010) *Handbook of Phonetic Sciences* (2nd edn). Oxford: Wiley-Blackwell.

Harmegnies, Bernard (1987) *Contribution à la Caractérisation de la Qualité Vocale: Analyses Plurielles de Spectres Moyens à Long Terme de Parole*. Doctoral dissertation, Université de l'Etat à Mons.

Harmegnies, Bernard, John H. Esling, and Véronique Delplancq (1989) Quantitative study of the effects of setting changes on the LTAS. In J. P. Tubach and J. J. Mariani (eds.), *European Conference on Speech Communication and Technology*, vol. 2. Edinburgh: CEP Consultants, 139–142.

Harmegnies, Bernard, Véronique Delplancq, John H. Esling, and Marielle Bruyninckx (1994) Effets sur le signal vocal de changements délibérés de qualité globale en anglais et français. *Revue de Phonétique Appliquée* 111, 139–153.

Harrington, Jonathan (2012) The coarticulatory basis of diachronic high back vowel fronting. In Solé and Recasens (eds.), 103–122.

Harrington, Jonathan, Felicity Cox, and Zoe Evans (1997) An acoustic phonetic study of broad, general and cultivated Australian English vowels. *Australian Journal of Linguistics* 17, 155–184.

Harris, Jimmy G. (1987) *Linguistic Phonetic Notes (1969–1979)*. Bangkok: Craftsman Press.

(1999) States of the glottis for voiceless plosives. In Ohala et al. (eds.), 2041–2044.

Harris, Katherine S., Eric Vatikiotis-Bateson, and Peter J. Alfonso (1992) Muscle forces in vowel vocal tract formation. In John J. Ohala, Terrance M. Nearey, Bruce L. Derwing, Megan M. Hodge, and Grace E. Wiebe (eds.), *ICSLP 92 Proceedings.* Edmonton: University of Alberta, 879–881.

Hartl, Dana M., Ollivier Laccourreye, Jacqueline Vaissière, and Daniel Brasnu (2003) Acoustic analysis of autologous fat injection versus thyroplasty in the same patient. *Annals of Otology, Rhinology & Laryngology* 112, 987–992.

Hartl, Dana M., Lise Crevier-Buchman, Jacqueline Vaissière, and Daniel Brasnu (2005) Phonetic effects of paralytic dysphonia. *Annals of Otology, Rhinology & Laryngology* 114, 792–798.

(2009) Long-term acoustic comparison of thyroplasty versus autologous fat injection. *Annals of Otology, Rhinology & Laryngology* 118, 827–832.

Hassan, Zeki Majeed, John H. Esling, Scott R. Moisik, and Lise Crevier-Buchman (2011) Aryepiglottic trilled variants of /ʕ, ħ/ in Iraqi Arabic. In Lee and Zee (eds.), 831–4.

Haudricourt, André-Georges (1946) Les mutations consonantiques des occlusives initiales en mon-khmer. *Bulletin de la Société de Linguistique de Paris* 43, 82–92.

Hayward, Katrina and Richard J. Hayward (1989) 'Guttural': Arguments for a new distinctive feature. *Transactions of the Philological Society* 87, 179–193.

Heffner, Roe-Merrill S. (1950) *General Phonetics.* Madison: University of Wisconsin Press.

Hejná, Michaela (2015) *Pre-Aspiration in Welsh English: A Case Study of Aberystwyth.* Doctoral dissertation, University of Manchester.

Hejná, Michaela, Pertti Palo, and Scott R. Moisik (2016) Glottal squeaks in VC sequences. *Interspeech 2016*, San Francisco, 1136–1140.

Henderson, Eugénie J. A. (1971) *The Indispensable Foundation: A Selection from the Writings of Henry Sweet.* London: Oxford University Press.

Henrich, Nathalie (2006) Mirroring the voice from Garcia to the present day: Some insights into singing voice registers. *Logopedics Phoniatrics Vocology* 31, 3–14.

Herzallah, Rukayyah S. (1990) *Aspects of Palestinian Arabic Phonology: A Non-Linear Approach.* Doctoral dissertation, Cornell University.

Herzel, Hanspeter, David Berry, Ingo R. Titze, and Marwa Saleh (1994) Analysis of vocal disorders with methods from nonlinear dynamics. *Journal of Speech, Language, and Hearing Research* 37, 1008–1019.

Heselwood, Barry (2007) The 'tight approximant' variant of the Arabic *'ayn. Journal of the International Phonetic Association* 37, 1–32.

Heselwood, Barry and Reem Maghrabi (2016) Variation in realizations of /r/ in Saudi Arabian Arabic. Paper presented at *BAAP 2016*, Lancaster.

Hess, Susan A. (1998) *Pharyngeal Articulations.* Doctoral dissertation, UCLA.

Heyne, Matthias and Donald Derrick (2015) The influence of tongue position on trombone sound: A likely area of language influence. In Scottish Consortium (ed.), paper 547.

Hillel, Allen D. (2001) The study of laryngeal muscle activity in normal human subjects and in patients with laryngeal dystonia using multiple fine-wire electromyography. *Laryngoscope* 111, 1–47.

Hillenbrand, James M. and Robert A. Houde (1996) Role of F_0 and amplitude in the perception of intervocalic glottal stops. *Journal of Speech, Language, and Hearing Research* 39, 1182–1190.

Hirano, Minoru (1974) Morphological structure of the vocal cord as a vibrator and its variations. *Folia Phoniatrica* 26, 89–94.

(1975) Phonosurgery: Basic and clinical investigations. *Otologia (Fukuoka)* 21, 239–440.

(1977) Structure and vibratory behavior of the vocal folds. In Masayuki Sawashima and Franklin S. Cooper (eds.), *Dynamic Aspects of Speech Production*. Tokyo: University of Tokyo Press, 13–27.

Hirano, Minoru and Yuki Kakita (1985) *Cover-body theory of vocal fold vibration*. In Raymond G. Daniloff (ed.), *Speech Science: Recent Advances*. San Diego: College-Hill Press, 1–46.

Hirano, Minoru and John Ohala (1969) Use of hooked-wire electrodes for electromyography of the intrinsic laryngeal muscles. *Journal of Speech and Hearing Research* 12, 362–373.

Hirano, Minoru, Shigejiro Kurita, and Tadashi Nakashima (1981) The structure of the vocal folds. In Stevens and Hirano (eds.), 33–41.

Hirano, Minoru, Kensuke Kiyokawa, and Shigejiro Kurita (1988) Laryngeal muscles and glottic shaping. In Osamu Fujimura (ed.), *Vocal Physiology: Voice Production, Mechanisms and Functions*. New York: Raven Press, 49–65.

Hirose, Hajime (1995) Imaging the larynx: Past and present. In Bell-Berti and Raphael (eds.), 247–257.

(1996) Voicing distinction in esophageal speech. *Acta Oto-Laryngologica Suppl.* 524, 56–63.

(2010) Investigating the physiology of laryngeal structures. In Hardcastle, Laver, and Gibbon (eds.), 130–152.

Hockett, Charles F. (1958) *A Course in Modern Linguistics*. New York: The Macmillan Company.

Holder, William (1669) *Elements of Speech*. London: T. N. for F. Martyn Printer.

Hollien, Harry (1972) Three major vocal registers: A proposal. In Rigault and Charbonneau (eds.), 320–331.

(1974) On vocal registers. *Journal of Phonetics* 2, 125–143.

Hollien, Harry and John F. Michel (1968) Vocal fry as a phonational register. *Journal of Speech and Hearing Research* 11, 600–604.

Hollien, Harry, Paul Moore, Ronald W. Wendahl, and John F. Michel (1966) On the nature of vocal fry. *Journal of Speech and Hearing Research* 9, 245–247.

Honda, Kiyoshi (1996) Organization of tongue articulation for vowels. *Journal of Phonetics* 24, 39–52.

(2004) Physiological factors causing tonal characteristics of speech: From global to local prosody. Paper presented at *Speech Prosody*, Nara, Japan.

Honda, Kiyoshi, Hiroyuki Hirai, Jo Estill, and Yoh'ichi Tohkura (1995a) Contributions of vocal tract shape to voice quality: MRI data and articulatory modeling. In Fujimura and Hirano (eds.), 23–38.

Honda, Kiyoshi, Tomoyoshi Kurita, Yuki Kakita, and Shinji Maeda (1995b) Physiology of the lips and modeling of lip gestures. *Journal of Phonetics* 23, 243–254.

Honda, Kiyoshi, Hiroyuki Hirai, Shinobu Masaki, and Yasuhiro Shimada (1999) Role of vertical larynx movement and cervical lordosis in F_0 control. *Language and Speech* 42, 401–411.

Honda, Kiyoshi, T. Kitamura, H. Takemoto, S. Adachi, P. Mokhtari, S. Takano, et al. (2010) Visualisation of hypopharyngeal cavities and vocal-tract acoustic modelling. *Computer Methods in Biomechanics and Biomedical Engineering* 13, 443–453.

Honikman, Beatrice (1964) Articulatory settings. In David Abercrombie, Dennis B. Fry, P. A. D. McCarthy, N. C. Scott, and J. L. M. Trim (eds.), *In Honour of Daniel Jones*. London: Longmans, 73–84.

Honjow, Iwao and Nobuhiko Isshiki (1971) Pharyngeal stop in cleft palate speech. *Folia Phoniatrica* 23, 347–354.

Hsu, Hui-Chin, Alan Fogel, and Rebecca Cooper (2000) Infant vocal development in the first 6 months: Speech quality and melodic complexity. *Infant and Child Development* 9, 1–16.

Huffman, Franklin E. (1976) The register problem in fifteen Mon-Khmer languages. *Oceanic Linguistics Special Publications* 13, *Austroasiatic Studies Part I*, 575–589.

Ikekeonwu, Clara I. (1999) Igbo. In IPA (1999), 108–110.

Infante Ríos, Patricia and Carolina Pérez Sanz (2011) Creak and creaky voice: Similar sounds, different meanings. Poster presented at Phonetics and Phonology in Iberia 2011, Tarragona.

IPA (1989) *Chart of the International Phonetic Alphabet.*

(1999) *Handbook of the International Phonetic Association: A Guide to the Use of the International Phonetic Alphabet.* Cambridge: Cambridge University Press.

(2005) *Chart of the International Phonetic Alphabet.*

Iwata, Ray, Masayuki Sawashima, Hajime Hirose, and Seiji Niimi (1979) Laryngeal adjustments of Fukienese stops. *Ann. Bull. RILP* 13, 61–81.

Jacobsen, William H. Jr. (1969) Origin of the Nootka pharyngeals. *International Journal of American Linguistics* 35, 125–153.

Jacobson, Leon C. (1980) Voice-quality harmony in Western Nilotic languages. In Robert M. Vago (ed.), *Issues in Vowel Harmony*. Amsterdam: John Benjamins, 183–200.

Jakobson, Roman (1941/1968) *Child Language, Aphasia and Phonological Universals.* The Hague: Mouton.

Jones, Daniel (1956) *An Outline of English Phonetics* (8th edn). Cambridge: W. Heffer & Sons.

Jones, Stephen (1934) Somali [ħ] and [ʕ]. *Le maître phonétique* 49, 8–9.

Kahane, Joel C. (1986) *Anatomy and Physiology of the Speech Mechanism*. Austin: Pro-Ed.

Kawahara, Hideki, Alain de Cheveigné, and Roy D. Patterson (1998) An instantaneous-frequency-based pitch extraction method for high quality speech transformation: Revised TEMPO in the STRAIGHT-suite. In *Proceedings ICSLP'98*, Sydney.

Kedrova, Galina E. and Constantine Leo Borissoff (2013) The concept of 'basis of articulation' in Russia in the first half of the 20th century. *Historiographia Linguistica* 40, 151–197.

Kent, Raymond D. (1981) Articulatory-acoustic perspectives on speech development in language behavior in infancy and early childhood. In Rachel E. Stark (ed.),

Language Behavior in Infancy and Early Childhood. New York: Elsevier North Holland, 105–126.

Kent, Raymond D. and Martin J. Ball (eds.) (2000) *Voice Quality Measurement.* San Diego: Singular Publishing.

Kent, Raymond D. and Houri K. Vorperian (1995) Development of the craniofacial-oral-laryngeal anatomy: A review. *Journal of Medical Speech-Language Pathology* 3, 145–190.

Keyser, Samuel Jay and Kenneth N. Stevens (1994) Feature geometry and the vocal tract. *Phonology* 11, 207–236.

Khan, Sameer ud Dowla and Constanze Weise (2013) Upper Saxon (Chemnitz dialect). *Journal of the International Phonetic Association* 43, 231–241.

Kimura, Miwako, Ken-Ichi Sakakibara, Hiroshi Imagawa, Roger Chan, Seiji Niimi, and Niro Tayama (2002) Histological investigation of the supra-glottal structures in humans for understanding abnormal phonation. *Journal of the Acoustical Society of America* 112(5), https://doi.org/10.1121/1.4780065.

Kingston, John (2005) The phonetics of Athabaskan tonogenesis. In Sharon Hargus and Keren Rice (eds.), *Athabaskan Prosody.* Amsterdam: John Benjamins, 137–184.

Kirby, James P. (2011) Vietnamese (Hanoi Vietnamese). *Journal of the International Phonetic Association* 41, 381–392.

Knowles, Gerald O. (1974) *Scouse: The Urban Dialect of Liverpool.* Doctoral dissertation, University of Leeds.

Kodzasov, Sandro V. (1987) Pharyngeal features in the Daghestan languages. In *Proceedings of the XIth International Congress of Phonetic Sciences*, vol. 2. Tallinn: Academy of Sciences of the Estonian SSR, 142–144.

Koike, Minako, Noriko Kobayashi, Hajime Hirose, and Yuki Hara (2002) Speech rehabilitation after total laryngectomy. *Acta Otolaryngologica Suppl.* 547, 107–112.

Koopmans-van Beinum, Florien J. and Jeannette M. van der Stelt (1986) Early stages in the development of speech movements. In Björn Lindblom and Rolf Zetterström (eds.), *Precursors of Early Speech.* Basingstoke: Macmillan, 279–308.

Koufman, James A. and P. David Blalock (1991) Functional voice disorders. *Otolaryngologic Clinics of North America* 24, 1059–1073.

Kreiman, Jody and Bruce Gerratt (2000) Measuring voice quality. In Kent and Ball (eds.), 73–101.

Kreiman, Jody and Diana Sidtis (2011) *Foundations of Voice Studies: An Interdisciplinary Approach to Voice Production and Perception.* Oxford: Wiley-Blackwell.

Kröger, Bernd J., Phil Hoole, Robert Sader, Christian Geng, Bernd Pompino-Marschall, and Christiane Neuschaefer-Rube (2004) MRT-Sequenzen als Datenbasis eines visuellen Artikulationsmodells. *HNO* 52, 837–843.

Labov, William (1963) The social motivation of a sound change. *Word* 19, 273–309.

(1972) *Sociolinguistic Patterns.* Philadelphia: University of Pennsylvania Press.

(1994) *Principles of Linguistic Change: Internal Factors*, vol. 1. Oxford: Blackwell.

(2001) *Principles of Linguistic Change: Social Factors*, vol. 2. Oxford: Blackwell.

Labov, William and Ronald Kim (2015) Peripherality as an organizing principle of West Germanic phonology. Paper presented at Oxford University, 1 Dec 2015.

Laccourreye, Henri, Jean Lacau St. Guily, Alain Fabre, Daniel Brasnu, and Madeleine Menard (1987) Supracricoid hemilaryngopharyngectomy: Analysis of 240 cases. *Annals of Otology, Rhinology & Laryngology* 96, 217–221.

Laccourreye, Henri, Ollivier Laccourreye, Madeleine Menard, Gregory Weinstein, and Daniel Brasnu (1990) Supracricoid laryngectomy with cricohyoidoepiglottopexy: A partial laryngeal procedure for glottic carcinoma. *Annals of Otology, Rhinology & Laryngology* 99, 421–426.

Laccourreye, Ollivier, Lise Crevier-Buchman, Véronique Jouffre, Henri Laccourreye, Daniel Brasnu, and Gregory Weinstein (1995a) Acoustic parameters and speech analysis after supracricoid hemilaryngopharyngectomy. *Laryngoscope* 105, 1223–1226.

Laccourreye, Ollivier, Lise Crevier-Buchman, Gregory Weinstein, Bernard Biacabe, Henri Laccourreye, and Daniel Brasnu (1995b) Duration and frequency characteristics of speech and voice following supracricoid partial laryngectomy. *Annals of Otology, Rhinology & Laryngology* 104, 516–521.

Laccourreye, Ollivier, Lise Crevier-Buchman, F. Bou-Malhab, Stéphane Hans, Bernard Biacabe, and Daniel Brasnu (1998a) Injection intra-cordale de graisse autologue et paralysie récurrentielle unilatérale. *Ann. Otolaryngol. Chir. Cervicofac.* 115, 264–270.

Laccourreye, Ollivier, Lise Crevier-Buchman, Françoise Le Pimpec-Barthes, Dominique Garcia, Marc Riquet, and Daniel Brasnu (1998b) Recovery of function after intracordal autologous fat injection for unilateral recurrent laryngeal nerve paralysis. *Journal of Laryngology & Otology* 112, 1082–1084.

Laccourreye, Ollivier, Natacha Bély, Lise Crevier-Buchman, Stéphane Hans, Daniel Brasnu, and Philippe Halimi (1999) Computerized tomography of the glottis after intracordal autologous fat injection. *Journal of Laryngology & Otology* 112, 971–972.

Laccourreye, Ollivier, Jean-François Papon, Madeleine Menard, Lise Crevier-Buchman, Daniel Brasnu, and Stéphane Hans (2001) Treatment of recurrent unilateral paralysis with thyroplasty with Montgomery implant. *Annales de Chirurgie* 126, 768–771.

Laccourreye, Ollivier, Jean-François Papon, Romain Kania, Lise Crevier-Buchman, Daniel Brasnu, and Stéphane Hans (2003) Intracordal injection of autologous fat in patients with unilateral laryngeal nerve paralysis: Long-term results from the patient's perspective. *Laryngoscope* 113, 541–545.

Ladefoged, Peter (1964) *A Phonetic Study of West African Languages: An Auditory-Instrumental Survey.* Cambridge: Cambridge University Press.

(1975) *A Course in Phonetics.* New York: Harcourt Brace Jovanovich (2nd edn 1982).

Ladefoged, Peter and Ian Maddieson (1996) *The Sounds of the World's Languages.* Oxford: Blackwell.

Ladefoged, Peter, Joseph DeClerk, Mona Lindau, and George Papçun (1972) An auditory-motor theory of speech production. *Working Papers in Phonetics (UCLA)* 22, 48–75.

Laitman, Jeffrey T. and Raymond C. Heimbuch (1982) The basicranium of Plio-Pleistocene hominids as an indicator of their upper respiratory systems. *American Journal of Physical Anthropology* 59, 323–344.

Laitman, Jeffrey T. and Joy S. Reidenberg (2009) Evolution of the human larynx: Nature's great experiment. In Marvin P. Fried and Alfio Ferlito (eds.), *The Larynx*, vol. 1. San Diego: Plural Publishing, 19–38.

Lama, Ziwo 拉玛兹偓 (1991) 试论彝语次高调产生的原因 [A preliminary study on the origin of Yi second-high-level-tone]. 民族语文 *[Minzu Yuwen]* 5, 35–38.

(2012) *Subgrouping of Nisoic (Yi) Languages: A Study from the Perspective of Shared Innovation and Phylogenetic Estimation*. Doctoral dissertation, University of Texas at Arlington.

Lammert, Adam, Michael I. Proctor, and Shrikanth S. Narayanan (2010) Data-driven analysis of real-time vocal tract MRI using correlated image regions. In *Proceedings of Interspeech*. Makuhari, Chiba, Japan, 1572–1575.

Laradi, W. J. (1983) *Pharyngealisation in Libyan (Tripoli) Arabic*. Doctoral dissertation, University of Edinburgh.

Laufer, Asher (1996) The common [ʕ] is an approximant and not a fricative. *Journal of the International Phonetic Association* 26, 113–117.

Laufer, Asher and Thomas Baer (1988) The emphatic and pharyngeal sounds in Hebrew and in Arabic. *Language and Speech* 31, 181–205.

Laufer, Asher and Iovanna D. Condax (1979) The epiglottis as an articulator. *Journal of the International Phonetic Association* 9, 50–56.

Laver, John (1968) Voice quality and indexical information. *British Journal of Disorders of Communication* 3, 43–54.

(1974) Labels for voices. *Journal of the International Phonetic Association* 4, 62–75.

(1975) *Individual Features in Voice Quality*. Doctoral dissertation, University of Edinburgh.

(1979) *Voice Quality: A Classified Bibliography*. Amsterdam: John Benjamins.

(1980) *The Phonetic Description of Voice Quality*. Cambridge: Cambridge University Press.

(1991) *The Gift of Speech: Papers in the Analysis of Speech and Voice*. Edinburgh: Edinburgh University Press.

(1994) *Principles of Phonetics*. Cambridge: Cambridge University Press.

Laver, John and Janet Mackenzie Beck (2007) *Vocal Profile Analysis Scheme – VPAS*. Queen Margaret University College – QMUC, Speech Science Research Centre, Edinburgh.

Laver, John and Peter Trudgill (1979) Phonetic and linguistic markers in speech. In Klaus R. Scherer and Howard Giles (eds.), *Social Markers in Speech*. Cambridge: Cambridge University Press, 1–32.

Laver, John, Sheila Wirz, Janet Mackenzie, and Steven M. Hiller (1991) A perceptual protocol for the analysis of vocal profiles. In Laver, 265–280.

Laver, John, Steven M. Hiller, and Janet Mackenzie Beck (1992) Acoustic waveform perturbations and voice disorders. *Journal of Voice* 6, 115–126.

Lawson, Eleanor, James M. Scobbie, and Jane Stuart-Smith (2015) The role of anterior lingual gesture delay in coda /r/ lenition: An ultrasound tongue imaging study. In Scottish Consortium (ed.), paper 332.

Lee, Wai-Sum and Eric Zee (eds.) (2011) *Proceedings of the XVIIth International Congress of Phonetic Sciences*. Hong Kong.

Lennon, Robert, Rachel Smith, and Jane Stuart-Smith (2015) An acoustic investigation of postvocalic /r/ variants in two sociolects of Glaswegian. In Scottish Consortium (ed.), paper 1019.

Lewis, Paul (1968) Akha phonology. *Anthropological Linguistics* 10, 8–18.

Li, Charles N. and Sandra A. Thompson (1977) The acquisition of tone in Mandarin-speaking children. *Journal of Child Language* 4, 185–199.

Lieberman, Daniel E., Robert C. McCarthy, Karen M. Hiiemae, and Jeffrey B. Palmer (2001) Ontogeny of postnatal hyoid and larynx descent in humans. *Archives of Oral Biology* 46, 117–128.

Lieberman, Philip (1984) *The Biology and Evolution of Language.* Cambridge, MA: Harvard University Press.

Lieberman, Philip and Edmund S. Crelin (1971) On the speech of Neanderthal man. *Linguistic Inquiry* 2, 203–222.

Lindau, Mona (1975) Features for vowels. *UCLA Working Papers in Phonetics* 30, 1–55.

(1978) Vowel features. *Language* 54, 541–563.

(1979) The feature expanded. *Journal of Phonetics* 7, 163–176.

(1985) The story of /r/. In Victoria Fromkin (ed.), *Phonetic Linguistics: Essays in Honor of Peter Ladefoged.* Orlando: Academic Press, 157–168.

Lindblom, Björn (1963) Spectrographic study of vowel reduction. *Journal of the Acoustical Society of America* 35, 1773–1781.

(2009) Laryngeal mechanisms in speech: The contributions of Jan Gauffin. *Logopedics Phoniatrics Vocology* 34, 149–156.

Lindestad, Per-Åke, Maria Södersten, Björn Merker, and Svante Granqvist (2001) Voice source characteristics in Mongolian 'throat singing' studied with high-speed imaging technique, acoustic spectra, and inverse filtering. *Journal of Voice* 15, 78–85.

Lindqvist, Jan (1969) Laryngeal mechanisms in speech. *Speech Transmission Laboratory: Quarterly Progress and Status Reports* 2–3, 26–32.

Lindqvist-Gauffin, Jan (1972) A descriptive model of laryngeal articulation in speech. *Speech Transmission Laboratory: Quarterly Progress and Status Reports* 13, 1–9.

Lloyd, John E., Ian Stavness, and Sidney Fels (2012) ArtiSynth: A fast interactive biomechanical modeling toolkit combining multibody and finite element simulation. In Yohan Payan (ed.), *Soft Tissue Biomechanical Modeling for Computer Assisted Surgery.* Berlin: Springer-Verlag, 355–394.

Lowie, Wander and Sybrine Bultena (2007) Articulatory settings and the dynamics of second language speech production. *Proceedings of the 2007 PTLC Conference.* London: UCL.

Luchsinger, Richard and Godfrey E. Arnold (1965) *Voice – Speech – Language. Clinical Communicology: Its Physiology and Pathology.* London: Constable.

Mackenzie Beck, Janet (1988) *Organic Variation and Voice Quality.* Doctoral dissertation, University of Edinburgh.

(2005) Perceptual analysis of voice quality: The place of Vocal Profile Analysis. In Hardcastle and Mackenzie Beck (eds.), 285–322.

Mackenzie Beck, Janet and Felix Schaeffler (2015) Voice quality variation in Scottish adolescents: Gender versus geography. In Scottish Consortium (ed.), paper 737.

Mackenzie Beck, Janet, John Laver, and Steven M. Hiller (1991) Structural pathologies of the vocal folds and phonation. In Laver, 281–318.

MacNeilage, Peter F. (1998) The Frame/Content Theory of evolution of speech production. *Behavioral and Brain Sciences* 21, 499–511.

(2008) *The Origin of Speech*. Oxford: Oxford University Press.

MacNeilage, Peter F. and Barbara L. Davis (2001) The role of rhythmic cyclicities in infant action development. *Developmental Science* 4, 79–83.

(2005) A cognitive-motor syllable frame for speech production: Evidence from neuropathology. In Hardcastle and Mackenzie Beck (eds.), 129–144.

MacNeilage, Peter F., Barbara L. Davis, Ashlynn Kinney, and Christine L. Matyear (2000) The motor core of speech: A comparison of serial organization patterns in infants and languages. *Child Development* 71, 153–163.

Martínez-Celdrán, Eugenio, Ana Ma. Fernández-Planas, and Josefina Carrera-Sabaté (2003) Castilian Spanish. *Journal of the International Phonetic Association* 33, 255–259.

Mathworks® (2011) File Exchange by user Peter Hammer, August 11, 2011; www.mathworks.com/matlabcentral/fileexchange/32506-marching-cubes.

Matisoff, James A. (1968) *A Grammar of Lahu*. Berkeley: University of California Press.

MATLAB and Statistics Toolbox Release (R2009a) The MathWorks, Inc., Natick, MA.

McCarthy, John J. (1988) Feature geometry and dependency: A review. *Phonetica* 45, 84–108.

(1991) *Semitic gutturals and distinctive feature theory*. Manuscript, University of Massachusetts, Amherst. Retrieved from http://works.bepress.com/cgi/viewcontent.cgi?article=1068&context=john_j_mccarthy.

(1994) The phonetics and phonology of Semitic pharyngeals. In Patricia Keating (ed.), *Papers in Laboratory Phonology III*. Cambridge: Cambridge University Press, 191–233.

McCune, Lorraine, Marilyn M. Vihman, Liselotte Roug-Hellichius, Diane Delery, and Lakshmi Gogate (1996) Grunt communication in human infants (Homo sapiens). *Journal of Comparative Psychology* 110, 27–37.

McGowan, Richard S. (1992) Tongue-tip trills and vocal-tract wall compliance. *Journal of the Acoustical Society of America* 91, 2903.

Mennen, Ineke, James M. Scobbie, Esther de Leeuw, Sonja Schaeffler, and Felix Schaeffler (2010) Measuring language-specific phonetic settings. *Second Language Research* 26, 13–41.

Michel, François, Stéphane Hans, Lise Crevier-Buchman, Daniel Brasnu, Madeleine Menard, and Ollivier Laccourreye (2003) Thyroplastie avec implant de Montgomery sous anesthésie locale dans les paralysies laryngées unilatérales. *Ann. Otolaryngol. Chir. Cervicofac.* 120, 259–267.

Michel, John F. and Harry Hollien (1968) Perceptual differentiation in vocal fry and harshness. *Journal of Speech and Hearing Research* 11, 439–443.

Miller, Amanda L. (2007) Guttural vowels and guttural coarticulation. *Journal of Phonetics* 35, 56–84.

Miller, Amanda L., Johanna Brugman, Bonny Sands, Levi Namaseb, Mats Exter, and Chris Collins (2009) Differences in airstream and posterior place of articulation among N|uu clicks. *Journal of the International Phonetic Association* 39, 129–161.

Miller-Ockhuizen, Amanda (2003) *The Phonetics and Phonology of Gutturals: A Case Study from Juǀ'hoansi* (Outstanding Dissertations in Linguistics). New Haven, CT: Routledge.

Mills, Timothy (2009) *Speech Motor Control Variables in the Production of Voicing Contrasts and Emphatic Accent.* Doctoral dissertation, University of Edinburgh.

Moerman, Mieke, Jean-Pierre Martens, Lise Crevier-Buchman, Virginie Woisard, and Philippe Dejonckere (2005) Evaluation perceptive des voix de substitution: l'échelle I (I) NFVo. *Revue de Laryngologie Otologie Rhinologie* 126, 323–325.

Moisik, Scott R. (2008) *A Three-Dimensional Model of the Larynx and the Laryngeal Constrictor Mechanism: Visually Synthesizing Pharyngeal and Epiglottal Articulations Observed in Laryngoscopy.* Master's thesis, University of Victoria.

(2012) Harsh voice quality and its association with blackness in popular American media. *Phonetica* 69, 193–215.

(2013) *The Epilarynx in Speech.* Doctoral dissertation, University of Victoria.

Moisik, Scott R. and Dan Dediu (2019) Does morphological variation influence click learning and production? Evidence from a phonetic learning and imaging study. In Bonny Sands (ed.), *The Handbook of Clicks.* Leiden: Brill.

Moisik, Scott R. and John H. Esling (2007) 3-D auditory-articulatory modeling of the laryngeal constrictor mechanism. In Trouvain and Barry (eds.), vol. 1, 373–376.

(2011) The 'whole larynx' approach to laryngeal features. In Lee and Zee (eds.), 1406–1409.

(2014) Modeling the biomechanical influence of epilaryngeal stricture on the vocal folds: A low-dimensional model of vocal-ventricular fold coupling. *Journal of Speech, Language, and Hearing Research* 57, S687–S704.

Moisik, Scott R. and Bryan Gick (2017) The quantal larynx: The stable regions of laryngeal biomechanics and implications for speech production. *Journal of Speech, Language, and Hearing Research* 60, 540–560.

Moisik, Scott R. and John H. Esling, and Lise Crevier-Buchman (2010) A high-speed laryngoscopic investigation of aryepiglottic trilling. *Journal of the Acoustical Society of America* 127, 1548–1559.

Moisik, Scott R., Hua Lin, and John H. Esling (2014) A study of laryngeal gestures in Mandarin citation tones using simultaneous laryngoscopy and laryngeal ultrasound (SLLUS). *Journal of the International Phonetic Association* 44, 21–58.

Moisik, Scott R., John H. Esling, Lise Crevier-Buchman, Angélique Amelot, and Philippe Halimi (2015) Multimodal imaging of glottal stop and creaky voice: Evaluating the role of epilaryngeal constriction. In Scottish Consortium (ed.), paper 247.

Moisik, Scott R., Ewa Czaykowska-Higgins, and John H. Esling (2019) Phonological potentials and the lower vocal tract. *Journal of the International Phonetic Association* 49. Published online, 16 April 2019, https://doi.org/10.1017/S0025100318000403.

Monsen, Randall B. and A. Maynard Engebretson (1977) Study of variations in the male and female glottal wave. *Journal of the Acoustical Society of America* 62, 981–993.

Montler, Timothy (1998) The major processes affecting Klallam vowels. In *Papers for the 33rd International Conference on Salish and Neighboring Languages.* Seattle: University of Washington, 366–373.

Moolenaar-Bijl, A. J. (1957) Laryngeal whistle. *Folia Phoniatrica* 9, 164–168.

Morrison, Murray D., Hamish Nichol, and Linda Rammage (2013) *The Management of Voice Disorders*. Boston: Springer US.

Munhall, Kevin, Eric Vatikiotis-Bateson, and Yoh'ichi Tohkura (1995) X-ray film database for speech research. *Journal of the Acoustical Society of America* 98, 1222.

Nair, Angelika, Garyth Nair, and Gernot Reishofer (2016) The low mandible maneuver and its resonential implications for elite singers. *Journal of Voice* 30, 128. e13–128.e32.

Namdaran, Nahal (2006) *Retraction in St'át'imcets: An Ultrasonic Investigation*. Master's thesis, University of British Columbia.

Narayanan, Shrikanth, Erik Bresch, Prasanta Ghosh, Louis Goldstein, Athanasios Katsamanis, Yoon Kim, et al. (2011) A multimodal real-time MRI articulatory corpus for speech research. In *Proceedings of Interspeech*, Florence, Italy, 837–840.

Nathani, Suneeti, D. Kimbrough Oller, and Alan B. Cobo-Lewis (2003) Final syllable lengthening (FSL) in infant vocalizations. *Journal of Child Language* 30, 3–25.

Nathani, Suneeti, David J. Ertmer, and Rachel E. Stark (2006) Assessing vocal development in infants and toddlers. *Clinical Linguistics and Phonetics* 20, 351–369.

Nearey, Terrance M. (1978) *Phonetic Feature Systems for Vowels*. Bloomington: Indiana University Linguistics Club. IU Ling club reprint 78 thesis.

Negus, Victor E. (1949) *The Comparative Anatomy and Physiology of the Larynx*. London: William Heinemann Medical Books Ltd (reprinted 1962).

Ng, Manwa L., Yang Chen, and Ellen Y. K. Chan (2012) Differences in vocal characteristics between Cantonese and English produced by proficient Cantonese-English bilingual speakers: A long-term average spectral analysis. *Journal of Voice* 26, e171–e176.

Nishimura, Takeshi, Akichika Mikami, Juri Suzuki, and Tetsuro Matsuzawa (2006) Descent of the hyoid in chimpanzees: Evolution of face flattening and speech. *Journal of Human Evolution* 51, 244–254.

Nishiyama, Koichiro, Hajime Hirose, Yoshiaki Iguchi, Hiromi Nagai, Jun Yamanaka, and Makito Okamoto (2002) Autologous transplantation of fascia into the vocal fold as a treatment for recurrent nerve paralysis. *Laryngoscope* 112, 1420–1425.

Nissenbaum, Jon, John E. Kirsch, Morris Halle, James B. Kobler, Hugh D. Curtin, and Robert E. Hillman (2002) High-speed MRI: A new means for assessing hypotheses concerning the phonetic control of voice and F0. *North East Linguistic Society* 33, MIT, November 11, 2002.

Nolan, Francis J. (1983) *The Phonetic Bases of Speaker Recognition*. Cambridge: Cambridge University Press.

(2005) Forensic speaker identification and the phonetic description of voice quality. In Hardcastle and Mackenzie Beck (eds.), 385–411.

Nouwen, Johan, Stéphane Hans, Erwan De Mones, Daniel Brasnu, Lise Crevier-Buchman, and Ollivier Laccourreye (2004) Thyroplasty type I without arytenoid adduction in patients with unilateral laryngeal nerve paralysis: The Montgomery implant versus the Gore-Tex implant. *Acta Otolaryngologica* 124, 732–738.

Novikova, K. A. (1960) *Ocherki Dialektov Evenskogo Jazyka: Ol'skij Govor* (vol. 1). Moscow/Leningrad: Akademija Nauk.

Ohala, John J. (1972) How is pitch lowered? *Journal of the Acoustical Society of America* 52, 124.

(1983) The origin of sound patterns in vocal tract constraints. In Peter F. MacNeilage (ed.), *The Production of Speech*. New York: Springer, 189–216.

(1990) There is no interface between phonology and phonetics: A personal view. *Journal of Phonetics* 18, 153–171.

(1993) The phonetics of sound change. In Charles Jones (ed.), *Historical Linguistics: Problems and Perspectives*. London: Longman, 237–278.

(1994) Towards a universal, phonetically-based theory of vowel harmony. In *ICSLP 94*. Yokohama: Acoustical Society of Japan, 491–494.

(2005) Phonetic explanations for sound patterns: Implications for grammars of competence. In Hardcastle and Mackenzie Beck (eds.), 23–38.

(2011) Accommodation to the aerodynamic voicing constraint and its phonological relevance. In Lee and Zee (eds.), 64–67.

(2012) The listener as a source of sound change: An update. In Solé and Recasens (eds.), 21–35.

Ohala, John J. and Brian W. Eukel (1987) Explaining the intrinsic pitch of vowels. In Robert Channon and Linda Shockey (eds.), *In Honor of Ilse Lehiste*. Dordrecht: Foris, 207–215.

Ohala, John J., Y. Hasegawa, Manjiri Ohala, D. Granville, and A. C. Bailey (eds.) (1999) *Proceedings of the 14th International Congress of Phonetic Sciences*. Berkeley: University of California.

Oller, D. Kimbrough (1978) Infant vocalization and the development of speech. *Allied Health and Behavioral Sciences* 1, 523–549.

(1980) The emergence of the sounds of speech in infancy. In Yeni-Komshian et al. (eds.), 93–112.

(2000) *The Emergence of the Speech Capacity*. Mahwah, NJ: Lawrence Erlbaum.

(2004) Underpinnings for a theory of communicative evolution. In D. Kimbrough Oller and Ulrike Griebel (eds.), *Evolution of Communication Systems*. Cambridge, MA: MIT Press, 49–65.

Oller, D. Kimbrough, Rebecca E. Eilers, A. Rebecca Neal, and Alan B. Cobo-Lewis (1998) Late onset canonical babbling: A possible early marker of abnormal development. *American Journal on Mental Retardation* 103, 249–263.

Oller, D. Kimbrough, Rebecca E. Eilers, A. Rebecca Neal, and Heidi K. Schwartz (1999) Precursors to speech in infancy: The prediction of speech and language disorders. *Journal of Communication Disorders* 32, 223–245.

Ota, Mitsuhiko (2003) The development of lexical pitch accent systems: An autosegmental analysis. *Canadian Journal of Linguistics* 48, 357–383.

Padayodi, Cécile M. (2008) Kabiye. *Journal of the International Phonetic Association* 38, 215–221.

Painter, Colin (1973) Cineradiographic data on the feature 'covered' in Twi vowel harmony. *Phonetica* 28, 97–120.

(1986) The laryngeal vestibule and voice quality. *Archives of Oto-Rhino-Laryngology* 243, 329–337.

Panconcelli-Calzia, Giulio (1924) *Die Experimentelle Phonetik in ihrer Anwendung auf die Sprachwissenschaft*. Berlin: W. de Gruyter & Co.

Perez, Kathe S., Lorraine Olson Ramig, Marshall E. Smith, and Christopher Dromey (1996) The Parkinson larynx: Tremor and videostroboscopic findings. *Journal of Voice* 10, 354–361.

Peterson, Gordon E. and Harold L. Barney (1952) Control methods used in a study of the vowels. *Journal of the Acoustical Society of America* 24, 175–184.

Pettorino, Massimo and Antonella Giannini (1984) F1 locus and place of articulation. In *Proceedings of the 10th International Congress of Phonetic Sciences*. Utrecht, 201–204.

Pike, Kenneth L. (1947) *Phonemics: A Technique for Reducing Languages to Writing*. Ann Arbor: University of Michigan Press.

(1967) *Language in Relation to a Unified Theory of the Structure of Human Behavior*. The Hague: Mouton de Gruyter.

Podesva, Robert J. (2007) Phonation type as a stylistic variable: The use of falsetto in constructing a persona. *Journal of Sociolinguistics* 11, 478–504.

(2013) Gender and the social meaning of non-modal phonation types. In Chundra Cathcart, I-Hsuan Chen, Greg Finley, Shinae Kang, Clare S. Sandy, and Elise Stickles (eds.), *Proceedings of the 37th Annual Meeting of the Berkeley Linguistics Society*. Berkeley: BLS, 427–448.

Podesva, Robert J. and Patrick Callier (2015) Voice quality and identity. *Annual Review of Applied Linguistics* 35, 173–194.

Pompino-Marschall, Bernd and Marzena Żygis (2011) Glottal marking of vowel-initial words in German. In Lee and Zee (eds.), 1626–1629.

Pratt, Teresa and Annette D'Onofrio (2017) Jaw setting and the California Vowel Shift in parodic performance. *Language in Society* 46(3), 283–312.

Pressman, Joel J. (1954) Sphincters of the larynx. *Archives of Otolaryngology* 59: 221–236.

Preston, Dennis R. (1992) Talking black and talking white: A study in variety imitation. In Joan H. Hall, Nick Doane, and Dick Ringler (eds.), *Old English and New: Studies in Language and Linguistics in Honor of Frederic G. Cassidy*. New York: Garland, 326–355.

(2006) Perceptual dialectology. In Keith Brown (ed.), *Encyclopedia of Language and Linguistics* (2nd edn). Oxford: Elsevier, vol. 4, 258–265.

Pulleyblank, Douglas (2006) Minimizing UG: Constraints upon constraints. In *Proceedings of the 25th West Coast Conference on Formal Linguistics*. Somerville, MA: Cascadilla Proceedings Project, 15–39.

Ramanarayanan, Vikram, Louis Goldstein, Dani Byrd, and Shrikanth S. Narayanan (2011) An MRI study of articulatory settings of L1 and L2 speakers of American English. In *Proc. International Seminar on Speech Production (ISSP'11)*, June 2011.

(2013) An investigation of articulatory setting using real-time magnetic resonance imaging. *Journal of the Acoustical Society of America* 134, 510.

Redi, Laura and Stefanie Shattuck-Hufnagel (2001) Variation in the realization of glottalization in normal speakers. *Journal of Phonetics* 29, 407–429.

Rees, Maryjane (1958) Some variables affecting perceived harshness. *Journal of Speech and Hearing Research* 1, 155–168.

Reidenbach, Martina M. (1997) Anatomical considerations of closure of the laryngeal vestibule during swallowing. *European Archives of Oto-Rhino-Laryngology* 254, 410–412.

(1998a) Aryepiglottic fold: Normal topography and clinical implications. *Clinical Anatomy* 11, 223–235.

(1998b) The muscular tissue of the vestibular folds of the larynx. *European Archives of Oto-Rhino-Laryngology* 255, 365–367.

Remacle, Marc, Hans E. Eckel, Antonio Antonelli, Daniel Brasnu, Dominique Chevalier, Gerhard Friedrich, et al. (2000) Endoscopic cordectomy: A proposal for a classification by the Working Committee, European Laryngological Society. *European Archives of Oto-Rhino-Laryngology* 257, 227–231.

Remacle, Marc, Christophe Van Haverbeke, Hans E. Eckel, Patrick Bradley, Dominique Chevalier, Votko Djukic, et al. (2007) Proposal for revision of the European Laryngological Society classification of endoscopic cordectomies. *European Archives of Oto-Rhino-Laryngology* 264, 499–504.

Remijsen, Bert and D. Robert Ladd (2008) The tone system of the Luanyjang dialect of Dinka. *Journal of African Languages and Linguistics* 29, 173–213.

Rice, Keren (2011) Consonantal place of articulation. In van Oostendorp et al. (eds.), 519–549.

Rigault, André and René Charbonneau (eds.) (1972) *Proceedings of the 7th International Congress of Phonetic Sciences* (Montreal, 1971). (*Janua Linguarum*, Series Major, 57). The Hague: Mouton.

Roach, Peter J. (1979) Laryngeal-oral coarticulation in glottalized English plosives. *Journal of the International Phonetic Association* 9, 2–6.

(2004) British English: Received Pronunciation. *Journal of the International Phonetic Association* 34, 239–245.

Rose, Phil (1989) Phonetics and phonology of Yang tone phonation types in Zhenhai. *Cahiers de Linguistique Asie Orientale* 18, 229–245.

Rose, Sharon (1996) Variable laryngeals and vowel lowering. *Phonology* 13, 73–117.

Rothenberg, Martin (1992) A multichannel electroglottograph. *Journal of Voice* 6, 36–43.

Roug, Liselotte, Ingrid Landberg, and Lars-Johan Lundberg (1989) Phonetic development in early infancy: A study of four Swedish children during the first eighteen months of life. *Journal of Child Language* 16, 19–40.

Rousselot, Abbé Pierre-Jean (1904) *Principes de phonétique expérimentale* (2 vols.). Paris: Didier.

Russell, G. Oscar (1931) *Speech and Voice*. New York: The Macmillan Company.

(1936) Etiology of follicular pharyngitis, catarrhal laryngitis, or so-called clergyman's throat; and singer's nodes. *Journal of Speech Disorders* 1, 113–122.

Saeed, J. I. (1999) *Somali*. Amsterdam: Benjamins.

Sagey, Elizabeth C. (1986) *The Representation of Features and Relations in Non-Linear Phonology*. Doctoral dissertation, MIT.

Sakakibara, Ken-Ichi, Leonardo Fuks, Hiroshi Imagawa, and Niro Tayama (2004a) Growl voice in ethnic and pop styles. *Proceedings of the International Symposium on Musical Acoustics* (ISMA2004), Nara, Japan.

Sakakibara, Ken-Ichi, Miwako Kimura, Hiroshi Imagawa, Seiji Niimi, and Niro Tayama (2004b) Physiological study of the supraglottal structure. Paper presented at the *International Conference on Voice Physiology and Biomechanics*, Marseille, 2004.

San Segundo, Eugenia, Peter French, Paul Foulkes, Vincent Hughes, and Philip Harrison (2016) Voice quality analysis in forensic voice comparison: Developing the Vocal Profile Analysis Scheme. *IAFPA 25, University of York, 2015.*

San Segundo, Eugenia, Paul Foulkes, Peter French, Philip Harrison, Vincent Hughes, and Colleen Kavanagh (2018) The use of the Vocal Profile Analysis for speaker characterization: Methodological proposals. *Journal of the International Phonetic Association*, 1–28. doi: https://doi.org/10.1017/S0025100318000130.

Sapir, Edward and Morris Swadesh (1939) *Nootka Texts: Tales and Ethnological Narratives with Grammatical Notes and Lexical Materials.* Philadelphia: Linguistic Society of America; University of Pennsylvania.

Sasaki, Clarence T., Paul A. Levine, Jeffrey T. Laitman, and Edmund S. Crelin (1977) Postnatal descent of the epiglottis in man. *Archives of Otolaryngology* 103, 169–171.

Sato, Kiminori, Minoru Hirano, and Tadashi Nakashima (2000) Comparative histology of the maculae flavae of the vocal folds. *Annals of Otology, Rhinology & Laryngology* 109, 136–140.

Saussure, Ferdinand de (1916) *Cours de linguistique générale.* Lausanne & Paris: Librairie Payot & Cie.

(1960) *Course in General Linguistics*, ed. C. Bally and A. Sechehaye in collaboration with A. Reidlinger, trans. W. Baskin, London, Peter Owen (rev. edn 1974). First published in 1916.

Sawashima, Masayuki, Hajime Hirose, and Osamu Fujimura (1967) Observation of the larynx by a fiberscope inserted through the nose. *Journal of the Acoustical Society of America* 42, 1208.

Schaeffler, Sonja and James M. Scobbie (2010) An ultrasound and Vicon study of articulatory settings in German-English bilinguals. Presentation at the *5th Ultrafest Conference*. New Haven: Haskins Laboratories.

Schaeffler, Sonja, James M. Scobbie, and Ineke Mennen (2008) An evaluation of inter-speech postures for the study of language-specific articulatory settings. Paper presented at the 8th ISSP.

Scherer, Klaus R. (2003) Vocal communication of emotion: A review of research paradigms. *Speech Communication* 40, 227–256.

Scottish Consortium for ICPhS 2015 (ed.) (2015) *Proceedings of the 18th International Congress of Phonetic Sciences.* Glasgow: University of Glasgow.

Shahin, Kimary (2011) Pharyngeals. In van Oostendorp et al. (eds.), 604–637.

Sheppard, W. C. and H. L. Lane (1968) Development of the prosodic features of infant vocalizing. *Journal of Speech and Hearing Research* 11, 94–108.

Shewell, Christina (1998) The effect of perceptual training on ability to use the Vocal Profile Analysis Scheme. *International Journal of Language & Communication Disorders* 33, 322–326.

Shi, Rushen and Janet F. Werker (2001) Six-month-old infants' preference for lexical words. *Psychological Science* 12, 70–75.

Singer, Mark I. and Eric D. Blom (1980) An endoscopic technique for restoration of voice after laryngectomy. *Annals of Otology, Rhinology & Laryngology* 89, 529–533.

Snow, David and Heather L. Balog (2002) Do children produce the melody before the words? A review of developmental intonation research. *Lingua* 112, 1025–1058.

Solé, Maria-Josep (2002) Aerodynamic characteristics of trills and phonological patterning. *Journal of Phonetics* 30, 655–688.

Solé, Maria-Josep and Daniel Recasens (eds.) (2012) *The Initiation of Sound Change.* Amsterdam: John Benjamins.

Solé, Maria-Josep, Daniel Recasens, and Joaquin Romero (eds.) (2003) *Proceedings of the 15th International Congress of Phonetic Sciences.* Barcelona: Universitat Autònoma de Barcelona.

Sprouse, Ronald L., Maria-Josep Solé, and John J. Ohala (2010) Tracking laryngeal height and its impact on voicing. *12th Conference on Laboratory Phonology,* University of New Mexico, Albuquerque.

Stark, Rachel E. (1980) Prespeech segmental feature development. In Yeni-Komshian et al. (eds.), 73–92.

Stark, Rachel E., Susan N. Rose, and Margaret McLagen (1975) Features of infant sounds: The first eight weeks of life. *Journal of Child Language* 2, 205–221.

Stark, Rachel E., Lynne E. Bernstein, and Marilyn E. Demorest (1993) Vocal communication in the first 18 months of life. *Journal of Speech and Hearing Research* 36, 548–558.

Stavness, Ian, John E. Lloyd, Yohan Payan, and Sidney Fels (2011) Coupled hard-soft tissue simulation with contact and constraints applied to jaw-tongue-hyoid dynamics. *International Journal for Numerical Methods in Biomedical Engineering* 27, 367–390.

Stavness, Ian, Mohammad Ali Nazari, Pascal Perrier, Didier Demolin, and Yohan Payan (2013) A biomechanical modeling study of the effects of the orbicularis oris muscle and jaw posture on lip shape. *Journal of Speech, Language, and Hearing Research* 56, 878–890.

Steinhauer, Kimberly M. and Jo Estill (2008) The Estill Voice Model: Physiology of emotion. In Krzysztof Izdebski (ed.), *Emotions in the Human Voice: Volume II Clinical Evidence.* San Diego: Plural Publishing, 83–99.

Steriade, Donca (1987) Locality conditions and feature geometry. *Proceedings of NELS* 17, 595–618.

Stevens, Kenneth N. and Minoru Hirano (eds.) (1981) *Vocal Fold Physiology.* Tokyo: University of Tokyo Press.

Stewart, J. M. (1967) Tongue root position in Akan vowel harmony. *Phonetica* 16, 185–204.

Story, Brad H. and Ingo R. Titze (1995) Voice simulation with a body-cover model of the vocal folds. *Journal of the Acoustical Society of America* 97, 1249.

Stuart-Smith, Jane (1999) Glasgow: Accent and voice quality. In Paul Foulkes and Gerard Docherty (eds.), *Urban Voices: Accent Studies in the British Isles.* London: Arnold, 203–222.

(2007) A sociophonetic investigation of postvocalic /r/ in Glaswegian adolescents. In Trouvain and Barry (eds.), 1449–1452.

Sundberg, Johan (2013) Perception of singing. In Diana Deutsch (ed.), *The Psychology of Music* (3rd edn). San Diego: Elsevier Academic Press, 69–105.

Sundberg, Johan and P.-E. Nordström (1976) Raised and lowered larynx: The effect on vowel formant frequencies. *STL-QPSR* 17, 35–39 (Stockholm: KTH).

Sweet, Henry (1877) *A Handbook of Phonetics*. Oxford: Clarendon Press.

(1890) *A Primer of Phonetics*. Oxford: Clarendon Press.

(1906) *A Primer of Phonetics* (3rd edn, revised). Oxford: Clarendon Press.

Święciński, Radosław (2013) An EMA study of articulatory settings in Polish speakers of English. In Ewa Waniek-Klimczak and Linda R. Shockey (eds.), *Teaching and Researching English Accents in Native and Non-Native Speakers*. Berlin: Springer, 73–82.

Takano, Sayoko and Kiyoshi Honda (2007) An MRI analysis of the extrinsic tongue muscles during vowel production. *Speech Communication* 49, 49–58.

Teshigawara, Mihoko (2003) *Voices in Japanese Animation: A Phonetic Study of Voices of Heroes and Villains in Japanese Culture*. Doctoral dissertation, University of Victoria.

Teshigawara, Mihoko and Emi Zuiki Murano (2004) Articulatory correlates of voice qualities of good guys and bad guys in Japanese anime: An MRI study. In *Proceedings of INTERSPEECH 2004 – ICSLP*. Jeju, Korea.

Thelen, Esther (1991) Motor aspects of emergent speech: A dynamic perspective. In Norman A. Krasnegor, Duane M. Rumbaugh, Richard L. Schiefelbusch, and Michael Studdert-Kennedy (eds.), *Biological and Behavioral Determinants of Language Development*. Hillsdale, NJ: Lawrence Erlbaum Associates, 339–362.

Thurgood, Ela (2017) The use of distribution of laryngealization for low tone differentiation: A case study of Iu-Mien tones. Paper presented at *LSA 2017*, Austin, TX.

Tiede, Mark K. (1996) An MRI-based study of pharyngeal volume contrasts in Akan and English. *Journal of Phonetics* 24, 399–421.

Titze, Ingo R. (1973) The human vocal cords: A mathematical model, part I. *Phonetica* 28, 129–170.

(1991) Mechanisms underlying the control of fundamental frequency. In Jan Gauffin and Britta Hammarberg (eds.), *Vocal Fold Physiology: Acoustic, Perceptual, and Physiological Aspects of Voice Mechanisms*. San Diego: Singular Publishing Group, 129–148.

(2006) *The Myoelastic Aerodynamic Theory of Phonation*. Iowa City: National Center for Voice and Speech.

(2008) Nonlinear source-filter coupling in phonation: Theory a. *Journal of the Acoustical Society of America* 123, 1902–1915.

Titze, Ingo R. and Brad H. Story (1997) Acoustic interactions of the voice source with the lower vocal tract. *Journal of the Acoustical Society of America* 101, 2234.

Torcy, Tiphaine de, Agnès Clouet, Claire Pillot-Loiseau, Jacqueline Vaissière, Daniel Brasnu, and Lise Crevier-Buchman (2014) A video-fiberscopic study of laryngopharyngeal behaviour in the human beatbox. *Logopedics Phoniatrics Vocology* 39, 38–48.

Traill, Anthony (1985) *Phonetic and Phonological Studies of !Xóõ Bushman* (*Quellen zur Khoisan-Forschung* 1). Hamburg: Helmut Buske Verlag.

(1986) The laryngeal sphincter as a phonatory mechanism in !Xóõ Bushman. In Ronald Singer and John K. Lundy (eds.), *Variation, Culture and Evolution in African Populations: Papers in Honour of Dr Hertha de Villiers*. Johannesburg: Witwatersrand University Press, 123–131.

Traissac, Louis (1992) *Réhabilitation de la voix et de la déglutition après chirurgie partielle ou totale du larynx*. (*Rapport de la Société Française d'Oto-Rhino-Laryngologie et de Chirurgie Cervico-Faciale*). Paris: Ed. Arnette.

Trent, Sonja A. (1995) Voice quality: Listener identification of African-American versus Caucasian speakers. *Journal of the Acoustical Society of America* 98, 2936.

Trigo, Loren (1987) *Voicing and Pharyngeal Expansion*. Manuscript, MIT, Cambridge, MA.

(1991) On pharynx-larynx interactions. *Phonology* 8, 113–136.

Trouvain, Jürgen and William J. Barry (eds.) (2007) *Proceedings of the 16th International Congress of Phonetic Sciences*. Saarbrücken: Universität des Saarlandes.

Trudgill, Peter (1974) *The Social Differentiation of English in Norwich*. Cambridge: Cambridge University Press.

(2010) *Investigations in Sociohistorical Linguistics: Stories of Colonisation and Contact*. Cambridge: Cambridge University Press.

Tsai, C.-G., L.-C. Wang, S.-F. Wang, Y.-W. Shau, T.-Y. Hsiao, and W. Auhagen (2010) Aggressiveness of the growl-like timbre: Acoustic characteristics, musical implications, and biomechanical mechanisms. *Music Perception* 27, 209–222.

Tucker, Archibald N. (1975) Voice quality in African languages. In Sayyid H. Hurreiz and Herman Bell (eds.), *Directions in Sudanese Linguistics and Folklore*. Khartoum: Khartoum University Press, 44–76.

Tur-Sinai (Turchiner), H. N. (1937) *Ha-mivta ha-aliz* ('The Joyful Pronunciation'). Jerusalem: The Committee of the Hebrew Language (in Hebrew).

UCLA (2009) *UCLA Phonetics Lab Archive*. archive.phonetics.ucla.edu.

Uffmann, Christian (2011) The organization of features. In van Oostendorp et al. (eds.), 643–668.

van den Berg, Janwillem (1955) On the role of the laryngeal ventricle in voice production. *Folia Phoniatrica* 7, 57–69.

(1968) Mechanism of the larynx and the laryngeal vibrations. In Bertil Malmberg (ed.), *Manual of Phonetics*. Amsterdam: North-Holland, 278–308.

van den Berg, Janwillem, J. T. Zantema, and P. J. Doornenbal (1957) On the air resistance and the Bernoulli Effect of the human larynx. *Journal of the Acoustical Society of America* 29, 626–631.

van den Berg, Janwillem, William Vennard, D. Burger, and C. C. Shervanian (1960) *Voice Production: The Vibrating Larynx*. Groningen University, Medical Physics Department. Utrecht: Stichting Film en Wetenschap, Universitaire Film.

van Oostendorp, Marc, Colin J. Ewen, Elizabeth V. Hume, and Keren Rice (eds.) (2011) *The Blackwell Companion to Phonology*, vol. 1. Oxford: Wiley-Blackwell.

Van Riper, Charles and John V. Irwin (1958) *Voice and Articulation*. Englewood Cliffs, NJ: Prentice-Hall.

Vaux, Bert (1996) The status of ATR in feature geometry. *Linguistic Inquiry* 26, 175–182.

Vihman, Marilyn M. (2014) *Phonological Development: The First Two Years* (2nd edn). Oxford: Wiley-Blackwell.

Vihman, Marilyn M., Marlys A. Macken, Ruth Miller, Hazel Simmons, and Jim Miller (1985) From babbling to speech: A re-assessment of the continuity issue. *Language* 61, 397–445.

Vilkman, Erkki, Aatto Sonninen, Pertti Hurme, and Pentti Körkkö (1996) External laryngeal frame function in voice production revisited: A review. *Journal of Voice* 10, 78–92.

Vorperian, Houri K., Raymond D. Kent, Lindell R. Gentry, and Brian S. Yandell (1999) Magnetic resonance imaging procedures to study the concurrent anatomic development of vocal tract structures: Preliminary results. *International Journal of Pediatric Otorhinolaryngology* 49, 197–206.

Wallet, Lucille, Lise Crevier-Buchman, Stéphane Hans, and Jacqueline Vaissière (2009) Etude perceptive des modalités interrogatives et assertives après laryngectomies partielles verticales. *Revue de Laryngologie Otologie Rhinologie* 130, 1–5.

Walton, Chloe, Erin Conway, Helen Blackshaw, and Paul Carding (2017) Unilateral vocal fold paralysis: A systematic review of speech-language pathology management. *Journal of Voice* 31, 509.e7–509.e22.

Weinstein, Gregory S., Ollivier Laccourreye, Daniel Brasnu, and Henri Laccourreye (2000) *Organ Preservation Surgery for Laryngeal Cancer*. San Diego: Singular Publishing Group.

Weir, N. F. (1973) Theodore Billroth: The first laryngectomy for cancer. *Journal of Laryngology & Otology* 87, 1161–1169.

Weiss, Michael S., Grace H. Yeni-Komshian, and John M. Heinz (1979) Acoustical and perceptual characteristics of speech produced with an electronic artificial larynx. *Journal of the Acoustical Society of America* 65, 1298–1308.

Welmers, William E. (1946) A descriptive grammar of Fanti. *Language* 22, 3–78.

Wernicke, Carl (1874) *Der aphasische Symptomencomplex: eine psychologische Studie auf anatomischer Basis*. Breslau: Max Cohn & Weigert.

Westerberg, Fabienne E. (2016) *An Auditory, Acoustic, Articulatory and Sociophonetic Study of Swedish Viby-i*. MPhil thesis, University of Glasgow.

Whalen, Doug H. and Andrea G. Levitt (1995) The universality of intrinsic F_0 of vowels. *Journal of Phonetics* 23, 349–366.

Whalen, Doug H., Bryan Gick, Masanobu Kumada, and Kiyoshi Honda (1998) Cricothyroid activity in high and low vowels: Exploring the automaticity of intrinsic F0. *Journal of Phonetics* 27, 125–142.

Whalen, Doug H., Andrea G. Levitt, and Louis M. Goldstein (2007) VOT in the babbling of French- and English-learning infants. *Journal of Phonetics* 35, 341–352.

Wilkins, John (1668) *An Essay Towards a Real Character and a Philosophical Language*. London: John Martyn.

Williams, Gareth T., I. Malcolm Farquharson, and James K. F. Anthony (1975) Fibreoptic laryngoscopy in the assessment of laryngeal disorders. *Journal of Laryngology and Otology* 89, 299–316.

Wilson, Ian L. (2006) *Articulatory Settings of French and English Monolingual and Bilingual Speakers*. Doctoral dissertation, University of British Columbia.

Wilson, Ian and Bryan Gick (2006) Ultrasound technology and second language acquisition research. In Mary Grantham O'Brien, Christine Shea, and John Archibald (eds.), *Proceedings of the 8th Generative Approaches to Second Language Acquisition Conference (GASLA 2006).* Somerville, MA: Cascadilla Proceedings Project, 148–152.

(2014) Bilinguals use language-specific articulatory settings. *Journal of Speech, Language, and Hearing Research* 57, 361–373.

Wormald, Jessica (2016) *Regional Variation in Panjabi-English.* Doctoral dissertation, University of York.

Wyss, Peter (1976) Akha. In William A. Smalley (ed.), *Phonemes and Orthography: Language Planning in 10 Minority Languages of Thailand.* Canberra: Australian National University, 239–257.

Xu, Yi, Albert Lee, Wing-Li Wu, Xuan Liu, and Peter Birkholz (2013) Human vocal attractiveness as signaled by body size projection. *PLoS ONE* doi.org/10.1371/journal.pone.0062397.

Yamada, Michihisa, Minoru Hirano, and Hiroshi Ohkubo (1983) Recurrent laryngeal nerve paralysis: A 10-year review of 564 patients. *Auris Nasus Larynx* 10, S1–S15.

Yanagisawa, Eiji, Jo Estill, Steven T. Kmucha, and Steven B. Leder (1989) The contribution of aryepiglottic constriction to 'ringing' voice quality: A videolaryngoscopic study with acoustic analysis. *Journal of Voice* 3, 342–350.

Yanushevskaya, Irena and Daniel Bunčić (2015) Russian. *Journal of the International Phonetic Association* 45, 221–228.

Yeni-Komshian, Grace H., James F. Kavanaugh, and Charles A. Ferguson (eds.) (1980) *Child Phonology.* New York: Academic Press.

Zangger Borch, Daniel, Johan Sundberg, Per-Åke Lindestad, and Margareta Thalén (2004) Vocal fold vibration and voice source aperiodicity in 'dist' tones: A study of a timbral ornament in rock singing. *Logopedics Phoniatrics Vocology* 29, 147–153.

Zemlin, Willard R. (1968) *Speech and Hearing Science: Anatomy and Physiology.* Englewood Cliffs, NJ: Prentice-Hall.

Zeroual, Chakir, John H. Esling, and Lise Crevier-Buchman (2008) The contribution of supraglottic laryngeal adjustments to voice: Phonetic evidence from Arabic. *Logopedics Phoniatrics Vocology* 33, 3–11.

Zhu, Hua and Barbara Dodd (2000) The phonological acquisition of Putonghua (Modern Standard Chinese). *Journal of Child Language* 27, 3–42.

Zolotas, Kostas and Sonya Bird (2010) An ultrasound investigation of didgeridoo articulations. *Canadian Acoustics* 38, 198–199.

Multimedia References

Alanna (2012) *How to Do an Australian Accent.* AwesomeAlanna.

Antonsen, Ole Edvard (1997) 'The Honeymooners'. Bjørn Nessjø, *Read My Lips*, EMI Records.

Armstrong, Louis (1926) 'Heebie Jeebies'. Boyd Atkins, OKeh.

(1929) 'When You're Smiling'. Mark Fisher, Larry Shay, Joe Goodwin, OKeh.

(1931) 'Lazy River'. Sidney Arodin and Hoagy Carmichael, OKeh.

(1967) 'What a Wonderful World'. Bob Thiele & George Weiss, ABC.

Atkinson, Rowan (1992) Mr Bean. John Birkin, Richard Curtis, *Merry Christmas, Mr Bean*, Tiger Television / Thames Television.

Barber, Jill (2008) 'Chances'. Jill Barber and Ron Sexsmith, *Chances*, Outside Music.

BBC (1971) *English with a Dialect, and Irish, Scottish and Welsh Accents* (LP). BBC Records.

Bean, Sean (1993–97) Richard Sharpe. Tom Clegg, *Sharpe*, ITV series.

Bee Gees (1977a) 'Stayin' Alive'. Barry, Robin and Maurice Gibb, *Saturday Night Fever*, RSO.

(1977b) 'More Than a Woman'. Barry, Robin and Maurice Gibb, *Saturday Night Fever*, RSO.

(1977c) 'How Deep Is Your Love'. Barry, Robin and Maurice Gibb, *Saturday Night Fever*, RSO.

Beglin, Jim (2007–12) Football commentator. ITV Sports (later BT and RTÉ).

Berle, Milton (1966) *Henny Youngman heckles Milton Berle. The Hollywood Palace*, ABC.

Bidisha (2011) *The Countertenor*. BBC Radio 4, 26 Nov 2011.

Blanc, Mel (1937–89) Sylvester, Daffy Duck. *Looney Tunes, Merrie Melodies*, Warner Bros.

Bland, Bobby 'Blue' (1961) 'Cry Cry Cry'. Don D. Robey, *Two Steps from the Blues*, Duke/MCA.

Brando, Marlon (1972) Don Vito Corleone. Francis Ford Coppola, *The Godfather*, Paramount Pictures.

Brandt, Paul (2001) 'Small Towns and Big Dreams'. Paul Brandt, *Small Towns and Big Dreams*, Brand-T Records.

Brown, Bryan (1981) Joe Harman. David Stevens, *A Town Like Alice*, Seven Network.

Brown, James (1966) 'It's a Man's Man's Man's World'. James Brown and Betty Jean Newsome, *It's a Man's Man's Man's World*, King Records.

Brown, June (1985) Dot. *EastEnders*, BBC TV.

Bruce, Fiona (2011) *The Queen's Palaces: Buckingham Palace*. BBC TV.

Candy, John and Eugene Levy (1982–83) The Schmenge Brothers, *SCTV*. CBC TV.

Canyon, George (2008) 'Just Like You'. George Canyon, Richard Marx, Gary Harrison, *What I Do*, 604 Records.

Capstick, Tony (1981) *Capstick Comes Home* (LP). Air.

Caro, Francisco José (2013) *TVE Telediario 2*, RTVE.

Carrey, Jim (2000) The Grinch. Ron Howard, *How the Grinch Stole Christmas*, Universal Pictures.

Carson, Johnny (1989) Jimmy Stewart Interview. *The Tonight Show*, NBC.

CBC Northern Service (1984) *Traditional Inuit Music*. QCS 1442, CBC Northern Service Broadcast Recording, 7'''' vinyl, 33⅓ RPM.

Christie, Lou (1963) 'Two Faces Have I.' Twyla Herbert and Lou Christie, *Lou Christie*, Roulette Records.

(1965) 'Lightnin' Strikes'. Lou Christie and Twyla Herbert, *Lightnin' Strikes*, MGM.

Clapper, Mike (2011) Washington Wizards/Mystics PA Announcer.

Cohen, Sacha Baron (2018) Col. Erran Morad. *Who Is America?* SHOWTIME.

Connery, Sean (1962) James Bond, 007. Terence Young, *Dr No*, Eon Productions.
   (1983) James Bond, 007. Irvin Kershner, *Never Say Never Again*, TaliaFilm II
   Productions.

Connolly, Billy (1982) *Billy Connolly Live 1982*. YouTube.

Cooper, Bradley (2015) Craig Kristofferson. Don Roy King, *The Californians, Saturday Night Live 40th Anniversary Special*, NBC.

Cooper, Gary (1943) Robert Jordan. Sam Wood, *For Whom the Bell Tolls*, Paramount
   Pictures.

Davies, Ray (1964a) 'You Really Got Me'. *The Kinks*, Pye/Reprise.
   (1964b) 'All Day and All of the Night'. *The Kinks*, Pye/Reprise.

Dawson, Michael (2013) *England's Stuart Broad Nets with Tottenham Hotspur
   Defender Michael Dawson.* ecb.co.uk.

de Hoog, Ariane (2012) Talk mit DW Moderatorin Ariane de Hoog. *Typisch deutsch*,
   Deutsche Welle.

Dench, Judi (1998) Queen Elizabeth I. John Madden, *Shakespeare in Love*, Universal
   Pictures/ Miramax.

Diamantopoulos, Chris (2013) Mickey Mouse. Chris Savino, *Bad Ear Day*, Disney.

Donnelly, Deirdre (1996–2001) Siobhan Mehigan. *Ballykissangel*, BBC TV series.

Dylan, Bob (1963) 'Blowin' in the Wind'. *The Freewheelin' Bob Dylan*, Columbia.
   (1965) 'Mr. Tambourine Man'. *Bringing It All Back Home*, Columbia.

E.R.T. (2013) Last news E.R.T. Greek National TV, 11 June 2013.

Esgueva, Mónica (2014) *La Sociedad Líquida. Para Todos La 2*, TVE Entrevista,
   RTVE.

Ferguson, Craig (2014) *The Late Late Show*. CBS.

Fish Symboled Stamp (2013) Загасан Ширээт Тамга. YouTube: Chonos
   Entertainment.

Foggy Hogtown Boys (2010) 'Little Sadie'. *Scotch and Sofa*, cdbaby.

Franklin, Gretchen (1985) Ethel. *EastEnders*, BBC TV.

Fujimoto, Momoko (2011) *Momone Momo* UTAU voice. Christopher Torres,
   'Saraj00n' and 'daniwell', *Nyan Cat*. GIF animation and song.

Glenister, Robert (2004) Ash Morgan. *Hustle*, BBC TV.

Goodland, Norman (1981) *My Old Chap: Norman Goodland Reads His Wessex Verse*
   (LP). Saydisc.

Gresky, Julia (2016) 'Ritual Holes Cut in Human Skulls 6,000 Years Ago'. *Quirks &
   Quarks, with Bob McDonald*. CBC Radio, 7 May 2016.

Grünwald, Günter (2009) *Sprachprobleme im Biergarten. Grünwald Freitagscomedy*
   16 Oct 2009, Bayerisches Fernsehen.
   (2011) *Bayrisch Menthol. Grünwald Freitagscomedy* 16 Sep 2011.
   (2013) *Monika Gruber beschimpft Danilo aus Sachsen*. YouTube.

Helm, Levon (1968) 'The Weight'. Robbie Robertson, The Band, *Music from Big Pink*,
   Capitol.

Henley, Larry (1964) 'Bread and Butter'. Larry Parks and Jay Turnbow, The Newbeats,
   Bread and Butter, Hickory Records.

Henson, Jim (1955–90) Kermit the Frog. *Sam and Friends* (WRC TV), *Sesame Street* (NET), *The Muppet Show* (ITV).

(1975–90) Swedish Chef. *The Muppet Show*, ITV.

Henshaw, John (2002–05) Wilf Bradshaw. *Born and Bred*, BBC TV.

Hopkins, Anthony (1991) Dr Hannibal Lecter. Jonathan Demme, *Silence of the Lambs*, Orion Pictures.

Iglesias, Julio (1978) 'Pobre Diablo'. Julio Iglesias, Ramón Arcusa and Manuel de la Calva, *Emociones*, Sony.

Ionda, Cristina Serban (2014–17) Gina Kadinsky. Chris Bailey, *The Brokenwood Mysteries*, South Pacific Pictures.

Irons, Jeremy (2011–13) Rodrigo Borgia. Neil Jordan, *The Borgias*, Showtime.

Jackman, Hugh (2008) Drover. Baz Luhrmann, *Australia*, 20th Century Fox.

Jackson, Gordon (1981) Noel Strachan. David Stevens, *A Town Like Alice*, Seven Network.

Jagger, Mick (1966) 'Under My Thumb'. Mick Jagger and Keith Richards, *Aftermath*, Decca.

(1968) 'Sympathy for the Devil'. Mick Jagger and Keith Richards, *Beggars Banquet*, Decca.

(1978) 'Beast of Burden'. Mick Jagger and Keith Richards, *Some Girls*, Rolling Stones.

Jaumandreu, Marta (2013) *TVE Telediario 2*, RTVE.

Johnson, Robert (1937) 'Hell Hound on My Trail'. Vocalion.

Kane, Harry (2015) Tottenham Hotspur (interviews). BeanymanSports.

Kardashian, Kim (2007–16) Kim Kardashian. *Keeping Up with the Kardashians*, Ryan Seacrest, Eliot Goldberg, Bunim-Murray Productions (BMP), Ryan Seacrest Productions.

Katter, Bob (2013) *Viewpoint*. Sky News National, 7 Apr 2013.

Kavner, Julie (1989–2016) Marge Simpson. James Brooks, Matt Groening, Sam Simon, *The Simpsons*, FOX.

Kharitonov, Leonid (1965) 'Song of the Volga Boatmen'. Red Army Choir, Tchaikovsky Hall, Moscow.

Kirwan, Dervla (1996–2001) Assumpta Fitzgerald. *Ballykissangel*, BBC TV series.

Kotierk, Apayata (2001) Kumaglak. Zacharias Kunuk, *Atanarjuat: The Fast Runner*, Aboriginal Peoples Television Network.

Kraśko, Piotr (2009) 'Pytajnik Piotr Kraśko o swoich studiach'. Dziennik.pl and *Wiadomości*, TVP.

LaMarche, Maurice (1993) The Godpigeon. *Animaniacs*, Warner Bros.

Le Borgne, Jean-Yves (2014) Discours du bâtonnier. Rentrée de l'EFB Paris 2014.

Lecluyse, Guy (2008) Yann Vandernoout. Dany Boon, *Bienvenue Chez Les Ch'tis*, Pathé.

Leighton, Ralph (1996) *Deep in the Heart of Tuva: Cowboy Music from the Wild East*. New York: Ellipsis Arts (CD).

Lewis, Jerry (1961) 'Jerry Lewis – 1961 – Standup Comedy'. *The Ed Sullivan Show*, CBS.

Lukschy, Wolfgang (1952) Marshal Will Kane (German voice-over for Gary Cooper). Fred Zinnemann, *Zwölf Uhr mittags (High Noon)*, United Artists.

Mandel, Howie (1981) Howie Mandel. Marty Callner, *The 6th Annual Young Comedians*, HBO.

Mansbridge, Peter (1988–2017) *The National*. CBC Television.

Marsden, Gerry (1963) 'You'll Never Walk Alone'. Richard Rodgers and Oscar Hammerstein, George Martin, *The Best of Gerry and the Pacemakers*, Columbia (EMI).

Mercer, Jack (1935–45, 1947–84) Popeye. *Popeye the Sailor Man* (over 450 episodes). Paramount Pictures.

Mercer, Rick (2001) *Talking to Americans: The Special. This Hour Has 22 Minutes*, CBC Television.

Meriman, Bill (1979) Boxing ring announcer. Danny Lopez vs. Mike Ayala championship fight.

Miodek, Jan (2012) *Prof. Miodek o desce*. www.wroclove2012.com.

Monroe, Marilyn (1959) 'I Wanna Be Loved By You'. Herbert Stothart, Harry Ruby and Bert Kalmar, 1928; Billy Wilder, *Some Like It Hot*, United Artists.

Morse, Helen (1981) Jean Paget. David Stevens, *A Town Like Alice*, Seven Network.

Nabors, Jim (1965) Gomer Pyle. Aaron Ruben, *Gomer Pyle: U.S.M.C.*, CBS.

Najdek, Paweł (2001) World Weightlifting Championships. 250kg Clean and Jerk @2001 Worlds (YouTube).

Newton, Robert (1954) Long John Silver. Byron Haskin, Martin Rackin, *Long John Silver*, Treasure Island Pictures Pty. Ltd.

Nighy, Bill (2014) Johnny Worricker. David Hare, *Salting the Battlefield*, BBC Two.

Nilsson, Cecilia (2006) Anja. Henning Mankell, *Wallander*, TV4 Sweden.

Ocora (1968) *Musique du Burundi* (LP). OCR 40. France.

(1988) *Burundi: Musiques Traditionelles* (CD, RE, RM). C559003. France.

O'Malley, Daragh (1993–2006) Sgt. Harper. *Sharpe's Rifles*, ITV series.

Ondar, Kongar-ool, (1996) *Medley of Throat-Singing Styles Accompanied by Doshpuluur*. In Leighton, track 1.

Osborne Brothers (1967) 'Rocky Top'. Felice and Boudleaux Bryant, Decca/MCA.

Oz, Frank (1975–2000) Sam the Eagle. *The Muppet Show*, ABC, ITV.

(1980) Yoda. George Lucas, *The Empire Strikes Back*, 20th Century Fox.

Page, Steven (1992) 'If I Had $1000000', 'New Kid (On the Block)'. The Barenaked Ladies, *Gordon*, Sire/Reprise.

Palin, Michael (1969) *Monty Python's Flying Circus* (Gumby sketches). BBC TV.

Pesci, Joe (1990) Tommy DeVito. Martin Scorsese, *Goodfellas*, Warner Bros.

Price, Vincent (1982) Voice overs. *Michael Jackson's Thriller*. Epic Records, Vestron Video.

Putin, Vladimir (2012) Victory Day speech, 9 May 2012.

Radner, Gilda (1978a) Lisa Loopner. *The Nerds & The Norge, Saturday Night Live*, NBC.

(1978b) Roseanne Rosannadanna. *Saturday Night Live*, NBC.

Ratzenberger John (1982–93) Cliff Claven. *Cheers*, Paramount, CBS TV.

Ravenscroft, Thurl (1953–2004) Tony the Tiger. *Kellogg's (Sugar) Frosted Flakes*, Kellogg Company.

Red Dwarf (1997) 'Beyond a Joke'. *Red Dwarf VII, 42*. Robert Llewellyn and Doug Naylor, BBC TV.

Reyes, Nicolas (1987) 'Bamboléo'. Tonino Baliardo, Chico Bouchiki, Nicolas Reyes, *Gipsy Kings*, Elektra.

Reynolds, Jack (1970) 'Country Comforts' (backing vocals to Rod Stewart). Elton John and Bernie Taupin, *Gasoline Alley*, Mercury/Vertigo.

Rinaldi, Benedetta (2013) Intervista ad Andrea Cavalieri. RAI Italia TV, 21 Nov 2013.

Robinson, Edward G. (1948) Johnny Rocco. John Huston, *Key Largo*, Warner Bros.

Rock, Chris (1996) *Chris Rock – Bring The Pain* (VHS, DVD 2002). DreamWorks.

Rogers, Kenny (1969) 'Ruby, Don't Take Your Love to Town'. Mel Tillis, Kenny Rogers and the First Edition, Reprise.

    (1978) 'The Gambler'. Don Schlitz, *The Gambler*, United Artists.

Romano, Chris (2014) Slow Mobius. Justin Roiland and Dan Harmon, *Rick and Morty, Ricksy Business*, TOON TV.

Salie, Faith (2013) 'Faith Salie on Speaking with "Vocal Fry"'. *CBS Sunday Morning*, 12 Sep 2013.

Salmond, Alex (2014) 2014 Scottish National Party Conference: Alex Salmond farewell speech, BBC News, 14 Nov 2014.

Segovia, Bricio (2012) *Raphael – Entrevista RT* (Moscú, Noviembre 2012). RT Actualidad.

Serling, Rod (1959–64) *The Twilight Zone*. CBS.

Soggy Bottom Boys (2000) 'I Am a Man of Constant Sorrow'. Dick Burnett, Mercury Nashville.

Somerville, Jimmy (1990) 'Read My Lips (Enough Is Enough)'. Jimmy Somerville, *Read My Lips*, London Recordings.

Steimle, Uwe (2015) *Mission@Home: Steimles sächsischer Sahnekuchen*. Dresden Fernsehen.

Stewart, Jimmy (1946) George Bailey. Frank Capra, *It's a Wonderful Life*, Liberty Films.

Stewart, Rod (1970a) 'Only a Hobo'. Bob Dylan, *Gasoline Alley*, Mercury/Vertigo.

    (1970b) 'My Way of Giving'. Ronnie Lane and Steve Marriott, *Gasoline Alley*, Mercury/Vertigo.

    (1970c) 'Country Comforts'. Elton John and Bernie Taupin, *Gasoline Alley*, Mercury/Vertigo.

Stumph, Wolfgang (1989) *Werktätige in der DDR 1989*. YouTube.

Suárez, Luis (2014) Luis Suárez Interview: On Racism, Biting and the Future. GuardianFootball, 24 Oct 2014.

Sutton, Frank (1965) Sgt. Vince Carter. Aaron Ruben, *Gomer Pyle: U.S.M.C.*, CBS.

Tamiroff, Akim (1943) Pablo. Sam Wood, *For Whom the Bell Tolls*, Paramount Pictures.

Tautou, Audrey (2010) Interview Audrey Tautou: Audrey Tautou tournage 2010. (re: *Amélie & De Vrais Mensonges*), aufemininTV.

Taylor, Koko (1969) '29 Ways'. Willie Dixon, Arc/BMI, *Koko Taylor*, Chess Producing Corp.

Tsipras, Alexis (2015) Greek Prime Minister Alexis Tsipras Speaks at the UN, 27 Sep 2015. GreekReporter.com.

Ulayuruluk, Abraham (2001) Tuurngarjuak. Zacharias Kunuk, *Atanarjuat: The Fast Runner*, Aboriginal Peoples Television Network.

US Army (2012) *Defy Expectations: Drill Sergeant* advertisement. Army Future Soldier Center.

Valli, Frankie (1962a) 'Sherry'. Bob Gaudio, *The Four Seasons*, Vee-Jay Records.
  (1962b) 'Big Girls Don't Cry'. Bob Crewe and Bob Gaudio, *The Four Seasons*, Vee-Jay Records.
  (1963) 'Walk Like a Man'. Bob Crewe and Bob Gaudio, *The Four Seasons*, Vee-Jay Records.
Welker, Frank (1983) Dr Claw. Dave Cox, Edouard David, *All That Glitters, Inspector Gadget*, LBS Communications.
Willerslev, Eske (2011) 'Ice Age Animals'. *Science in Action*, BBC World Service, 3 Nov 2011.
  (2013) 'New North American Ancestors'. *Quirks & Quarks, with Bob McDonald*. CBC Radio, 30 Nov 2013.
Wilson, Rt. Hon. Harold (1970) *BBC Election 1970*, David Dimbleby interview with Harold Wilson. BBC TV.
Worsley, Lucy (2013) *Tales from the Royal Bedchamber*. Nick Gillam-Smith, BBC Four.
  (2014) *Tales from the Royal Wardrobe*. Nick Gillam-Smith, BBC Four.
Youngman, Henny (1966) Henny Youngman Heckles Milton Berle. *The Hollywood Palace*, ABC.

Author/Artist Index

Subject Index

CPSIA information can be obtained
at www.ICGtesting.com
Printed in the USA
LVHW020352051022
730012LV00008B/303